INFORMED CHOICE IN MATERNITY CARE

Also by Mavis Kirkham

Birth Centres: A Social Model for Maternity Care
The Midwife–Mother Relationship*
Developments in the Supervision of Midwives

* *Also published by Palgrave Macmillan*

Informed Choice in Maternity Care

Edited by

Mavis Kirkham

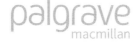

First published 2004 by
PALGRAVE MACMILLAN
Houndmills, Basingstoke, Hampshire RG21 6XS and
175 Fifth Avenue, New York, N.Y. 10010
Companies and representatives throughout the world

PALGRAVE MACMILLAN is the global academic imprint of the Palgrave
Macmillan division of St. Martin's Press, LLC and of Palgrave Macmillan Ltd.
Macmillan® is a registered trademark in the United States, United Kingdom
and other countries. Palgrave is a registered trademark in the European
Union and other countries.

ISBN 0–333–99843–X

This book is printed on paper suitable for recycling and made from fully
managed and sustained forest sources.

A catalogue record for this book is available from the British Library.

10 9 8 7 6 5 4 3 2 1
13 12 11 10 09 08 07 06 05 04

Printed and bound in China

Contents

Acknowledgements

Many people have made this book possible. I am grateful to the authors for fitting this writing into their busy and committed lives.

I would like to thank all those who were involved in our study, the women and staff who gave so generously of their time, our collaborators in the University of York and the University of Glamorgan, and our funders, the Department of Health. I particularly wish to thank Helen Stapleton for her tremendously hard work, integrity, insight and support throughout that project and the production of this book. I thank the colleagues who stretch my thinking: Penny Curtis and the midwives of the Women's Informed Childbearing and Health Research Group, University of Sheffield, and Anna Fielder and the midwives of the Association of Radical Midwives. Last, but never least, I thank Jane Flint who has supported the production of this book with unfailing efficiency and good humour.

Mavis Kirkham

Notes on Contributors

Tricia Anderson trained as a midwife in Dorset and worked in hospital and community sittings before setting up in independent practice in 1997. She is currently a Senior Lecturer in Midwifery at Bournemouth University, where she is Course Leader for the MA in Advanced Midwifery Practice. Prior to this she was Editor of the *MIDIRS Midwifery Digest* and *The Practising Midwife* and Co-Editor of the *Informed Choice* Initiative. Tricia is widely published and leads workshops nationally and internationally for midwives on all aspects of normal birth.

Susan Bewley is a Consultant in obstetrics and maternal-fetal medicine and Clinical Director of Women's Services at Guy's and St Thomas' Hospitals NHS Trust, London, UK. She has extensive clinical experience in complicated and high-risk pregnancy. She trained in medical law and ethics and has written about legal and ethical problems in reproduction. Her research interests include the predictors and consequences of severe maternal morbidity, HIV, sickle cell and domestic violence in pregnancy.

Jayne Cockburn has been a Consultant in Obstetrics and Gynaecology with a special interest in High Risk Obstetrics at Frimley Park NHS Trust since 1995. She is also Secretary of the British Society of Psychosomatic Obstetrics, Gynaecology and Andrology. Since 1996 she has been a member of the Nixon Forum, organising training of doctors in psychological aspects of Obstetrics and Gynaecology and aiming to get this aspect of care recognised formally by the Royal College of Obstetrics and Gynaecology. She is passionate about empowering women to access health care and working to understand their needs in a holistic way. As a long-standing feminist she is interested in gender issues in health care. She has interests in post-traumatic stress disorder after labour and postnatal depression.

Jill Demilew has been a Consultant Midwife at King's College Hospital London for 25 years working in inner-city practice including NHS and previously independent practice. She is passionate about supporting women to make continuing decisions about themselves and their children. During the late 1990s she project-managed the clinical governance framework into a Community Trust, learning how organisational systems enable or hinder effective clinical practice. She is working with women experiencing problematic addiction and how to navigate making their choices in a stigmatising system.

Nadine Pilley Edwards completed a PhD at the University of Sheffield on women's experiences of home births in 2001 and is researching the experiences of lay members on Maternity Services Liaison Committees. She is the Vice Chair of the Association for Improvements in the Maternity Services (AIMS), and trained as a childbirth educator in 1982. She is the co-founder of the Scottish Birth Teachers Association and of the Birth Resource Centre in Edinburgh.

Nicky Ellis is a Community Midwife in Leicester. She currently works in a Sure Start area. Her particular interests are in promoting culturally sensitive midwifery care with minority ethnic groups especially with refugees and asylum seekers. She has developed a local support network for breast-feeding mothers and has experience in teaching and research.

Barbara Hewson is a barrister called in 1985, based in Hardwicke Building, Lincoln's Inn, London. She is a member of the Bars of Ireland and Northern Ireland. She has a special interest in women's reproductive health and in 1998 received the first 'Barrister of the Year' award from *The Lawyer* magazine for her work promoting pregnant women's autonomy. She has acted in test cases in Ireland on the right to a home birth and the rights of domiciliary midwives.

Mavis Kirkham is Professor of Midwifery in the WICH Research Group at the University of Sheffield. She has been involved in clinical midwifery and midwifery research since 1971 and works in a rural birth centre as well as booking a small number of women for home births in Sheffield each year.

Valerie Levy has recently retired after a long career teaching and researching midwifery practice. Her most recent post was as Professor (Midwifery) at the Chinese University of Hong Kong; prior to that she was Principal Lecturer in Midwifery Studies at the Royal College of Nursing. Valerie's research interests include management of the third stage of labour, psychological aspects of childbirth and the making and facilitation of informed choices during pregnancy.

Mary Newburn is Head of Policy Research at the National Childbirth Trust (NCT), the largest and best-known childbirth and early parenting charity in Europe. As a senior manager in the NCT, Mary contributes to the direction and development of the charity, which offers information and support services and publications, carries out research on new parents' experiences, and maintains informal parents' networks through its 400 branches. The NCT champions user involvement in the maternity services and lobbies and campaigns for women-centred, family-focused policies and care, based on the best available evidence of effectiveness.

Alicia O'Cathain is an MRC Fellow in Health Services Research at the Medical Care Research Unit, School of Health and Related Research, University of Sheffield, UK. Her research interests include the evaluation of new health technologies and services such as decision aids for patients and NHS Direct, users' views of services, and the development of mixed methods in health services research.

Julia Simpson is a Senior Lecturer in Nursing at the School of Health and Social Care, University of Teesside. As a clinical practitioner she practised in the area of theatre and anaesthetic nursing. As an academic she has teaching and research experience, having been awarded an NHS Executive Northern and Yorkshire Research Training Fellowship in 1996 to explore the topic of Caesarean section. She is particularly interested in how professionals' and users' perspectives inform health policy and has undertaken an ethnographic study of Caesarean section that will form the basis of a sociological PhD.

Helen Stapleton is a midwifery researcher in the Department of Midwifery and Children's Nursing, University of Sheffield. Prior to her academic career, she worked as an independent midwife and medical herbalist in London. Areas of interest include qualitative methodologies, sociological and anthropological perspectives on childbirth and parenting, and complementary and alternative therapies. Her current PhD research focuses on the experiences of teenagers making the transition to parenthood.

Meg Wiggins is a Senior Research Officer at the Social Science Research Unit, Institute of Education, University of London. Prior to this, she worked in the Policy Research department of the UK's National Childbirth Trust and the Women's Health Project in Johannesburg, South Africa. Her research has concentrated on a variety of aspects of women's health, including their experiences of pregnancy and the postnatal period. She is researching the best ways of supporting teenage parents.

Introduction

MAVIS KIRKHAM

Philosophies of maternity care have moved in recent years from requiring clients' consent to treatment to a more complex notion of informed choice. Evidence has existed for many years to show that childbearing women want more information and choices in their care (Cartwright, 1979; Perkins 1991) and there are well established links between perceived control and improved emotional outcomes (Green, Coupland and Kitzinger, 1988). There are, however, dilemmas with increasing the power of clients relative to that of health professionals as the latter may then perceive their expert knowledge as being undermined. Redefinition of the concept of expertise is possible but is unlikely to happen without radical changes in the philosophy and organisation of care (Guilliland and Pairman, 1995). Whilst 'Patient Partnership' has been an NHS Executive medium-term priority for some years (NHS Executive, 1996), the achievement of such partnership would involve unprecedented change in the power relationships, organisation and delivery of maternity services. At the same time, the development of increasingly sophisticated ante-natal screening services, increased emphasis on evidence-based care and professional nervousness with regard to litigation all serve to focus attention on professional expertise and technology rather than on women's choices.

In 1993, *Changing Childbirth* (Department of Health, 1993), a policy document for England, charged providers of maternity care to work towards making the service more woman-focused. It particularly emphasised the need for women to have information made easily available so that they could make informed choices about their care. Since then debate has ranged over what informed choice means in maternity care and to what extent it is either possible or desirable. The policy of informed choice, and the ensuing debate, has certainly changed the language of maternity service providers.

This book aims to examine different aspects of informed choice and consider the issues from differing viewpoints, grounded throughout in the context of contemporary maternity care. It therefore includes a number of projects using different research methods to shed light upon the experience of childbearing women and the professionals within the maternity services. The authors come from very different backgrounds and are therefore able to bring different bodies of knowledge and experience to focus upon informed choice.

It is right that the book starts with individual women and their decision-making. Nadine Edwards is honorary vice-chair of the Association for

Improvements in the Maternity Services. In Chapter 1 she presents part of her research on the decision-making of women who chose home birth.

Barbara Hewson (Chapter 2) presents a legal viewpoint. As a barrister she is able to draw out legal, as well as ethical, dilemmas within maternity services' policies and practice with regard to informed consent and informed choice.

Valerie Levy is a midwife and she presents part of her research in Chapter 3. Her work focuses upon midwives and their dilemmas in facilitating informed choice during pregnancy.

Chapters 4 to 8 concern the MIDIRS *Informed Choice* leaflets; a unique initiative to make research evidence available to childbearing women and midwives in a concise and clear format.

In 1994, the Department of Health made funding available for MIDIRS (Midwives Information and Resource Service) and the NHS Centre for Reviews and Dissemination to collaboratively produce evidence-based leaflets on ten discrete, pregnancy-related topics. This collaboration resulted in the production of series 1–5 of the *Informed Choice* leaflets, which were published in 1996; series 6–10 were published in 1997. (See Chapter 4 for the full titles of the leaflets.) The leaflets were updated towards the end of 1999 and redesigned in 2002. In 2003 they are to be relaunched, with five new titles, in a resource pack. They are now available on line (http://www.midirs.org/nelh/nelh.nsf/welcome?openform)

Chapters 4, 5 and 6 are drawn from our research (Kirkham and Stapleton, 2001) to evaluate the MIDIRS *Informed Choice* leaflets. Alicia O'Cathain reports the randomised controlled trial (RCT) where the leaflets were introduced into normal NHS practice. They were not found to increase informed choice (Chapter 4). Chapters 5 and 6 are drawn from the qualitative research conducted within the RCT sites and elsewhere. Helen Stapleton compares ethnographic studies of maternity units which had purchased the leaflets and used them for some time, and those which used them within the RCT. No strategy for achieving informed choice was found within either group of maternity units; staff simply equated the presence of the leaflets in the units with informed choice (Chapter 5). Thus it was scarcely surprising that the presence of leaflets alone did not change either attitudes or clinical practice. The culture of the service was such that informed compliance was the norm, though it was called informed choice by staff.

Chapter 6 extends our work on the culture of maternity services by contrasting the culture of the large maternity units with smaller ones where staff were able to relate more directly with women. These units were not included in the RCT because their small size could have made no impact upon that large study. Yet the qualitative data from those sites set up a real contrast and suggest possible ways forward.

It is important to consider a situation, contrasting to the one we found in our research, where real strategic planning took place in a maternity unit before the MIDIRS leaflets were introduced. Jill Demilew describes this process in Chapter 8 and demonstrates how great a cultural change was needed as well as the scope and extent of professional skills and competencies that are required in order to facilitate informed choice.

When doing our research we were aware of other research which used the MIDIRS leaflets differently and found them to be of real use to women in informing their decision-making. Chapter 7 is an example of such work. Mary Newburn and Meg Wiggins report their study, which introduced the MIDIRS *Informed Choice* leaflets and created opportunities for groups of women to discuss them. This is a useful example of research on how services could work better, coming from a service user group, the National Childbirth Trust.

Chapters 9 and 10 address the topical issue of choice around Caesarean section. Susan Bewley and Jayne Cockburn, both consultant obstetricians, discuss the complexities of both the state of our knowledge and the ethics surrounding 'request' Caesarean sections. Julia Simpson, a nurse and social scientist, analyses the team narrative where senior obstetricians discuss with a new obstetric senior house officer and medical students the dilemmas around requests for Caesarean sections. Through analysis of the language and how it is used, and following the threads of the narrative, the values of participants and their concerns are examined.

In Chapter 11, Nicky Ellis, a community midwife in Leicester, reports a small study of the birth experiences of South Asian Muslim women. By choosing to study women who were educated in the UK, she separates the issues of ethnicity and language. For these women, 'the problems in communication did not spring from a lack of a common language with their carers but from the manner in which they were cared for.'

In Chapter 12, Tricia Anderson tells the story of three women who did not make the right choices as defined by the maternity services with which they were involved. She examines what was 'allowed' within the NHS and what the women achieved in the care of independent midwives.

In Chapter 13 I endeavour to pull together the key issues and examine the links and tensions between client choice and service organisation.

In many ways this book makes sad reading. Informed choice is unusual in maternity care and compliance is common. Equal information on different options is not usually offered as staff tend to steer women towards professionally defined 'right' choices. Yet, despite the pressures of bureaucracy and professional status, which lead staff to ensure women's compliance, there are other possibilities. This book shows many aspects of what is possible in maternity care as well as the scale of the cultural change which would be required to make informed choice real.

References

Cartwright, A. (1979) *The Dignity of Labour?* London: Tavistock.

Department of Health (1993) *Changing Childbirth: Report of the Expert Maternity Group.* London: HMSO.

Green, J.M., Coupland, V.A. and Kitzinger, J.V. (1988) *Great Expectations: A Prospective*

Study of Women's Expectations and Experiences of Childbirth. Child Care and Development Unit, University of Cambridge.

Guilliland, K. and Pairman, S. (1995) *The Midwifery Partnership: A Model for Practice.* Department of Nursing and Midwifery, Victoria University of Wellington.

Kirkham, M. and Stapleton, H. (eds) (2001) *Informed Choice in Maternity Care: An evaluation of evidence-based leaflets.* NHS Centre for Reviews and Dissemination, University of York. Report no 20.

NHS Executive (1996) *Patient Partnership.* London: HMSO.

Perkins, E.R. (1991) *Persuasion or Education? Health service methods of communication with parents.* Unpublished PhD thesis, Faculty of Education, University of Nottingham.

CHAPTER 1

Why Can't Women Just Say No? And Does It Really Matter?

NADINE PILLEY EDWARDS

Chapter Contents

■ Introduction

■ What do we know about choice in maternity care?

■ Women's experiences of constraints to choice

■ Limiting impacts of maternity services

■ Women's ways of being in the world

■ In what rhetorical space does choice arise?

■ How much does choice really matter?

■ Could the rhetoric of choice be transformed into one of ethical decision-making?

Introduction

This chapter is based on an in-depth qualitative study of 30 women's experiences of planning home births in Scotland (Edwards, 2001). While that study discussed how women viewed safety and risk, their relationships with midwives (see also Edwards, 2000) and the ethical impact of the medical model of birth, the following discussion focuses on choice (and thus rights, control and power). I attempt to provide a framework based on an interaction between what these women said, and some of the postmodernist/feminist theoretical constructs about decision-making. This enables a fuller debate about why choice is a potentially problematic concept. I focus on the limitations to decision-making experienced by the women I interviewed, and why the notion of choice (and even rights) is inadequate. Drawing on critiques of modernity's health care ethics, feminist ethics of care and its critics, feminist interpretations of relational autonomy and feminist political theory, I suggest why decision-making is integral to self-esteem and thus why and how it could be supported. The theories I use explain how the current construction of choice and its use within maternity care has been divorced from morality. The rhetoric of choice is thus somewhat empty, leading (at best) to confusion. The separation of choice from morality leaves it wide open to being used coercively by professionals who believe they know best and those who put the professionals' ideology into practice. Choice can thus only be given meaning again if it is reintegrated as part of a network of aspects of ethical decision-making based on individual concerns. In the next section I give a brief overview of some of the debates on choice in childbearing.

What do we know about choice in maternity care?

Choice is considered to be fundamental

We know that, in current western culture based on libertarian values, choice is considered to be fundamental to responsible personhood. While maternity care policies from 1904 to 1990 suffered from paternalism (see for example Inter-Departmental Committee, 1904; Maternity Services Advisory Committee, 1982, 1984, 1985; Ministry of Health, 1930, 1932, 1954, 1956, 1959, 1961, 1970, 1979), libertarian values were much more evident in the more recent Cumberlege Report (Department of Health, 1993), where choice was seen to be integral to the provision of maternity services. The medical profession in particular was criticised for its paternalistic attitudes and all professionals involved in childbearing were urged to provide comprehensive information, a range of services to meet the needs of different women, and respect for individual choice.

Choice is culturally constructed

However, from a general socio/cultural perspective, we also know that choice is constructed. Wendy Trevathan (1997, p. 80) commented that, 'only in rare circumstances can a woman act and behave exactly as she wishes during the birth process', because social norms usually dictate where and how women give birth, what 'artifacts' are used, and who receives the baby. In global terms, cross-cultural analyses (Davis-Floyd and Sargent, 1997; DeVries *et al.*, 2001; Jordan, 1993) demonstrate particularly clearly that choices are constructed through belief systems and resources. For example, in some cultures, home birth is an almost impossible 'choice' to make, whereas in others, it would be just as unthinkable to 'choose' otherwise. A number of sociologists, midwives and others have pointed out that women in western cultures make choices that are not only limited by intersections of class, race and other factors, but that the intersection between ideology and resources results in a predetermined, medically oriented menu over which women have limited control to define or change (Browner and Press, 1997; Cartwright and Thomas, 2001; Kitzinger, 1990; Lazarus, 1997; Mander, 1993, 1997; Mason, 1998; Ralston, 1994; Wagner, 1994). This has led to claims by some feminists that choice is a 'social construction that makes people feel free even in the context of oppression' (Gregg, 1995, p. 27).

Choice is potentially coercive

In our own culture, obstetric ideology is particularly coercive. The medical definition of safety and risk means that while minor choices exist, conceptual choices cannot. As Shelley Romalis (1985) pointed out, the coercive contract implies that the woman should privilege professional opinion over her own:

> The 'final say' clause in the doctor–patient contract is negotiated relatively early in the pregnancy relationship. 'You can have your baby any way you like as long as you understand that I must step in when the safety of you and the baby is involved.' (p. 190)

More recently, this was spelt out more clearly still:

> the obstetrician must respect the wishes of the mother and father, but only as far as it can be done without risking the health of the mother or the baby. Finally the obstetrician must be the expert who dares to set limits on 'experience hunting' and take full responsibility for the birth. (Rutanen and Ylikorkala, in Viisainen, 2000a, p. 796)

While these views starkly express the assumption that obstetric ideology has a monopoly on safety (and thus any decisions arising from this), coercion has many different faces, and control can be exerted in many different ways (Kirkham and Stapleton, 2001; Levy, 1999a, 1999b, 1998; Lukes, 1974; Shapiro, 1983).

For example, Romalis' (1985) research in Canada suggested that the influence of practitioners is such that, 'when the doctor is reluctant, drags his feet, or does not heartily encourage innovative practices, most patients will hesitate to take the initiative' (p. 194). In Josephine Green and colleagues' (1998) study, women made different 'choices' in different areas and hospitals serving similar populations, depending on the policies and practices in use. In another area 4 per cent of women used waterpools during labour and/or birth in one hospital, but 22 per cent used them in another hospital only 15 miles away (Scottish Health Feedback, 1993). Roseline Barbour (1990) described what happened when some men attempted to advocate for their partners, 'one expectant father told me: "We've come to see the consultant about Helen being induced ... and, frankly, it'll be over my dead body." Both this man and another attending for the same reason later revealed that the inductions were to take place as the doctor had satisfied them with the medical explanation he had provided' (p. 203).

David Machin and Mandy Scamell (1997) suggested that whatever women's views during pregnancy, the medical model in a hospital setting during labour is irresistible. It is irresistible because the basis for coercion is maternal responsibility and the promise of a live baby if women co-operate, and unbearable censure and blame if they do not (Gregg, 1995, p. 127; Murphy-Lawless, 1998). Choice is predicated on an obstetric definition of safety and the frequently held assumption that the baby's physical health must take precedence over women's choices (Dimond, 1993).

Bridget McAdam-O'Connell (1998, p. 122) suggests that choices are limited, not only by obstetric regimes, but that even within these regimes choices are largely meaningless, because women are unlikely to understand the value systems on which choices are based. They are systematically denied knowledge about and control over technological and pharmacological interventions, which remain 'in the realm of professional or specialist knowledge', leaving them ill-informed or mis-informed. Thus choice is firmly located within the 'power/knowledge system of obstetrics' (Murphy-Lawless, 1998, p. 23).

Even when practitioners are overtly committed to providing information and choice, Elizabeth Smythe (1998, p. 173) found that women were encouraged to make their own decisions only until there was a decision to be reached on something that the midwife felt strongly about. More often, as Valerie Levy (1998) suggests, practitioners may be unaware of their own agendas and, as she describes, may feel caught on a tightrope, balancing women's needs, those of their midwifery, medical and Trust colleagues, and perhaps even their own, as well as the potential conflict between (dominant) 'scientific' and (subordinate) experiential knowledges. Those who dare to do otherwise often find themselves ostracised, and victims of horizontal violence (Hadikin and O'Driscoll, 2000; Leap 1997).

Choice is based on subjectivities

If in addition to the above we consider individuals and their 'personal biographies' (Weiner *et al.*, 1997): that is, their different contexts, different abilities, faced with different concerns and constraints, choice unravels rather rapidly into a series of complex processes, rather than the unproblematic, 'thin', linear 'shopping list' approach criticised by Helen Stapleton (1997). In this view information is never unbiased. Those gathering and providing it, do so from their own interests and constraints. Thus the vacuum assumed by a rhetoric of choice is filled with a complex interaction of concerns. Decision-making occurs as these (unstable) interests are negotiated or suppressed, and is thus an ongoing dialogue within the self and between the self and others. Yet, as Carolyn McLeod and Susan Sherwin (2000, p. 267) comment:

> Patients' autonomy is generally reduced to the exercise of 'informed choice' in which the information provided is restricted to that deemed relevant by the health-care provider (and by the health-care system, which has determined what information is even available

by pursuing certain sorts of research programs and ignoring others). Even in 'ideal' cases in which patients have strong autonomy skills and full access to all the available information, it is important to recognize the influence that oppression may have on the information base and, thereby, on the meaningful options available to patients.

I come back to the issue of information, but first turn to what the woman in my study said about the decisions they wanted to make and how these were supported or undermined.

Women's experiences of constraints to choice

What makes choice more or less viable

Joseph Raz (in Brison, 2000, p. 286) suggests that:

If having an autonomous life is an ultimate value, then having a sufficient range of accept-able options is of intrinsic value, for it is constitutive of an autonomous life that it is lived in circumstances where acceptable alternatives are present.

The women in my study made very similar comments:

NPE: 'I just wondered what that means for you, what it means to be in control?'
'Well, to have a choice first of all, and the means to do it. Yeh, just being aware of all your options as well, so you know basically what's best for you.'

In a hegemonous system, lack of choice (what remains off the menu) often remains invisible and leaves obstetrics free to bend terminology to accommodate and reflect its own beliefs. It oversees the location, structure and content of most maternity care, and as the women in my study pointed out, basic choices about engaging with maternity services, how care is provided, who might attend birth, and the environment for birth are almost entirely missing. They provided insights into why choice is messier and potentially life-changing than generally understood and explained why they felt unable to put some of their decisions into practice. Their reasons included conflicting ideology, lack of information, fragile relationships between them and their midwives, lack of support for and/or alternatives to medical birth and practices, and the difficulty of asserting themselves in an unsympathetic environment.

Limiting impacts of maternity services

Place of birth

The women in the study suggested that fundamental choices were unavailable or constrained. For example, with few exceptions, the women repeatedly commented that the information about home birth is unforthcoming, and that it is a difficult option to choose because of a medicalised cultural assumption that it is unsafe. Having planned to have a home birth they then suggested that this option is heavily constrained by a risk discourse that reflects a medicalised, rather than a social/midwifery view of birth:

> 'They [midwives] were speaking in one way, but there was another agenda. And the other agenda was to my mind – if I could be persuaded to go to hospital, I would be. And I felt that we were talking about my life and what I was entitled to and what I could get and birth plans etc, etc. But there was something subtly discouraging in the whole line that was being taken that made me believe that there would have to be a very, very small – only very small problems – before I would end up in hospital. So I felt it was a wee bit dishonest really. I didn't feel that there was the support there for actually being at home.'

Continuity

In terms of the structure of care on offer, most women wanted a greater level of continuity than was provided by teams of six to eight midwives (Edwards, 1998, 2000), but found they were unable to exert any control over this. Because of the midwives' workloads and the on-call rota system in operation, neither women nor midwives appeared to have any choice about which midwife attended them during labour and birth. Even during pregnancy, this seemed impossible:

> 'I actually saw [the community midwifery manager]. I had an appointment with her because I had strong feelings about the fact that I would like to get to know, and I would want the person delivering the baby to get to know me prior to the birth so that we could be fairly clear about my wants and needs, and opinions on various forms of intervention and drug use. And she agreed that three midwives would be allocated to my case. She couldn't guarantee who would be at the birth, but she could guarantee that one of three midwives would be at the birth and that I could get to know the three over the forthcoming months. This arrangement broke down almost immediately, with appointments being kept by completely strange midwives without any prior notice being given to me. So it seems clear that they are unable to accommodate me – well they are unable to accommodate me. But they're even unable to accommodate the compromise that they suggested to try and make me feel more comfortable.'

Attendants

While some women felt concerned about the level of medicalisation even within community midwifery, the idea that it could be 'your [the woman's] choice to get her [midwife] in' seemed inconceivable, given the current assumptions and legalities concerning the management of birth. And yet, while women appreciated the existence of a community midwifery service and observed the ways in which midwives attempted to provide a good service despite the constraints they faced, some pointed out the coerciveness of a system that recognises only 'qualified' midwives:

> 'part of me says that there shouldn't be a law that says that you must have a midwife with you and if there's anyone else with you, they're subject to prosecution, because that means that by having women with knowledge or lay midwives or whatever, with a woman that puts that person in danger of prosecution. And I think that's *outrageous*. Women know what they need and I find it ridiculous that the law puts itself in the way of that. They seem to have some kind of belief in the medical system – that it is appropriate.'

> 'the feeling I got [was] I should do as I was told. You will adhere to this ... I think I was going to say that I thought it [the home birth service] was a way of controlling. Yeh, I think it's just almost like a form of controlling people and reminding people that, you know, it's dangerous to go alone and that it would be illegal to, you know, to have a birth without a midwife. And, yeh, I don't think there's a great deal of choice about it is there? There's not any variety. It is just a monitoring service, It doesn't allow you any opportu- nities to get to know a midwife, or trust a midwife. It's just about monitoring you and doing all the things they do in hospital but doing it in the community ... I do feel that your knowledge is totally overridden ... I do find it totally unbelievable, and I don't think I appreciated that until I had a baby at home and realised that even, you know, even although you're in your own home you still don't have great deal of control.'

Environment

Many women also commented from previous experiences of hospital births on the lack of appropriate options for normal birth within a medicalised/hospital setting:

> 'How can you make a good choice out of five bad choices? And I just sort of thought – now let's think. Where would I want to give birth here. And I thought – nowhere. Not on this horrible plastic chair. Not on this horrible high plastic bed. You know, none of these were in any way inviting for me to lie on, or sit on, or squat on – and the bed was too high. You couldn't kneel on the floor, you know. It was just, I thought, this is not a good place to have a baby, you know.'

Spatial, temporal and material arrangements for birth in hospital constrained women's choice, by constraining their abilities to put decision-making into practice. This was one of the key reasons many planned to have their babies at home. The current spatial layout of hospital, and temporal arrangements for birth has bodies in mind, only so far as institutionally managing those bodies. As Moira Gatens (1996) pointed out, the body tends to be organised around culture rather than vice versa, and as Barbara Adams commented, clock time has taken precedence over nature's time. As one woman who felt constrained by restrictions on space and time in hospital commented:

'If you're in hospital and sometime in the past you've thought, this is what I'd really like to do. This is really how I'd like my labour managed, it just goes completely out of the window once you're actually in hospital. And being told what to do by staff, because they think it's best. So it's only, you know, after a couple of months when you've been home, that you think, oh, it was like it was a different world when you said, or wrote down, I wanted to do that. It bears no relation to what actually goes on. So, I see, and I don't know how this is going to work, but I see being at home as a way of joining up what you thought when you were pregnant and what you wanted when you were pregnant, and what actually happens in the labour.'

Routine procedures

All the women in the study questioned some of the routine procedures during pregnancy and labour, for example, the use of ultrasound and tests in pregnancy, vaginal examinations, fetal heart monitoring and blood pressure examinations during labour, the giving of Syntometrine for the birth of the placenta and the use of Vitamin K after birth. While they experienced some choice with some procedures, they felt that others were understood by practitioners to be requirements. While some women appreciated what they called 'checking' and 'monitoring' during labour, others found it interfered with their focus on giving birth:

'I was assured that they would only do them [vaginal examinations] out of necessity, but I still don't understand why they're necessary. I can't clearly see that myself. And the same with the blood pressure, somehow I have the feeling that they can't observe women and feel that things are alright and that she's alright without having to use physical monitors all the time. That is what I find slows me down, interferes with me and made me feel that I had to be checked.'

While there were exceptions, it seemed difficult for these questions even to be raised within a medicalised framework. Midwives are so afraid of not adhering to routine practices that they continued with painful vaginal examinations and other procedures despite women's explicit expressions of pain and/or instructions to stop. Where these questions were raised during pregnancy, women were mainly steered towards practices midwives felt obliged to follow and away from those that might challenge the boundaries within which they practised. Consider the following for example from the first and second interviews with one of the women in my study:

'I did consider not having the Syntometrine injection, and they're not keen on that at all. I'm finding more opposition against that than having the home birth. So I said well we'll just see how it goes, but I mean if everything goes the way I'm hoping it's going and everything's natural then I'm just going to carry on. I don't see why I should get some intervention then, when everything's going so fine.'

NPE: 'How have your discussions gone about the Syntometrine?'
'Ah, I've given in to that I must admit, I have. I've given in. My GP wasn't happy about it … and all the midwives. I've spoken to a few of them and because I've seen different midwives I've asked them all, just to find out, you know, what their opinion is and they're all very for it – everybody. Yeh, they're not keen for me not to have it so I've sort of given in.'

The final irony was that the woman researched the subject further and decided not to have Syntometrine unless it was needed, but received it because her decision was not amended in her birth plan.

Information/steering

This leads to the problematic nature of information giving which I alluded to earlier, which is clear in the quotations above and which Jo Green and colleagues (1998, p. 178) suggests is an essential ingredient for decision-making:

'Information is in many ways a pre-requisite for "external" control since having adequate information forms part of the basis upon which decisions can be made.'

A number of women commented on the difficulty of getting specific information that might support their own needs and beliefs, but might also lead them to make informed decisions that would challenge their midwives' policies and practices. Sometimes, midwives seemed vague or evasive about providing information:

'Most of the questions I had I wouldn't get a satisfactory answer to, so I stopped bothering asking them, and just found out myself really – although that does leave you with a lot of gaps. It means you're going in blind. I could find out a lot about the physiology of birth without asking a professional, but I can't find out about their procedures without asking them. And when they're not very forthcoming – I wouldn't say that they were deliberately vague. I don't know. Somehow it all stayed vague, just like my questions.'

'they [midwives] proclaimed the baby breech and then insisted the baby would turn and they wouldn't talk about what the implications were and they wouldn't say what their procedures were or what hospital policy was if the baby stayed that way.'

Women whose babies were in a breech position towards the later months of their pregnancies reported that they were unable to engage their midwives in conversations about the possibility of continuing with their plans to give birth at home. They were told that breech births are medical cases that take place in hospital and that they would discontinue being involved in the woman's care.

All in all, there were many examples of women's decisions bending to external power. They were also aware that their wills could be shaped in such a way that it appeared that all parties apparently concurred. They were aware that information could enable or disable their autonomy and that it was extremely difficult to break through the 'layers of medical expertise' and aware that they were persuaded to comply with a style of care that did not necessarily meet their needs to be autonomous. Concurring with the reality described by Robin Gregg (1995) and Jo Murphy-Lawless (1998), women frequently drew on 'little strategies' (and described their midwives as doing the same) to exert minor influence on a system that largely erases their subjectivity and agency prior to their engagement with it.

Skills

To provide information that might support women to make decisions that lie outside medical policies, midwives require the skills to make these a reality. But lack of midwifery skills was frequently referred to by the women in this study. In forfeiting 'unusual' but potentially normal births to obstetrics, midwives have also forfeited the skills they had and the potential for developing these, to help women safely through challenging normal births. While a few midwives have retained these skills (see, for example, Cronk. 1992, 1998a, 1998b; Warmsley, 1999) and understand that women's decision-making within a social midwifery approach to birth depends on the skills of the midwives providing it, this understanding seems generally lost. Decision-making, even rights, cut little ice if we lack the skills and resources to put these into practice. A woman who had a long labour at home resulting in an instrumental hospital birth reflected:

> 'I so much wanted this baby to come at home, and not to be interfered with. And it was like a terrible disappointment. But they [midwives] did realise that in time and in the end I felt they were really very supportive in their own way ... And I think some of them felt bitterly disappointed for me as well. One in particular was really disappointed. She really wanted me to be able to have the baby at home but didn't — maybe couldn't have — supported me in that way. They were very good to us afterwards, and they all came to visit us and were very kind and yeh, in a way they wanted to be supportive, they certainly did ... And I just always remembered thinking it was sad they didn't have more things included in their training that they could just feel more supportive. Cos they wanted to but ...'

Conflicting ideologies

Women were aware that midwives positioned themselves differently on the medical/midwifery spectrum. They also recognised that however much some midwives were prepared to 'stretch' their policies, and however skilled they were, there were differences between their ideologies and the ideology of the system in which these midwives practised. These created barriers to meaningful engagement, information exchange and decision-making:

'If there seems to be a problem, I don't want to hold out and have a bloody natural child-birth and a dead baby, or a really unhealthy baby. I'm just – I am really anxious that they'll kind of panic and want to take charge really quickly. And the other thing was about cutting the cord, where I didn't feel quite so happy, because I was saying that I wanted the cord to be left until it had stopped pulsating. And I do feel quite strongly about that. And she [midwife] was saying, oh well [said slightly severely], you know, if it comes out and it's round the neck and it's very tight and we can't get it off, then we'd want to cut it right then. Is that okay? [said slightly menacingly]. And I don't know. Yes, if the baby's in danger, then of course, do anything. But I suppose it's just if I don't know I'm coming from the same value basis as somebody, then I don't know if they're going to be making decisions on the same basis as I would.'

Often, conscientious midwives were in the impossible situation of making sure women complied with medical policies, as well as fulfilling their obligation to provide choice. The confusion generated by providing policy-guided information, overlaid with a rhetoric of choice was evident:

'One of the midwives that came round spoke to me about it [Vitamin K]. But again, it was one of these things that was sort of dumped in my lap – this has got to be your choice. Though she only told me the good side. She told me about the importance of the injection, and then said, this has got to be your choice. And I didn't understand if it was so good, why it needed to be my choice. So it's been up to me to find the other side. I don't feel I've got a sort of unbiased view on it yet. So again, I'm taking the advice of the medical people I have around me – which is the midwife – who advises it.'

'They [midwives] said that meconium staining ... they said that the baby was in distress and that they were going to phone the ambulance on those grounds. And then they said that the heart beat was a hundred and forty, which was as it had been from the very beginning, so it sounded as if they thought there was meconium, however the baby was well and the baby wasn't bothered. So the two of those things don't seem to combine for me. But anyway they said that it would be advisable to go into hospital ....They were very keen for us to make the decision *immediately*. The midwife came back in and she, you know, she came up to me and she was at the very most a foot away from me, and she was being very directive and saying, you know, that we should be going to hospital blah, blah, blah. And then she said at the end of all that, of course we'd be very happy to stay here and deliver you at home and I thought well if you are worried – in hindsight – if you are worried then surely you wouldn't be saying that. Surely you should be saying something else. So although I felt that they'd tried to indicate that there was a sense of urgency, I felt that that particular thing that they said meant that they weren't all that worried. That's what struck me about saying that to me .... One of the things I said was I really feel we have no choice and she said, oh yes but you do have a choice, oh yes but you do.'

Consider the contrast between the above quotation and the one below, where the midwife knew the views of the woman she was attending, shared a similar ideology and practised autonomously on a one-to-one basis:

'I knew that she [midwife] would tell me if there was anything wrong and if she was ever really worried about the baby you know – because it was a long labour and, you know I did have meconium staining at one point and we carried on. Whereas, definitely it seems to me that with the community midwives that's it, you're just into hospital. And she knew I didn't want it so she said, mm the heartbeat's fine, I think we're okay. And I thought, well we must be. I never thought that when I was in the bathroom that she would say to my partner, look another half an hour and that's it, we're going to have to go. I never felt there was any subterfuge. I knew that she was respecting me and telling me the truth the whole time which – I mean, later she said to me there were a few times when she was a little worried – but not much you know. So if you like it was good, cos she made me confident and she never lied to me. But she was able to manipulate that a little bit in a positive way you know. I trusted her so much that I let her take the worry, one or two times when there was a wee bit of worry. She absorbed that without me knowing, which is really good.'

As a result of conflicting ideology and mistrust, many women felt that not only did they need to develop their own confidence in their ability to give birth, and their knowledge about less medicalised approaches to birth, but that they had to find out as much as they possibly could about the medical model of birth, it's policies and practices, in order to have any hope of exerting at least some control over decision-making:

'I have to know everything about it. It feels that, you know, I can't just have the normal knowledge of a normal person to have a baby. I've got to have all the knowledge of all the nurses and all the obstetricians and all the rest of it because they won't advise me according to what they know I want. They will advise me according to their own set of rules and what they want. And that's not unbiased. They didn't give me unbiased information, and allow me to make my own decision. They specifically veered me towards their own outcome.'

'You've to know your stuff, which I think, that's not right. I shouldn't have to know my stuff. But I felt I had to read up so much because, they [midwives and doctors] could come across, you know, they could say something to me and I could say, oh really, oh dear, do I have that, oh gosh, my poor baby. Oh well yes, I'll have to go to hospital. So I felt I had to arm myself, basically.'

Telling not listening

There has tended to be an assumption that informed choice means informing women so that they will choose the choice being advised and that differences in opinion indicate a lack of understanding on the part of the woman (Kitzinger, 1990, p. 109). Thus a 'telling not listening' culture has emerged. Professional literature often urges midwives and doctors to improve their knowledge of evidence-based care along with their communication skills: as if communication forms a neutral bridge between information and choice. The women's quotations above suggest that this ignores power differentials between people and lacks awareness about or respect for different ideologies and concerns (see also Davis-Floyd, 1992; Davis-Floyd and Sargent, 1997; Jordan, 1993; Williamson, 1992; Young, 1990, 1997) and thus enhances the use of 'choice' as a powerful mechanism for control and manipulation, by rendering women irresponsible if they do not concur with dominant views:

> 'I found him [obstetrician] very insulting in his approach. He directly said I was being foolish. And when I went [to hospital] the second time, that was how he referred to me – three or four times in the conversation – I think you're being very foolish. And he implied that I didn't care about the safety of my baby. I don't know where you get your research from but if I thought home births were safe then I'd be advocating them. And he just gave me no credit for being an intelligent woman. He didn't give me credit for having read in the field or for the fact that it's me that's having the baby and of course the baby's safety is paramount to me.'

The women's observations that information, practices and policies arise from belief systems rather than absolute truths is well supported in sociological midwifery literature (Davis-Floyd and Sargent, 1997). Indeed, what we call 'facts' are largely underdetermined by the available evidence (Kuhn, 1970; Oakley, 2000) and are more closely aligned with beliefs.

There were therefore a number of connected reasons why the information/choice equation was problematic. Women need information as part of that equation, but the information available and provided is rarely contextualised and located in the power struggles between different ideologies and needs. Without acknowledging these issues, medical ideology continues a project which it names informed choice or consent, but in fact steers women into making 'correct' choices and providing the 'consent' needed by obstetrics to carry on business as usual. In other words, choice is a misnomer for compliance with obstetric hegemony. This is not to say that all interactions between women and practitioners are coercive or that choice is uniformly oppressive. What I do suggest is that the concept of choice within obstetric ideology is essentially oppressive because it tends towards maintaining a status quo which systematically deprives women of autonomy. It is predicated on a series of largely unacknowledged power structures that hold in place oppressive obstetric regimes which erase meaningful autonomy and responsibility. Predicating choice on a system that is resistant to ideological change and therefore changes in practice has less effect on its hegemony than we care to think, because choice is set within a much greater need to control women's behaviour. Of course choice is always constrained by intersections of concerns (race, class, resources, for example), but in obstetrics it masks power struggles between dominant ideology and normative practices and the attempts by individuals to exert a level of autonomy by making decisions that feel right for them. How has this linear notion of choice arisen – whereby individuals are considered to be equal and have been persuaded that 'truth' can only be produced through a constructed meaning of rationality?

Women's ways of being in the world

Women's ways of decision-making

Despite one or two counter-examples, most of the women in this study demonstrated patterns of decision-making that were located in ethics of care and relationality described by Carol Gilligan (1985) and Mary Belenky and colleagues (1986), rather than in choice and rights. These women, like those in the aforementioned studies, placed emphasis on relational ways of information-gathering, discussion and decision-making based on mutuality rather than control:

> NPE: 'Would you be able to say a bit more about control?
> 'Um … I wonder. I wonder, um … I mean, control isn't something that I would necessarily put lots of emphasis on. It's not that I want to be able to necessarily dictate so much what goes on. It's more that I don't want strong influence on me because I know that if I have that influence I bend to it, you know. And in the long run that's no good for me. It's much better if I'm doing what actually feels natural I think. But also I suppose it comes down to knowing what's going on. Knowing who's going to be there, you know … I suppose it's more dissipating control, you know. There's not so much of an issue of who is in control when it's at home, because it's not my wish to be pushy – but more just that there's no-one in control. That things can just flow and no-one feel that they're more or less part of things or so on, if that makes sense.'

The problem was that the rhetoric of choice, rights and control leaves little space for negotiation and relational decision-making in which control can be relinquished: if women did not take control, it was passed elsewhere. In other words, while they challenged the need for control during pregnancy, labour and birth, they often recognised the paradox that going with the flow might ultimately mean going with the flow of medical ideology. As Tess Cosslett (1994) pointed out, during the challenging experience of labour and birth, this led to an impossible internal conflict for women:

> 'It's a confusing one because I kind of want both ends of the spectrum. I want to be able to give up control completely and in terms of the process just be able to go with it. And I also want to have complete control over the space and what's happening in it, you know, who's doing what to me and who's doing what to the baby. And they don't feel very compatible, those two different kinds of states of being – completely surrendering to a very powerful process and also kind of going, hang on a minute, I don't like what you're doing there. So it feels like a funny balance.'

As for the women in Juliana van Olphen Fehr's (1999) study, ideally, choice would have meant making decisions as far as possible for an uncertain event and then responding to it in the context of broad philosophical agreement in dialogue with a trusted midwife. However, while trusting relationships are integral to social midwifery, these are not perceived as necessary for medically defined informed choice. The following comment was typical when women moved from fragmented medically based NHS care to one-to-one care from a midwife with a holistic philosophy:

> 'the difference of just knowing I'd have someone more in line with my thinking. I didn't feel that I needed a birth plan any more. I don't need these things any more. I don't need all these things because I trust her opinion and that way I don't have any fears. So I don't have to swot up so much and, you know, be so defensive.'

Decision-making was experienced as a dynamic dialogic process, based on their midwives' knowledges, the women's growing knowledge about child-bearing, and their changing minds and bodies (Diprose, 1994). They needed midwives who could move with them, so that issues could be discussed and left open. Individual women and midwives did their best, but they were hindered by lack of continuity and a definition of choice that involved isolated episodes of care whereby women were expected to make decisions 'on the spot' that would be documented and not usually revisited. Many women found their care to be lacking in flexibility and depth:

> 'Like I said to you before, all that time that you spend with them [midwives] and yet what do you do? You chat about the same things with each of them that comes. You never really scratch the surface.'

Why rights don't help ... much

Of course the increasing emphasis on human rights has had a profound impact on many areas of life, particularly in relation to minority groups and oppressed peoples. Campaigns for basic rights are crucial. However, talking to women about rights highlighted a number of problems in maternity care. A senior midwife once said to me that if women do not want an intervention, 'they just have to say no'. For the women in my study it was not so straightforward. An alternative was often unavailable. Thus, as Iris Marion Young (1990, 1997) suggested, inequalities between ideologies and peoples may be such that negative liberty (making a choice a right) needs to be replaced by positive liberty (where choice is well enough supported to become a reality). In addition, the notion of rights arises from the same oppressive discourse as choice, and the same barriers to exerting choice exist in relation to rights – perhaps even more so, as rights exist in an adversarial milieu. Women were usually aware of their rights, but many found that they did not want to appeal to these:

> 'I found out that I had a legal right [to a home birth], but I didn't really want to invoke that.'

> 'I'm not really very pushy. I don't like to feel I make waves.'

While some women felt that knowing their rights was of some benefit, appealing to these was a far cry from the supportive relationships they felt they needed. In Gilligan's terms (Hamer, 2000), the relatively simplistic, dualistic notion of rights cannot begin to address the complexities of procedural, circumstantial decision-making (Cornell, 1995; Shildrick, 1997):

> 'The most important thing to me was to feel supported. From what I could gather a home birth wasn't going to have much benefit if I wasn't with people who I felt were supportive.'

In practice, most women felt unable to appeal to their rights. In a very rare example of open conflict, the high cost of appealing to rights is evident. The effort required by the woman to maintain her position resulted in the potential undermining of that position and increased her sense of uncertainty and alienation from the very midwives she was relying on for support. In the quotation below, the woman had been told she could not have a home birth and had discussed this further with a community midwife and then written a letter reiterating her decision:

> 'I knew it was my choice and my right to have a home confinement. I thought no I'm not going to let you dissuade me, you know I'm not going to let you put me off. And I was quite adamant. I sort of met her match for match I think, for the more angry and adamant she got, the more adamant I got that this was my choice. But it's when you get home that you start to think, god what a big head to head I've had there and these are the women that are supposed to be coming and giving me care and if I alienate them I won't get the best care. Or perhaps I have made a bit of a silly choice you know .... She said ... that she didn't think that this was an appropriate decision for me to make and that I'd left it a bit late ... I mean I don't think that you've read up about all the facts here, you know. I think that you're not making a sensible decision. Really I think you should just go ahead with your hospital booking. And I said, look at the end of the day I know it's my right to choose a home confinement and I understand I've left it late but this is what I want and this is what I'm happy with. And she said, well I don't think I can support you in this decision. In my opinion I think you're making the wrong choice. I don't think that home is the best place for you to have your first child. You don't know what it's going to be like. You don't know what complications you're going to have and goodness knows anything could go wrong and you know, you could end up putting yourself and your child in danger. Do you want your unborn child to die? And of course I don't, but at the same time you know there's no reason why this unborn child should die, I've had a very low-risk pregnancy ... She did her very utmost to try and persuade me to change my booking back to the hospital ... It left me feeling very isolated and – why did I have to fight? ... I'm left with feelings of – what if something does go wrong, and am I going to get the told you so syndrome or, you know, the what do you expect you had a home confinement. That's not a nice feeling cos you end up with self-doubt – whether you are making the right decision or whether you are strong enough to actually go the whole way with it.'

Most women, however, were extremely reluctant to assert themselves if this meant jeopardising their relationships with the midwives they knew they would be dependent on during labour. These relationships were already seen as tenuous and fragile because of the lack of continuity and different mutually threatening ideologies.

Along with the difficulty in asserting themselves, women described a pull towards normality that was reflected in another study:

'I was just trying to be good and do everything as it was meant to be done. You know, according to the system. That's why I went to all these [parentcraft] classes in hospital [laughs]. Just trying to be a good parent, you know. Following all the rules.'

'it is easier to do what everybody else does, people do not want to step out from line, especially not Finns. They want to be like everybody else so that no one can say that they are different.' (Viisainen, 2000b)

Meantime, women had good reason to be cautious.

Being cautious

Jo Green and colleagues (1998, pp. 64–5) found that women wanted to be active decision-makers, and wanted control over what was done to them, but at the same time they noted hostility towards these women, which reconstructed the usually positively viewed well-educated, well-informed woman as problematic (pp. 19–24). Acts of control by professionals were particularly noticeable towards women who were seen to hold the strongest views – they were most likely to receive the opposite of what they wanted (p. 128). Similar findings (Jones *et al.*, 1998) showed that women with birth plans requesting as few interventions as possible received more interventions than similar women without birth plans. Diana Scully (1994) found that doctors in her study expected to be in control and disliked women who they experienced as non-compliant, questioning or 'difficult' (pp. 91–3). These women tended to be ignored or even cruelly treated (pp. 130–6).

When women speak out against obstetric ideology, they speak out in dangerous territory. We are obliged to protect ourselves and the social networks in which we exist and on which we depend. Sometimes this can involve relinquishing their own values in order to maintain relationships with practitioners:

'The first time round I'd had a scan done. And I actually didn't want to have it done, but I didn't realise I had a choice about it, and to be very honest, I felt so relieved that my doctor had agreed for a home birth for me, that I didn't want to push her. I thought, if I contest the scan, maybe she won't be so supportive of me. So that was at the back of my mind – I better do this to show that I'm willing to co-operate. And I didn't want to make waves.'

The need to be cautious was most evident in the interviews with the women who were most critical of obstetric ideology. While a degree of challenge/difference was tolerated, those who challenged most openly were well aware of the limits to 'choice':

> 'I'm not going in them stirrups, I'm not being cut, and I'm not having a Caesarean, I'm just going to let nature takes it course, and I remember the shocked look on his [obstetrician's] face, and he said to me, if you're going to take that tack, he said, you do realise that me and the other doctor will have you brought in for the Caesarean, on the grounds that you are not able to make the decision for yourself, yeh, basically, I'll be committed to hospital … So I have in the back of my head, that sort of big brother. And I feel that I'm complying, you know. I'm doing what I have to do.'

As Mary Belenky and colleagues (1986) and Elizabeth Debold and colleagues (1996) found, we cease to be ourselves in a myriad of ways, fragmenting what we think, what we say and what we do, working under cover (Hutchison, 1990; Levy, 1998), or as midwife Mary Cronk comments, 'doing good by stealth', imposing innumerable constraints on ourselves and others. Examining concepts of choice and rights suggested that women often felt unable to put their ethical judgements into practice, due to dominant medical ethics focused on the baby and responsible mothering, as well as an ethics of care focused on selflessness and nurturing. In other words both modernity's ethics and feminist ethics of care place constraints on women's autonomy. It is clear from the quotations that the cost is high, whether we assert or silence ourselves. Thus one could argue that accepting feminist ethics of care fails to acknowledge power differentials and how ethics of care and relationality may be constructed through oppressions. One could also argue as some feminists do (Debold *et al.*, 1996, Nicholson, 1999) that we need to consider how this serves oppression rather than challenges it, how it prevents women being themselves and making decisions they feel are right for themselves and their families and how this could be different.

In what rhetorical space does choice arise?

'Choice' has a fascinating history. It forms the external facet of a whole package of largely hidden assumptions about subjectivity: relationships between the person and itself, the person and its environment and the person and others. While some of the theories in this area are complex and located in diverse theoretical debates, if we engage with pregnant women, provide information, and support autonomous decision-making, we need to have more understanding about the nature of these interactions and why and how they can be profoundly empowering or disempowering.

Libertarian choice arises from the libertarian notions of the individual – often known as contract theory (see critiques by Carol Pateman, 1989 and

Young, 1990, 1997, for example). The idea is that the individual is (and always has been and will be) a pre-formed, self-contained, separate entity. The Cartesian edict is that this individual develops its rational abilities and strives to make objective (ethical) decisions that are free of other influences and desires – such as its own body, its emotions, the relationships it engages in, and the contexts in which its life is led. Decisions are thus assumed to be made in a vacuum – or in some sanitised, cerebral part of the mind. The ability to be rational is also attributed with certain values and beliefs. The dualistic thinking of Cartesian or modernistic thinking created a structure of hierarchical pairings based on the super-binary, male/female. *Male, rationality, science* were seen as dominant and *female, emotional, natural* for example, subordinate. In this way of thinking, women (and other subordinate peoples) are excluded from rationality and thus ethical decision-making. It is not difficult to extrapolate that 'patients' are considered to be subordinate and that providing limited choices has been assumed to be adequate (Shildrick, 1997). Any possibility of self-definition based on her own experience of herself (her body, habitat, experiences and knowledges) lies outside modernity's ethics. I am not suggesting that professionals and their clients necessarily, consciously engage with these assumptions, but that they exist nonetheless and thus shape how interactions occur. Not fully knowing or understanding the assumptions which direct our actions does not render them less powerful. On the contrary they may continue to undermine our efforts to change our practices.

Feminists' contributions have been particularly important in challenging this modernistic construction of decision-making and in examining the issues of power and knowledge involved. They also demonstrate how definitions of subjectivity influence how we respond to others. Theories that acknowledge relationality, difference and vulnerability, and the impact of diverse concerns show why informed choice/consent are problematic. But as one woman commented:

> 'It's very difficult to bring that sort of thing up with a midwife because they don't want to be seen like they're living in the bad old days. And of course, we won't do anything without your consent. Well, what sort of consent are you going to be giving at that point [in labour]. And that's not ever frankly discussed.'

How much does choice really matter?

Potential consequences of preventing decision-making

While planning a home birth in the 1970s, even in the last week of my pregnancy, my midwife attempted to lure me into hospital with the uncertain promise of a free layette if the child was born on Christmas day. I am sure that she was under considerable pressure from local GPs to persuade me to give birth in hospital – but it also demonstrated to me a profound misunderstanding about decision-making. What mattered to me could not be exchanged for a layette. To remove ethics from decision-making and call it choice is a form of violence: choice is not just skin-deep.

When we engage with women, we need to consider what it means when they feel pressurised or reluctantly coerced into decisions that feel wrong for them. As Carol Gilligan (Hamer, 1999) suggests, a system of rights is anathema to women who feel embedded in a rhetoric of guilt and blame, and situated in relationship networks which demand they consider others before themselves. They are likely to be pliable and unable to assert their own knowledge and needs. This is particularly acute in obstetrics, where risk becomes a powerful lever to ascertain compliance. The inadequacies and oppressive turns of both an ethics of care and modernity's reductionist ethics leave women without support and blaming themselves when they feel unable to forge their own meanings of birth. It may seriously impact on how they feel about themselves and how they feel they can relate to their babies, when they blame themselves for being ill-informed, unable to communicate, unassertive, and letting themselves and their children down as the woman's quotation below suggest:

> 'I mean it [birth] was just taken totally away from you. But it was in every sense. I was always really sort of a bit wary about the whole sort of thing about empowerment, and you know, the whole thing. But I mean it's just so true ... I just sort of lost every will to fight and confidence in my own body. Everything. It was just gone ... I mean I do feel incredibly robbed after the experience of childbirth. I find that really quite difficult to cope with [crying...] It's left me with a feeling that I didn't handle the situation very well ... feeling that I should have really handled the situation better. I should have been stronger you know. I should have sort of held out. I should not have given in. I should have been strong and sort of said, no I don't want to be induced, you know. But the pressures I was under at the time. I was sort of left with feeling, no, you know why didn't you just say no? Especially afterwards the midwife said you know, if you'd sort of made a fuss, they would have let you go back home. And I just turned round and said, why didn't I? You know. Why wasn't I just strong. Why didn't I? You know I could have avoided all that. And I mean, I know why I didn't ... But I didn't and I don't know, I just sort of feel I probably made the wrong decision although it's understandable why I made it. But you know it wasn't a good choice I made.'

Decreasing autonomy risks decreasing women's sense of self-worth, self-trust, self-esteem and confidence. It potentially violates their psyches, minds and bodies. There is a widely held view that all that matters is a live mother and baby. Women shared the view that their babies lives are paramount, but they also understood that the quality of life cannot be divorced from the bodily manifestations of being alive. Making decisions was one of the ways in which they attempted to shape the quality of their lives and the lives of their children. Thus choice reached down into the very fibres of their being. For them it formed part of an ethical stance which reflected their beliefs, values and life styles.

In this view autonomy cannot be separated from identity (Griffiths, 1995; Mackenzie and Stoljar, 2000), thus choice is deeply implicated with personhood. Threatening or undermining choice threatens and undermines autonomy. So as Margrit Shildrick (1997) and Elizabeth Smythe (1998) observe, medical encounters which undermine moral agency (or discount what matters) may undermine the self. As the women's quotations demonstrate, 'we cannot simply choose to abandon our cares or give up what matters to us. Or rather, we cannot do so without forfeit or loss' (Mackenzie 2000, p. 135). If we are distrusted and prevented from acting on our ethical stances, as I mentioned earlier, the effects can be devastating. And even though self-worth is complex, and (fortunately) women are resilient, Brison remarks that 'one assailant can undo a lifetime of self-esteem' (in Mackenzie 2000, p. 141), as birth accounts sometimes demonstrate.

The women in this study were perhaps more able and prepared than some women to exert autonomy. But even they felt hindered in a myriad of ways by the limitations of obstetric morality and its practices. It is infinitely more difficult for women who have had fewer opportunities to develop their beliefs and values, have received little support to put them into practice and may not even have felt able to articulate them (Mackenzie and Stoljar, 2000).

Potential consequences of enabling decision-making

Clinging to our own values and closing ourselves to those of others decreases dialogue, knowledge and trust. It increases silence, violence and oppression. Consider the difference when a woman feels support for her decision-making processes, and is able to develop a sense of herself as an able woman and a good mother:

> 'If I'm down about anything or I may have doubts about something I'm doing with [baby] you know. If I have a crisis of confidence, I think back to the birth and it's a very good anchor for me in that way. You know it makes me believe in my ability to make good choices and things like that, and I think it's made a tremendous impact on how I can make decisions ... It just feels pivotal and kind of a pivotal part of my politics really. It's almost like it drew together lots of things, lots of sides that I had already, and made them more cohesive as part of my life.'

Thus birth can be a crucial site for knowledge exchange, for mutual support between women and midwives, and for challenging dominant ideology which attempts to reduce ethical decision-making to an empty rhetoric of choice. As the women explained, the real issue is about trust. In the presence of trust between women and midwives, safe decision-making develops through the joint knowledges of both, in which the values of the woman are honoured.

Denying choice may deny a positive sense of self, while supporting it may contribute to a positive self-image. This is powerfully demonstrated by the quotations above, and by the one below in which a woman describes the contribution of her midwives to her reclaiming of autonomy after previous birth trauma:

> 'My daughter's birth was a true healing for me; both my body and my spirit were healed and put back together again. With the help of my midwives, I discovered the strength to reclaim my body and my baby.' (Noble, 2001, p. 113).

Could the rhetoric of choice be transformed into one of ethical decision-making?

Moving beyond the medical menu

Partial acceptance of limited diversity by current libertarianism suggests that women need more accurate, unbiased information and the right to choose the birth they want within a framework of medically defined risk. In practice, evidence-based information remains remarkably elusive (Kirkham and Stapleton, 2001). But even if it was widely distributed, this ignores my earlier claim that knowledge is intimately connected to social norms (Davis-Floyd and Sargent, 1997; DeVries *et al.*, 2001; Jordan, 1993). If we were to appeal to knowledge, it seems that women and babies (especially those living with poverty and exclusion) are best served by skilled midwives in out of hospital settings, where they receive fewer interventions and sustain fewer injuries (Chamberlain *et al.*, 1997; Rooks, 1997; Sandall *et al.*, 2001; Saunders *et al.*, 2000; Schlenzka, 1999). Jo Green and colleagues (1998, pp. 173–5), suggested that whatever views women held prior to birth, satisfaction rates were highest among those women who had fewest interventions. Some of the most positive childbearing accounts come from women who gave birth in out-of-hospital settings and/or had one or two trusted midwives during that period (Lemay, 1997; McCourt and Page, 1997; Noble, 2001; O'Connor, 1992; Ogden *et al.*, 1997a, 1997b; Sandall *et al.*, 2001; van Olphen Fehr, 1999). These are useful pointers, but if supporting women's abilities to make decisions is to avoid technological/natural polarities, then we need to listen more closely to the individual woman and provide support that is based on her values and beliefs, so that she can give birth in a way that most closely supports her autonomy and values and least betrays them. Without listening we risk imposing oppressive counter-cultural norms and replacing one set of rules and 'choices' with another: 'reduc[ing] 'plurality' to variations on the Same' (Code, 2000, p. 198).

As I also claimed, women's decision-making is more complex and relational than libertarianism choice can account for (Mackenzie and Stoljar, 2000). This suggests re-integrating the arbitrary division between choice and women's ethics so that their decision-making could be seen for what it is: a demonstration and development of their ethical stances. Moving beyond modernity's rights and choices, to postmodern diversity and multiplicity forges a different construction of ethics and decision-making. Women need support to develop their own moralities from which to make responsible decisions. While knowledge acquisition forms part of this process, it also involves facilitating the development of autonomy capacities. So the project of 'choice' becomes less about presenting a predetermined menu and more about providing opportunities which enhance women's autonomy potential as they engage with decisions about ongoing benefits and harms in the face of uncertainty: providing opportunities for decisions to be made and re-made where the focus is as much on dialogue as on the decisions made.

The women's accounts and feminist theory provided grounds to understand what contributes to, or detracts from autonomy/empowerment. The women's articulations about being listened to rather than controlled, trusted rather than surveilled, and feminist notions of relational autonomy confirmed that developing self-knowledge (Meyer, 2000), self-definition (Mackenzie, 2000; Meyer, 2000), self-trust (McLeod and Sherwin, 2000), self-esteem (Benson, 2000; Mackenzie, 2000) and self-reflection (Stoljar, 2000) contribute to meaningful autonomy.

Supporting midwives to support women's autonomy

At present informed choice masks an unethical situation in which women and midwives find themselves in a coercive framework that denies them autonomy. While women's ethics and choice remain divorced, and choice is predicated on obstetric ethics, women and midwives have been in an impossible situation where the midwife's need to remain within her policies are pitted against women's autonomy (Clarke, 1995; Kirkham, 1999). Supporting women to challenge policies could subject the midwife to stressful inquiries and threats of negligence in which her livelihood could be at risk. But protecting herself entails the equally problematic pursuit of distressing women and/or enforcing practices on women's vulnerable bodies, or causing women to withdraw from midwifery services.

Women's autonomy and integrity rested on being able to fulfil their own meanings of childbearing to the best of their abilities. This depended a great deal on midwives' support. As they explained, without this support they were less able to make decisions and less able to take responsibility for themselves and their families. This is not to say that midwives can wave a magic wand over women's lives that are adversely affected by poverty, abuse and other oppressions. As Carolyn McLeod and Susan Sherwin (2000, p. 276) point out:

> Health care by itself cannot, of course, correct all the evils of oppression. It cannot even cure all of the health-related effects of oppression. If health-care providers are to respond effectively to the problems, however, they must understand the impact of oppression on relational autonomy and make what efforts they can to increase the autonomy of their patients and clients.

Nor can they take sole responsibility for societal norms that attempt to negate women's autonomy over broad areas of life, especially when this involves any aspect of sexuality. We all share responsibility for these, but midwives (and other practitioners) can make a difference. As I have already suggested, midwives need a robust social midwifery ideology and the skills to provide women with material rather than theoretical alternatives to the prevalent medical model of birth. Without this there is no choice – part of saying 'no' depends on there being an alternative:

> 'You have no choice, you haven't really got any choice. The choice that I made was let's get this finished and over with or do what I had been doing for the past four hours, for another couple of hours. So okay, let's get this over with.'

Like women, midwives need a supportive milieu in which to develop their own knowledge, skills, and autonomy capacities during training, practice and supervision. But as Mavis Kirkham and Helen Stapleton (Kirkham, 1999; Kirkham and Stapleton, 2001) point out, the very skills needed to become autonomous may be lost in any or all of these situations. This is reinforced by a bullying, blaming culture (Hadikin and O'Driscoll, 2000; Levy, 1998).

Developing a reflexive turn: 'to lack self-awareness is to lack autonomy'

In order to influence maternity care so that childbearing may be a positive force in women's lives (a contribution maternity services purport to make) midwifery needs to develop a different level of consciousness based on the discussions above. Self-awareness underpins feminist practice – indeed any liberatory practices (Freire, 1972): 'to lack self-awareness is to lack autonomy' (Meyer, 2000, p. 157). Part of this involves being exposed to critical analyses of society in order to understand how they are captured as individuals and/or groups by ideologies and practices which reduce rather than enhance their autonomy (and thus that of women's). They need to understand how choice is located in a framework of ethical decision-making based on competing and complementary concerns. Self-awareness is also about understanding the impact of one upon another: the potential for benefit or harm located in rela- tionships. While this is less visible within a reductionist health care ethics, in which the subject is apparently constituted prior to relationship and unaf- fected by others (Colebrook, 1997), exchanges between women and midwives contribute to both empowerment and suffering: dialogic exchanges are influential. As Susan Brison (2000, p. 287) suggests:

> If we are 'second persons' – not just in the sense of having been formed by others in childhood, but also in that we continue to be shaped and sustained by others – then other's speech to and about us and ours to and about them are crucially important in the development and endurance of our autonomous selves.

Thus midwives need the human skills to engage with and trust women and themselves, as well as the ability to role model autonomous practices and accountability. The obstacles are formidable, but so too is the power of women and midwives' relationships based on mutual respect, shared knowledges and a willingness to listen ... and keep listening. And listening some more.

References

Barbour, Rosaline S. (1990) Fathers: the emergence of a new consumer group. In Jo Garcia, Robert Kilpatrick and Martin Richards (eds), *The Politics of Maternity Care: Services for Childbearing Women in Twentieth-Century Britain* (pp. 202–16). Oxford: Clarendon Press.

Belenky, Mary F., Clinchy, Blythe M., Goldberger, Nancy R. and Tarule, Jill M. (1986) *Women's Ways of Knowing: The Development of Self, Voice and Mind.* New York: Basic Books.

Benson, Paul (2000) Feeling crazy: self-worth and the social character of responsibility. In Catriona Mackenzie and Natalie Stoljar (eds), *Relational Autonomy: Feminist Perspectives on Autonomy, Agency and the Social Self* (pp. 72–93). Oxford and New York: Oxford University Press.

Brison, Susan J. (2000) Relational autonomy and freedom of expression. In Catriona Mackenzie and Natalie Stoljar (eds), *Relational Autonomy: Feminist Perspectives on Autonomy, Agency, and the Social Self* (pp. 181–209). Oxford and New York: Oxford University Press.

Browner, Carole H. and Press, Nancy (1997) The production of authoritative knowledge in American prenatal care. In Robbie E. Davis-Floyd and Carolyn F. Sargent (eds), *Childbirth and Authoritative Knowledge: Cross-Cultural Perspectives* (pp. 113–31). Berkeley, Los Angeles, London: University of California Press.

Cartwright, Elizabeth and Thomas, Jan (2001) Constructing risk. In Raymond DeVries, Cecilia Benoit, Edwin R. van Teijlingen and Sirpa Wrede (eds), *Birth by Design: Pregnancy, Maternity Care, and Midwifery in North America and Europe* (pp. 218–28). London and New York: Routledge.

Chamberlain, Geoffrey, Wraight, Ann and Crowley, Patricia (1997) *Home Births: The Report of the 1994 Confidential Enquiry by the National Birthday Trust Fund.* London: Parthenon Publishing Group.

Clarke, Rachel A. (1995) Midwives, their employers and the UKCC: an eternally unethical triangle. *Nursing Ethics,* **2(3)**: 247–53.

Code, Lorraine (2000) The perversion of autonomy and the subjection of women: discourses of social advocacy at century's end. In Catriona Mackenzie and Natalie Stoljar (eds), *Relational Autonomy: Feminist Perspectives on Autonomy, Agency, and the Social Self* (pp. 181–209). Oxford and New York: Oxford University Press.

Colebrook, Claire (1997) Feminism and autonomy: the crisis of the self-authoring subject. *Body and Society,* **3(2)**: 21–41.

Cornell, Drucilla (1995) What is Ethical Feminism? In Selya Benhabib, Judith Butler, Drucilla Cornell and Nancy Fraser (eds), *Feminist Contentions: A Philosophical Exchange* (pp. 75–106). London and New York: Routledge.

Cosslett, Tess (1994) *Women Writing Childbirth: Modern Discourses on Motherhood.* Manchester and New York: Manchester University Press.

Cronk, Mary (1992) A doubly difficult birth. *Nursing Times,* **88(47)**: 54–6.

Cronk, Mary (1998a) Hands off the breech. *The Practising Midwife*, **1(6)**: 13–15.

Cronk, Mary (1998b) Midwives and breech birth. *The Practising Midwife*, **1(7/8)**: 44–5.

Davis-Floyd, Robbie E. (1992) *Birth as an American Rite of Passage*. Berkeley, CA: University of California Press.

Davis-Floyd, Robbie E. and Sargent, Carolyn F. (eds) (1997) *Childbirth and Authoritative Knowledge: Cross-Cultural Perspectives*. Berkeley, Los Angeles, London: University of California Press.

Debold, Elizabeth, Tolman, Deborah and Brown, Lyn Mikel (1996) Embodying knowledge, knowing desire: authority and split subjectivities in girls' epistemological development. In Nancy Goldberger, Jill Tarule, Blythe Clinchy and Mary Belenky (eds), *Knowledge, Difference and Power: Essays Inspired By Women's Ways of Knowing* (pp. 85–125). New York: Basic Books.

Department of Health (1993) *Changing Childbirth: Report of the Expert Maternity Group* (Cumberlege Report), Part 1. London: HMSO.

DeVries, Raymond, Benoit, Cecilia, Teijlingen, Edwin R. van and Wrede, Sirpa (eds) (2001) *Birth by Design: Pregnancy, Maternity Care, and Midwifery in North America and Europe*. London and New York: Routledge.

Dimond, Bridgit (1993) Client autonomy and choice. *Modern Midwife*, **3(1)**: 15–16.

Diprose, Rosalyn (1994) *The Bodies of Women: Ethics, Embodiment and Sexual Difference*. London and New York: Routledge.

Edwards, Nadine P. (1998) Getting to know midwives. *MIDIRS Midwifery Digest*, **8(2)**: 160–3.

Edwards, Nadine P. (2000) Women planning home births: their own views on their relationships with midwives. In Mavis Kirkham (ed.), *The Midwife–Mother Relationship* (pp. 55–91). Basingstoke: Macmillan.

Edwards, Nadine P. (2001) *Women's Experiences of Planning Home Births in Scotland: Birthing Autonomy*. Unpublished PhD thesis, University of Sheffield.

Freire, Paulo (1972) *The Pedagogy of the Oppressed*. Harmondsworth: Penguin.

Gatens, Moira (1996) *Imaginary Bodies: Ethics Power and Corporeality*. London and New York: Routledge.

Gilligan, Carol (1985) *In a Different Voice: Psychological Theory and Women's Development*. Cambridge, MA and London: Harvard University Press.

Green, Josephine M., Coupland, Vanessa A., and Kitzinger, Jenny V. (1998) *Great Expectations: A Prospective Study of Women's Expectations and Experience of Childbirth* (2nd edn). Hale, Cheshire: Books for Midwives.

Gregg, Robin (1995) *Pregnancy in a High-Tech Age: Paradoxes of Choice*. New York and London: New York University Press.

Griffiths, Morwenna (1995) *Feminisms and the Self: The Web of Identity*. London and New York: Routledge.

Hadikin, Ruth and O'Driscoll, Muriel (2000) *The Bullying Culture: Cause, Effect, Harm Reduction*. Oxford, Auckland, Boston, Johannesburg, Melbourne, New Delhi: Books for Midwives.

Hamer, Mary (1999) Listen to the voice: an interview with Carol Gilligan. *Women: A Cultural Review*, **10(2)**: 173–84.

Hutchinson, Sally A. (1990) Responsible subversion: a study of rule-bending among nurses. *Scholarly Inquiry for Nursing Practice*, **4(1)**: 3–17.

Inter-Departmental Committee (1904) *Report of the Inter-Departmental Committee on Physical Deterioration*. London: HMSO.

Jones, M.H., Barik, S., Mangune, H.H., Jones, P., Gregory, S.J., and Spring, J.E. (1998) Do birth plans adversely affect the outcome of labour? *British Journal of Midwifery*, **6(1)**: 38–41.

Jordan, Brigitte (1993) *Birth in Four Cultures: A Cross-cultural Investigation of Childbirth in Yucatan, Holland, Sweden and the United States* (4th edn). Prospect Heights, IL: Waveland Press.

Kirkham, Mavis (1999) The culture of midwifery in the National Health Service in England. *Journal of Advanced Nursing*, **30(3)**: 732–9.

Kirkham, Mavis and Stapleton, Helen (2001) *Informed Choice in Maternity Care: An Evaluation of Evidence-Based Leaflets*. Women's Informed Childbearing and Health Research Group, School of Nursing and Midwifery, University of Sheffield; NHS Centre for Reviews and Dissemination, University of York.

Kitzinger, Jenny (1990) Strategies of the early childbirth movement: a case-study of the National Childbirth Trust. In Jo Garcia, Robert Kilpatrick and Martin Richards (eds), *The Politics of Maternity Care: Services for Childbearing Women in Twentieth-Century Britain* (pp. 61–91). Oxford: Clarendon Press.

Kuhn, Thomas S. (1970) *The Structure of Scientific Revolutions* (2nd edn). Chicago: University of Chicago Press.

Lazarus, Ellen (1997) What do women want? Issues of choice, control, and class in American pregnancy and childbirth. In Robbie E. Davis-Floyd, and Carolyn F. Sargent (eds), *Childbirth and Authoritative Knowledge: Cross-Cultural Perspectives* (pp. 132–58). Berkeley, Los Angeles, London: University of California Press.

Leap, Nicky (1997) Making sense of 'horizontal violence' in midwifery. *British Journal of Midwifery*, **5(11)**: 689.

Lemay, Celine (1997) *L'accouchement à la maison au Québec: les voix du dedans*. MSc., Université de Montréal.

Levy, Valerie (1998) *Facilitating and Making Informed Choices During Pregnancy: A Study of Midwives and Pregnant Women*. Unpublished PhD thesis, University of Sheffield.

Levy, Valerie (1999a) Midwives, informed choice and power: part 1. *British Journal of Midwifery*, **7(9)**, 583–6.

Levy, Valerie (1999b) Protective steering: a grounded theory study of the processes by which midwives facilitate informed choices during pregnancy. *Journal of Advanced Nursing*, **29(1)**: 104–12.

Lukes, Steven (1974) *Power: A Radical View*. London: Macmillan.

Machin, David and Scamell, Mandy (1997) The experience of labour using ethnography to explore the irresistible nature of the bio-medical metaphor during labour. *Midwifery*, **13**: 78–84.

Mackenzie, Catriona (2000) Imagining oneself otherwise. In Catriona Mackenzie and Natalie Stoljar (eds), *Relational Autonomy: Feminist Perspectives on Autonomy, Agency, and the Social Self* (pp. 124–50). Oxford and New York: Oxford University Press.

Mackenzie, Catriona and Stoljar, Natalie (eds) (2000) *Relational Autonomy: Feminist Perspectives on Autonomy, Agency and the Social Self*. Oxford and New York: Oxford University Press.

Mander, Rosemary (1993) Who chooses the choices? *Modern Midwife*, **3(1)**: 23–5.

Mander, Rosemary (1997) Choosing the choices in the USA: examples in the maternity area. *Journal of Advanced Nursing*, **25**: 1192–7.

Mason, Margaret (1998) Hospital-based childbirth education: In whose interests? In Patricia Kennedy and Jo Murphy-Lawless (eds), *Returning Birth to Women: Challenging Policies and Practices* (pp. 34–40). Dublin: Centre for Women's Studies TCD/WERRC.

Maternity Services Advisory Committee (1982) *Report to the Secretaries of State for Social Services and for Wales, Part I: Antenatal Care*. London: HMSO.

Maternity Services Advisory Committee (1984) *Report to the Secretaries of State for Social Services and for Wales, Part II: Care During Childbirth*. London: HMSO.

Maternity Services Advisory Committee (1985) *Report to the Secretaries of State for Social Services and for Wales, Part III: Care of the Mother and Baby*. London: HMSO.

McAdam-O'Connell, Bridget (1998) Risk, responsibility and choice: the medical model of birth and alternatives. In Patricia Kennedy and Jo Murphy-Lawless (eds), *Returning Birth to Women: Challenging Policy and Practices* (pp. 21–9). Dublin: Centre for Women's Studies TCD/WERRC.

McCourt, Christine and Page, Lesley (1997) *One-to-One Midwifery Practice: Report on the Evaluation of One-to-One Midwifery.* London: Thames Valley University and The Hammersmith Hospital NHS Trust.

McLeod, Carolyn and Sherwin, Susan (2000) Relational autonomy, self-trust, and health care for patients who are oppressed. In Catriona Mackenzie, and Natalie Stoljar (eds), *Relational Autonomy: Feminist Perspectives on Autonomy, Agency, and the Social Self* (pp. 259–79). Oxford and New York: Oxford University Press.

Meyer, Diana Tietjens (2000) Intersectional identity and the authentic self? Opposites attract! In Catriona Mackenzie and Natalie Stoljar (eds), *Relational Autonomy: Feminist Perspectives on Autonomy, Agency and the Social Self* (pp. 151–80). Oxford and New York: Oxford University Press.

Ministry of Health (1930) *Interim Report of Departmental Committee on Maternal Mortality and Morbidity.* London: HMSO.

Ministry of Health (1932) *Final Report of Departmental Committee on Maternal Mortality and Morbidity.* London: HMSO.

Ministry of Health (1954) *Report for the Year ended 31st December: Part II: On the State of the Public Health.* London: HMSO.

Ministry of Health (1956) *Report of the Committee of Enquiry into the Cost of the National Health Service.* London: HMSO.

Ministry of Health (1959) *Report of the Maternity Services Committee.* London: HMSO.

Ministry of Health (1961) *Human Relations in Obstetrics.* London: HMSO.

Ministry of Health (1970) *Domiciliary Midwifery and Maternity Bed Needs: The Report of the Standing Maternity and Midwifery Advisory Committee.* London: HMSO.

Ministry of Health (1979) *Royal Commission on the National Health Service.* London: HMSO.

Murphy-Lawless, Jo (1998) *Reading Birth and Death: A History of Obstetric Thinking.* Cork University Press.

Nicholson, Linda (1999) *The Play of Reason: From the Modern to the Postmodern.* Buckingham: Open University Press.

Noble, Carolyn (2001) *Birth Stories.* New Zealand: Ginninderra Press, PO Box 53, Charnwood, ACT 2615, www.ginninderrapress.com.au

O'Connor, Marie T. (1992) *Women and Birth: A National Study of Intentional Home Births in Ireland.* Dublin: Coombe Lying-in Hospital.

Oakley, Ann (2000) *Experiments in Knowing: Gender and Method in the Social Sciences.* Cambridge: Polity Press.

Ogden, Jane, Shaw, A. and Zander, Luke (1997a) Part 1: Women's memories of homebirth 3–5 years on. *British Journal of Midwifery,* **5(4)**: 208–11.

Ogden, Jane, Shaw, A. and Zander, Luke (1997b) Part 3: A decision with a lasting affect. *British Journal of Midwifery,* **5(4)**: 216–18.

Olphen Fehr, Juliana van (1999) *The Lived Experience of Being in a Caring Relationship with a Midwife during Childbirth.* Unpublished PhD thesis, George Mason University, Virginia, USA.

Pateman, Carol (1989) *The Disorder of Women.* Cambridge: Polity Press.

Ralston, Rossana (1994) How much choice do women really have in relation to their care? *British Journal of Midwifery,* **2(9)**: 453–6.

Romalis, Shelly (1985) Struggle between providers and the recipients: The case of birth practices. In E. Lewin and V. Olesen (eds), *Women, Health and Healing: Toward a New Perspective* (pp. 174–208). London: Tavistock.

Rooks, Judith (1997) *Midwifery and Childbirth in America*. Philadelphia: Temple University Press.

Sandall, Jane, Davies, Jacqueline and Warwick, Cathy (2001) *Evaluation of the Albany Midwifery Practice*. London: Kings College Hospital.

Saunders, Dawn, Boulton, Mary, Chapple, Jean, Ratcliffe, Julie and Levitan, Judith (2000) *Evaluation of the Edgeware Birth Centre*. North Thames Perinatal Public Health.

Schlenzka, Peter F. (1999) *Safety of Alternative Approaches to Childbirth*. Unpublished PhD thesis, Stanford University, California, USA.

Scottish Health Feedback (1993) *Lothian Maternity Survey 1992: A Report to Lothian Health Council*. Edinburgh: Lothian Health Council.

Scully, Diana (1994) *Men Who Control Women's Health*. New York and London: Teachers College Press.

Shapiro, M.C., Najam, J.M., Chang, A., Keeping, D., Morrison, J. and Western, J.S. (1983) Information control and the exercise of power in the obstetrical encounter. *Social Science and Medicine*, **17(3)**: 139–46.

Shildrick, Margrit (1997) *Leaky Bodies and Boundaries: Feminism, Postmodernism and (Bio)Ethics*. London and New York: Routledge.

Smythe, Elizabeth (1998) *'Being Safe' in Childbirth: A hermeneutic interpretation of the narratives of women and practitioners*. Unpublished PhD thesis, Massey University, New Zealand.

Stapelton, Helen (1997) Choice in the face of uncertainty. In Mavis J. Kirkham and Elizabeth R. Perkins (eds), *Reflections on Midwifery* (pp. 47–69). London, Philadelphia, Toronto, Sydney, Tokyo: Baillière Tindall.

Stapleton, Helen, Duerden, Jean and Kirkham, Mavis (1998) *Evaluation of the Impact of the Supervision of Midwives on Professional Practice and the Quality of Midwifery Care*. English National Board for Nursing, Midwifery and Health Visiting and the University of Sheffield.

Stoljar, Natalie (2000) Autonomy and the feminist intuition. In Catriona Mackenzie and Natalie Stoljar (eds), *Relational Autonomy: Feminist Perspectives on Autonomy, Agency and the Social Self* (pp. 94–111). Oxford and New York: Oxford University Press.

Trevathan, Wendy (1997) An evolutionary perspective on authoritative knowledge about birth. In Robbie E. Davis-Floyd and Carolyn F. Sargent (eds), *Childbirth and Authoritative Knowledge: Cross-Cultural Perspectives* (pp. 80–8). Berkeley, Los Angeles, London: University of California Press.

Viisainen, Kirsi (2000a) The moral dangers of home birth; parents' perceptions of risks in home birth in Finland. *Sociology of Health and Illness*, **22(6)**: 792–814.

Viisainen, Kirsi (2000b) *Choices in Birth Care: The Place of Birth*. Research Report 115. STAKES National Research and Development Centre for Welfare and Health, Department of Public Health, Faculty of Medicine, Helsinki University, Finland.

Wagner, Marsden (1994) *Pursuing the Birth Machine: The Search for Appropriate Birth Technology*. Ace Graphics, 10 Mallett St. (PO Box 366), Camperdown, N S W 2050, Australia.

Warmsley, Kate (1999) Caring for women during the latent phase of labour. *The Practising Midwife*, **2(2)**: 12–13.

Weiner, Carolyn, Strauss, Anselm, Fagerhaugh, Shzuko and Suczek, Barbara (1997) Trajectories, biographies, and the evolving medical technology scene. In Anselm Strauss and Juliet Corbin (eds), *Grounded Theory in Practice*. Thousand Oaks, London, New Delhi: Sage.

Williamson, Charlotte (1992) *Whose Standards? Consumer and Professional Standards in Health Care*. Oxford: Oxford University Press

Young, Iris Marion (1990) *Throwing Like a Girl and Other Essays in Feminist Philosophy and Social Theory*. Bloomington and Indianapolis: Indiana University Press.

Young, Iris Marion (1997) *Intersecting Voices*. Princeton, NJ: Princeton University Press.

CHAPTER 2

Informed Choice in Maternity Care

BARBARA HEWSON

'The fundamental principle, plain and incontestable, is that every person's body is inviolate.' (Lord Justice Robert Goff, 1984)

'The ability to make an informed choice is thus vital to the exercise of full autonomy.' (Seymour, 2000)

Background

According to MIDIRS: 'Pregnancy-related information has exploded into the media and pervades many aspects of every day life from health centre to high street, soap opera to newspaper. Despite this superabundance of 'information', many midwives would argue that there is still nothing even remotely comparable to Informed Choice' (*MIDIRS News*, 2001).

Why do we value choice so highly? One reason is that the right to accept or to refuse advice, examination, tests and treatment is a fundamental human right. Another is that examining, testing or treating a woman without her consent is unlawful. Therefore, consent is vital, not only for the woman's protection, but also for the protection of those caring for her. This raises the question, *What is the most appropriate way of obtaining consent?* Which takes us on to another important issue, that of information. *How can people make effective choices without the right information? And how much information has to be provided?* Whilst few would take issue with the idea of choice nowadays – a motherhood issue! – the questions just posed touch on some grey areas. Putting theory into practice is beset by a complex matrix of social factors.

The social context in which maternity care is provided has changed dramatically in the last few decades. The consumer health movement in general, and advances in women's rights – socially, politically, and in the workplace – have transformed women's expectations. Women no longer expect a highly paternalistic model of care and are more likely to question, or even to reject professional advice. There was a time when pregnant women were assumed to consent to whatever was done to them, when they came into hospital. That assumption no longer holds good in the United Kingdom.

It is salutary to recall that other countries still approach things differently: for example, the Republic of Ireland. The three main maternity hospitals in Dublin – the Coombe, the Rotunda, and the National Maternity Hospital in Holles Street – are among the largest maternity hospitals in Western Europe, and over 40 per cent of Irish births take place there (O'Connor, para. 57). As recently as August 2001 the Master of the Coombe, Dr Sean Daly, told the *Irish Times* that a woman signs a general consent form on admission to the labour ward. He said: 'You're supposed to seek consent. Tell them what you're doing and ask their permission to do it.' The Master of the National Maternity Hospital, Dr Declan Keane, said: 'Women are told in the antenatal classes that hospital policy is to break the waters. In labour, they are told: "you are now in labour. Our policy is to break the waters. We wish to rupture the membranes"'. He added, 'If they don't want it, we don't do it.' Dr Peter McKenna, the Master of the Rotunda, said that women's consent to procedures such as amniotomy 'would be covered by the general consent'. According to the *Irish Times,* he declined to explain how the 'general consent' operated at the Rotunda (*Irish Times*, 13 August 2001). Perhaps unsurprisingly, this approach to maternity care has been criticised in Ireland (O'Connor, *op.cit.* paras 46–71).

As a reaction to the highly organised and often interventionist models of care offered in larger centralised units, there has been a resurgence of interest in 'natural' childbirth: that is, physiological childbirth without interventions such as artificial rupture of membranes, Syntocinon, epidurals and forceps. For some women, EFM may also be experienced as unacceptably restrictive and invasive. One-to-one midwifery care has been shown to reduce the number of interventions during labour; but the NHS suffers from a shortage of midwives, and the Caesarean rate continues to rise. At the time of writing it is 21.5 per cent, while that in Northern Ireland is 23.9 per cent. (McGlynn, 2002). The UK's rate is said to be the third-highest in the world (*Observer*, 2002). Every percentage increase in the Caesarean rate costs the NHS an additional £5 million a year: which could pay for 167 midwives (O'Connor, *op.cit.*, para. 64). And the litigation bill for the NHS continues to rise. Some of the largest claims relate to the delivery of brain-damaged children, sometimes brought years after the birth in question.

Childbearing women tend to have job commitments, small families and are increasingly intolerant of morbidity. Thus, for example, women who have suffered third-degree tears during delivery may sue, alleging that they should have been offered the option of a Caesarean; and other women who have had Caesareans may allege that they were unnecessary. Parents of children born disabled may claim that an avoidable injury occurred before, during or after labour. Parents of a disabled child may allege that they should have been offered suitable screening beforehand, and offered the option of a termination. Even termination may be problematic. On 12 June 2002, a tearful anonymous woman gave an interview to Radio 4 claiming that, if she had been warned about the possibility of distress following an abortion, she would never have had one.

This incident illustrates a further problem: that of hindsight. To what extent are women and their carers supposed to consider the possible long-term ramifications of decisions taken, sometimes under conditions of urgency, during pregnancy or labour? If a labouring woman is in pain, distressed or exhausted, there is not the luxury of time to sit down and consider all possible options with her in depth. Some women may look back on their experience of labour with a jaundiced eye and conclude that it was awful; even though they had the best of care. Others may be happy with their care, despite a traumatic delivery. More work needs to be done to understand the psychology of labouring women and their perceptions of what is happening to them. Satisfactory follow-up might help to resolve problems of morbidity and unhappiness in new mothers.

Consent

The law on consent is straightforward, and can easily be understood by both professionals and users of health care services. In summary, the law says that adults have the right to decide whether to accept or to refuse care and treatment. Other aspects of health law – for example, the law regulating abortion, or artificial means of reproduction – have been framed by Parliament. But to date the law on consent remains largely judge-made: developing in a piecemeal, case-by-case fashion over the years. The law on children, mental patients and adults who lack capacity involves some statute law, which will be briefly described later in this chapter.

The fact that in recent years there has been a considerable amount of litigation about consent should not be taken to mean that the law is unclear, or that it is changing dramatically. No one consents to being treated negligently, and sometimes patients run a threefold attack on health professionals, alleging that what was done to them was done negligently, or done without consent, or that they did not give informed consent because certain risks were not brought to their attention.

In the United Kingdom's publicly funded healthcare system, both time and resources are limited. The National Health Service Act 1977 by section 1(1), imposes on the Secretary of State a very general duty:

'to continue the *promotion* in England and Wales of a comprehensive health service designed to secure *improvement (a)* in the physical and mental health of the people of those countries, and *(b)* in the prevention, diagnosis and treatment of illness, and for that purpose *to provide or secure the effective provision of services in accordance with this Act.'* [italic added]

The courts have accepted that 'a comprehensive health service may never, for human, financial and other resource reasons, be achievable. Recent history has demonstrated that the pace of developments as to what is possible by way of medical treatment, coupled with the ever increasing expectations of the public, mean that the resources of the NHS are and are likely to continue, at least in the foreseeable future, to be insufficient to meet demand' (*Reg.* v. *North and East Devon Health Authority*, 2000).

Section 3 of the 1977 Act deals with the provision of maternity care but the obligation on the Secretary of State is tempered by a wide discretion as to how such care is delivered:

'to provide . . . to such extent *as he considers necessary* to meet all reasonable requirements . . .(a) hospital accommodation;...(c) medical,...nursing and ambulance services; (d) such other facilities for the care of expectant and nursing mothers and young children *as he considers are appropriate* as part of the health service.' [italics added]

There is no mention of home births. Previously, the Midwives Act 1936 and then the National Health Service Act 1946 made express provision for a home birth service, to be provided by the local health authority (MA, 1936; NHSA, 1946). With the removal of that obligation, home birth services now constitute only 2 per cent of births (MIDIRS *Informed Choice* leaflet no 10).

According to the Expert Maternity Group, the demand for such a service remains unmet, with 22 per cent of women surveyed by MORI saying that they would like a home birth (HMSO, 1993). Some NHS authorities provide a home birth service, but for many women the choice is simply not available, unless they can afford the services of an independent midwife. Short of amending the existing 1977 Act to impose a statutory obligation on health authorities to provide such a service, there seems little prospect of this option becoming more widely available, unless purchasers and providers can be persuaded that home births are more economical.

When we go on to examine some of the recommendations made in relation to how informed consent should be sought, a pressing practical question will be – how to ensure that the consent process is effective, in the time available?

When the Human Rights Act 1998 was introduced, there was a certain amount of speculation about how this would affect the law on patients' rights generally. To date, it has had little impact, but that may be because it has only been in force since October 2000. Human rights issues will be considered last in this chapter.

Legal issues

Any intentional touching of a person without their consent, and without lawful justification, constitutes a legal wrong: in technical terms, the tort of trespass. An unauthorised procedure may also constitute a criminal offence, if it is invasive. Justice Cardozo ruled in an American case in 1914:

> 'Every human being of adult years and sound mind has a right to determine what shall be done with his own body; and a surgeon who performs an operation without his patient's consent commits an assault, for which he is liable in damages.' (*Schloendorff* v. *Society of New York Hospital*, 1914)

However, the chances of a prosecution for unwanted treatment are not great, unless the consequences for the patient have been really severe, involving loss of life or serious injury. On 25 June 2002, a judge directed the acquittal of two surgeons who were prosecuted for manslaughter, after removing the wrong kidney in a 69-year-old patient. Unlike a civil action, the responsibility for initiating a prosecution lies with the police and the Crown Prosecution Service. An example in 1993 concerned the gynaecologist Reginald Dixon. He had obtained consent for a hysterectomy from his patient, Barbara Whiten. During the operation, he found that she was pregnant. She was unaware of this. Nevertheless he continued the procedure, performing an abortion without her consent. In 1995, he was acquitted of unlawfully procuring a miscarriage. In 2002, the General Medical Council gave him a severe reprimand. That case illustrates the pitfalls where someone has consented to procedure 'A'; and whilst this is being performed, an unforeseen complication leads to a different procedure 'B' being carried out. It is unlikely that a prosecution would have been brought, if the termination of fetal life had not been involved. A more typical scenario might be where a woman consents to a Caesarean and – owing to complications – a hysterectomy and/or an oophorectomy is also performed. If she did not consent to the hysterectomy, she might bring a civil action for trespass – unless it could be shown that the hysterectomy was medically necessary (because of catastrophic haemorrhage, say). But it is unlikely that she could persuade the law enforcement agencies to mount a prosecution.

The civil courts have continued to maintain the importance of protecting individual autonomy – even when the interference is minimal. For instance, the House of Lords – the United Kingdom's highest court – ruled in 1972 that even a blood test (needed to prove paternity in that case) could not be forced on an adult without their consent. Lord Reid said:

'There is no doubt that a person of full age and capacity cannot be ordered to undergo a blood test against his will ... The real reason is that English law goes to great lengths to protect a person of full age and capacity from interference with his personal liberty. We have too often seen freedom disappear in other countries not only by coups d'état but by gradual erosion: and often it is the first step that counts. So it would be unwise to make even minor concessions.' (S v. McC)

This means that the law will not authorise an unwanted medical intervention on an adult. Adults are free to refuse treatment for reasons that are rational, irrational, or for no reason (*Sidaway* v. *Board of Governors of the Bethlem Royal Hospital and the Maudsley Hospital*, 1985). Various arguments have been put forward from time to time, to counter this approach. One is utilitarian: that society as a whole may benefit from curative treatments being imposed, if necessary. However, it is not obvious how society benefits as a whole, if the odd person is compelled to accept unwanted treatment. (Compare the possible wider social benefit if a treatment is prophylactic – such as a policy of universal vaccination for measles.) Another argument reflects the tyranny of the majority: as J. S. Mill put it, compelling each to live as seems good to the rest (Mill, 1975). To date, such counterarguments have not found favour.

Where children are concerned, the normal rule is that parents have the right to consent or to refuse treatment for their children. However, being a parent carries responsibilities as well as rights. The family courts have an inherent jurisdiction to protect children's welfare, as well as their powers under the Children Act 1989. Such courts have been willing to take the side of medical opinion, if a parental refusal of treatment is deemed to be harmful to the child's best interests. By contrast in Ireland, the Supreme Court recently upheld the constitutional right of parents to refuse a PKU test on their child (*North Western Health Board* v. *H.W.*, 2001, 3 IR 622). Mr Justice Hardiman commented:

'it is better to hesitate at the threshold of compulsion, even in its most benevolent form, than to adopt an easy but reductionist utilitarianism whose consequences may be unpredictable. Ample scope must be given to the fundamental values of human dignity, as well as those of positive logic … I do not see a conscientious disagreement with the health authorities as a failure of duty or an exceptional case justifying State intervention.' (ibid., 747, 757).

Under UK statute, 16- and 17-year-olds can consent to treatment in their own right (Family Law Reform Act 1969), and following the House of Lords' decision in the Gillick case, children under 16 can also consent in their own right to treatment, provided that they have sufficient maturity and understanding to understand the implications (*Gillick* v. *West Norfolk and Wisbech AHA*, 1986). But (and this may seem somewhat inconsistent), the law permits children's 'Gillick competent' refusals to be overridden – either by parental consent, or in extreme cases by a court, when treatment is in the child's best interests.

Saving life – to intervene or not?

The courts have had to consider various situations in which life-saving treatment ought to be discontinued. On each occasion, senior judges have stressed that, although our law respects the doctrine of the sanctity of life, this doctrine does not empower health professionals to impose unwanted life-saving treatment. The House of Lords has made it clear that if a person refuses life-saving treatment, she is not committing suicide (*Airedale NHS Trust* v. *Bland*, 1993). Therefore, it is wrong to see a health professional who accepts a refusal of treatment as aiding and abetting suicide. Even when someone is severely physically disabled, they are entitled to refuse treatment which would prolong life. For example, in the recent case of Ms B, the woman who wished her ventilator to be switched off, the President of the Family Division was critical of the doctors and the NHS Trust who tried to block her wishes. The President pointed out that the doctors had become emotionally involved, and that the Trust had failed to act promptly to break the impasse, which had occurred (*Ms B* v. *An NHS Trust*, 2002). Her judgment is interesting because it is the first time that a court has given detailed consideration to the importance of individual subjectivity in medical decision-making. The Court quoted a philosopher:

'If we accept that the subjective character of experience is irreducible and that it is grounded in the particularity of our points of view, then we are bound to realise that our respect for each other's differences and autonomy embodies a respect for the particularity of each other's points of view. Respect for autonomy is at the same time recognition of the irreducible differences that separate us as subjects … While we can imagine, we cannot know objectively 'what it is like to be' another person, no matter how many facts we are in possession of.' (Atkins, 2000)

Consent can be express or implied. A somewhat old-fashioned example of implied consent is where someone says 'I'm going to take some blood for testing, please can you roll up your sleeve', and the patient duly complies. (It is old-fashioned because nowadays one would expect some explanation of why blood is being sought, beforehand.) Clearly, the more invasive and uncomfortable the procedure – such as a vaginal examination – the more important it is to seek explicit consent beforehand, to avoid misunderstanding, and possible recriminations later on. I would argue that all interventions in labour which are invasive – such as ARM, EFM, the administration of drugs, episiotomies, and the use of operative delivery tools – require specific explanation and consent.

Recording consent

Does consent have to be in writing? No. A consent form is usually only used for major invasive procedures, including those done under a general anaesthetic. But the form itself is not a substitute for getting consent – at best, it is an evidential record only. If the patient has not in fact been given the information, which the form says has been given, the patient's signature carries little weight. Undue importance is sometimes attached to getting such forms signed in emergencies, with patients being asked to sign as they are being wheeled into the operating theatre (or even having a member of staff guiding the pen for them!). This is not desirable. Oral consent would suffice, provided it is carefully recorded in the patient's notes, afterwards. Since husbands or partners have no legal right to sign for their 'other half', it is also pointless asking them to sign a consent form.

It is Department of Health policy that written consent should be sought and obtained for any major surgical procedure or where a general anaesthetic is involved; similarly for any irreversible procedure, such as a sterilisation. But with any procedure which is invasive, and the consequences of which could be serious, good practice requires that the fact that consent has been sought and given should be recorded in the patient's notes. This would cover a range of procedures, from HIV-testing to performing an amniotomy.

What about 'birth plans'?

Birth plans are – ideally – a record of the woman's wishes for her treatment during labour, expressed in advance after discussions with a midwife. At that point, neither the woman nor the midwife can anticipate with certainty what may arise during labour. In preparing a birth plan, it is important to discuss the likely possibilities, and make it clear that the woman's wishes may not be achievable, if emergencies such as haemorrhage or severe fetal distress occur. She also needs to know that it is her right to change her mind during labour, so that a plan for (say) no pain relief can be scrapped without angst. These documents should be seen as an expression of preferences, without being unduly prescriptive. One risk of being too prescriptive is that something that hasn't been the subject of full discussion beforehand will occur. Equally, if the woman is known to be high-risk – e.g. hypertension, history of difficult labours, heart problems, drug addiction and so on – then her care will need to be planned, according to the anticipated risks which she faces.

Is the birth plan the same as an advance directive or 'living will'? No. An advance directive is a document, drawn up by someone whilst they are legally competent, expressing their wishes for treatment should they become incompetent: e.g. that they should not be resuscitated, for example. If that person later becomes unconscious, the directive is then binding on that person's carers. The courts have occasionally granted injunctions to patients seeking to ensure that their wishes with regard to future treatment were upheld. In the case of C, a mental patient in Broadmoor won an injunction to prevent his gangrenous leg being amputated (*Re C (Adult: Refusal of Treatment)*, 1994), even if he was rendered unconscious as a result of gangrenous infection. It was the first time an advance directive had been enforced by an injunction in England. The judge was satisfied that the patient had capacity, and fully appreciated the consequences of his refusal.

Pregnancy and advance refusals of treatment

There has been some debate here as to whether advance directives should be applied in the case of a pregnant woman who falls seriously ill. Suppose a pregnant woman has a serious accident, and an advance directive is produced, which states that she is not to be resuscitated. Should the fact that she is pregnant negate her written wishes? In some US states, legislation sets limits to the effectiveness of advance directives during a woman's pregnancy (Law Commission, 1995, para. 5.25). The Law Commission of England and Wales considered the question in 1995, and concluded:

> 'We do not ... accept that a woman's right to determine the sort of bodily interference which she will tolerate somehow evaporates as soon as she becomes pregnant.' (ibid.)

It pointed out that the only question could be whether the terms of the advance directive covered the woman's actual predicament. In its view, any uncertainty would be resolved in favour of keeping the foetus alive. Such a view is questionable, however, given that under UK law (as I shall explain in more detail later) a foetus has no right to life. There has been no decided case on this issue in the UK.

In 2001, an Irish hospital in Waterford refused to turn off a ventilator after a tourist from London suffered a brain haemorrhage and was pronounced brain dead. She had been married the previous year, and was fourteen weeks' pregnant. Interestingly, there was no suggestion that the woman's wishes were known or played any part in the hospital's decision. On the contrary, the hospital seems to have been exclusively concerned with the foetus. It kept the dead woman's body ventilated, until the foetus died two and a half weeks later. It had received legal advice that under no circumstances should the ventilator be turned off, without a court order. Yet it did not seek a court order. The hospital's position seems strangely inflexible: the woman was a visitor, and medical advice was that the foetus' chances of survival ranged extremely poor to nil. The Irish Attorney-General (whose role is to protect foetal interests) refused to be involved in any court action concerning the foetal 'right to life' in Article 40.3.3 of the Irish Constitution. He advised that life support could be discontinued (*Irish Times*, 15 and 16 June 2001). What the dead woman's husband made of all this is not known.

Re T

The only consideration of a pregnant woman's advance refusal to date was in *Re T* in 1993 (*Re T*, 1993). That concerned whether an advance refusal of blood products by a patient, T, was valid. Eventually the courts concluded that a relative, T's mother, had unduly influenced T. The background was that T who was heavily pregnant had been admitted to hospital, following a car crash. She developed pneumonia. She was given pethidine. T was an ex-Jehovah's Witness (JW). Her mother – who was estranged from the family – remained a committed JW. Whilst her mother was sitting with her, T suddenly told a nurse that she did not want any blood products, and later signed a refusal form to that effect. T was under the impression that alternative products were available. She was not aware that her situation could develop into a life-threatening emergency. Later she became unconscious. An emergency Caesarean was performed, but her baby was stillborn. The consultant advised a blood transfusion, but felt he could not administer blood in view of the form.

An extraordinary court battle then began between the hospital, and T's father and boyfriend. These family members insisted that the form should not be relied on. Initially, a doctor informed a judge by telephone that T had been under the influence of pethidine, and was not fully *compos mentis*. So the judge decided on an interim basis that T could be given blood, because she had lacked capacity to refuse it. At the full hearing, the doctor changed his evidence completely! This put the judge in an awkward position. He extricated himself from it by deciding that T's refusal was not fully informed, and that in any event she had not envisaged the emergency situation that arose after she became unconscious. In other words, the form did not cover the circumstances that had arisen. So he authorised a blood transfusion. The Court of Appeal agreed with the outcome, but gave other reasons. It decided that T's mother must have exerted undue influence over her, and that this invalidated her refusal. The Court made it clear in passing that the more important the medical decision, the greater the capacity that is required. The Court also recommended, that in cases of doubt, doctors should not hesitate to resort to the courts for guidance. Given the variety of answers that this case elicited, one wonders whether resort to the courts is as helpful as judges suggest.

Capacity

How can we know if a person has capacity, i.e. the ability to make decisions for herself? The first point is that every adult is presumed to be capable of decision-making – unless the facts prove otherwise. Examples of adults who lack capacity may include those suffering from long-term mental disability, those who are unconscious, or those suffering from temporary incapacitating factors, such as unconsciousness, shock, extreme exhaustion, or the impact of certain drugs. Incapacitated adults should be treated in their best interests (*Re F*, 1990). Any evidence of their previously expressed preferences should be taken into account.

Lady Justice Butler-Sloss has defined the circumstances in which the law regards a person as lacking capacity:

'A person lacks capacity if some *impairment or disturbance of mental functioning* renders the person unable to make a decision whether to consent to or to refuse treatment. That inability will occur when:

(a) The person is unable to *comprehend and retain* the information which is material to the decision, especially as to the likely consequences of having or not having the treatment in question;
(b) the patient is unable to *use the information* and *weigh it* in the balance as part of the process of arriving at a decision.' (*Re MB*, 1997) [emphasis added]

Whilst this formulation is intended to break down the decision-making process into its component parts, it may seem over-analytical and even cumbersome.

In 1995, the British Medical Association and the Law Society produced a useful handbook on assessment of mental capacity, in which it suggested the following checklist. Using their formulation, a person with capacity should be able to:

- understand in simple language what the medical treatment is, its purpose and nature and why it is being proposed;
- understand its principal benefits, risks and alternatives;
- understand in broad terms what will be the consequences of not receiving the proposed treatment;
- retain the information for long enough to make an effective decision; and
- make a free choice (i.e. free from pressure).

This shopping list is doubly useful, because it also summarises the main topics to be covered in order to ensure an informed choice.

What is a free choice?

Fraud, duress or undue influence can all render an apparent consent (or a refusal) invalid. In such situations, a person is no longer able to act independently. However, in practice, fraud or duress are unlikely. Fraud means deceit or dishonesty, and the courts will require compelling proof of such a serious allegation. (An accusation of fraud could also result in the professional's indemnity insurers avoiding liability.) Showing that a patient has been deliberately or recklessly misled is very difficult. Duress means force, or the threat of force, which again is unlikely in a maternity context. The BMA and the Law Society refer to someone making a choice free from pressure. So, just how much pressure can a professional apply, before they cross the line? It seems that the courts are loathe to interfere even when a professional is applying pressure, so long as a patient's independence has not been undermined. Thus, when a nurse persuaded an intelligent and educated man to change his mind about permitting use of sperm in fertility treatment after his death, the Court of Appeal decided that the nurse had not crossed the line (*Centre for Reproductive Medicine* v. *Mrs U*, 2002). By contrast, the Court of Appeal's concerns in *Re T* reflect a long-standing legal tradition, which regards religious influence as being particularly suspect.

Informed consent

Sadly, the law is not helpful in defining what we mean by an informed consent (or refusal). Courts in the United Kingdom do not accept that 'informed consent' means 'all the information that is available', since this might confuse or alarm patients. Lord Templeman in 1985 said that the information needed was 'information which is adequate to enable the patient to reach a balanced judgement' (*Sidaway, op. cit.*, p. 904). The Master of Rolls tweaked this formula in *Re T*:

> 'What is required is that the patient knew *in broad terms* the nature and effect of the procedure to which consent (or refusal) was given. There is indeed a duty on the part of doctors to give the patient *appropriately full* information as to the nature of the treatment proposed, the likely risks (including any special risks attaching to the treatment being administered by particular persons), but a failure to perform this duty sounds in negligence and does not, as such, vitiate a consent or refusal.' [emphasis added]

He continued:

'On the other hand, misinforming a patient, whether or not innocently, and the withholding of information which is expressly or impliedly sought by the patient may well vitiate either a consent or a refusal.'

It is axiomatic that if patients put specific questions, they must be answered; what is less clear is the idea of a patient *impliedly* seeking information. Possibly this means a situation where a reasonable patient would expressly seek the information, but this particular patient is inhibited from doing so for some reason (e.g. for reasons of embarrassment; lack of social competence); or a situation where it should be obvious what information the patient is looking for (so the patient doesn't have to spell it out).

In a more recent case, Lord Woolf has said that in the normal course health professionals should inform patients of 'a significant risk which would affect the judgement of a reasonable patient'. What constitutes a significant risk is unclear. Lord Woolf accepted that 0.1–0.2 per cent was not significant, but that 10 per cent was. However, he stressed that it was 'not possible to talk in precise percentages' (*Pearce* v. *United Bristol Health Care NHS Trust*, 1999).

The General Medical Council gives far more detailed guidance to doctors on what information they should provide (GMC, 1998):

'5. The information which patients want or ought to know, before deciding whether to consent to treatment or an investigation, may include:

- details of the diagnosis, and prognosis, and the likely prognosis if the condition is left untreated;
- uncertainties about the diagnosis including options for further investigation prior to treatment;
- options for treatment or management of the condition, including the option not to treat;
- the purpose of a proposed investigation or treatment; details of the procedures or therapies involved, including subsidiary treatment such as methods of pain relief; how the patient should prepare for the procedure; and details of what the patient might experience during or after the procedure including common and serious side effects;
- for each option, explanations of the likely benefits and the probabilities of success; and discussion of any serious or frequently occurring risks, and of any lifestyle changes which may be caused by, or necessitated by, the treatment;
- advice about whether a proposed treatment is experimental;
- how and when the patient's condition and any side effects will be monitored or re-assessed;
- the name of the doctor who will have overall responsibility for the treatment and, where appropriate, names of the senior members of his or her team;
- whether doctors in training will be involved, and the extent to which students may be involved in an investigation or treatment;
- a reminder that patients can change their minds about a decision at any time;

- a reminder that patients have a right to seek a second opinion;
- where applicable, details of costs or charges which the patient may have to meet.
...
8. You should raise with patients the possibility of additional problems coming to light during a procedure when the patient is unconscious or otherwise unable to make a decision. You should seek consent to treat any problems which you think may arise and ascertain whether there are any procedures to which the patient would object, or prefer to give further thought to before you proceed. You must abide by patients' decisions on these issues...'

The GMC emphasises that obtaining informed consent is not a one-off event, but a *process*. It says that, where appropriate, resort should be made to visual aids, written materials and accurate data. The ethical obligations required of doctors by their peers go well beyond what judges expect of them. Given the pressures that may arise on the labour ward, it is important to ensure that expectant women are given as much opportunity as possible to plan their care in advance.

Some screening issues

It is wrong to subject patients to screening without giving them an informed opportunity to reflect on the consequences of screening. As the website www.intellectualdisability.info points out, screening is not diagnosis, but is intended to identify those at risk of a disorder (which then has to be definitely established by some diagnostic test e.g. amniocentesis; CVS). It explains: 'Those considering screening need to make a number of decisions. Initially there are three: whether to be screened at all, for which specific disorders, and which test. For those screened and identified as high risk, there is the decision whether to undergo prenatal diagnosis. Following this, if the pregnancy is found to be affected a further decision will need to be made: whether to have a termination of pregnancy.' (See the section on Antenatal Screening.)

There is no point in offering a pregnant woman screening, if she prefers not to know whether or not she is carrying a foetus with a deformity. But though some women would not wish to have a termination, it may be important for the women and her partner to know in advance that she is carrying a disabled foetus, so that they can prepare themselves for this, before the birth. Failure to inform a pregnant woman of the results of a scan disclosing the likelihood that she would give birth to a Down's syndrome child is negligent (*Rand* v. *East Dorset HA*, 2000).

However, obtaining properly informed consent to screening poses significant problems. David Paintin notes that pregnant women and professionals have different expectations of screening: women want the reassurance that their baby is normal, while professionals are more concerned to identify fetal defects (Paintin, 1997). Screening also raises the problem of compliant behaviour. As Professor Richard Lilford says, 'Pregnant women tend not to use their right to opt out because the offer of screening by the clinic is perceived as an endorsement of screening – as a service the staff expect them to accept' (Lilford, in Paintin, Chapter 3, p. 19). Similarly, ultrasound scanning tends to be offered and accepted as routine, even though the case for routine scanning has not been established, and women might be less willing to use such technology, if they were given full information about its limitations in advance. In short, what are such technologies for, and why are they being offered to women, with so little thought being given to the practicalities involved in gaining women's informed consent beforehand?

The Department of Health (DoH) is now proposing that *all* pregnant women be offered screening for Down's syndrome, following an announcement by the Health Minister in April 2001, that 'all women would be offered antenatal screening for Down's syndrome by 2004'. The aim is to have a national screening programme to a basic standard of achieving a 60 per cent detection rate *for a 5 per cent false positive rate*. In a pregnant population of 600,000 every year, this would mean 30,000 false positives: an awful lot of 'worried well' to be counselled, and tested. The rationale for this proposal is not obvious. None is given in the DoH's recent consultation paper, beyond stating that, when finalised, the standards will be sent to the Clinical Negligence Scheme for Trusts for consideration. Interestingly, it also states that the forthcoming National Service Framework for children's services 'will incorporate maternity services' (DoH, 2002). Cynics will take this to mean that pregnant women are to be treated like children in future. In fact, as Dr Michael Fitzpatrick points out in *The Tyranny of Health*, this is typical of modern public health initiatives in general – they display a distinctly authoritarian dynamic, and they treat adults like children (Fitzpatrick, 2000). The fact that the DoH does not even bother to explain why such a measure is considered necessary is revealing in itself.

Getting informed consent in this context is undoubtedly challenging. As Dr Jenny Hewison has observed (Fitzpatrick, 2000, Ch. 7, pp. 44–7): 'Most people find the ideas of probability and risk difficult to understand'. She points out that for most people, risk means something like the risk of being run over when crossing a road; to give them the tools of thought required to understand the very different concept of risk involved in testing for (say) Down's syndrome is not straightforward, and takes time. The arithmetical calculations involved are unfamiliar, and may even be misunderstood by professionals. Here is a classic example, cited by Nassim Nicholas Taleb in his book *Fooled by Randomness: The Hidden Role of Chance in the Markets and in Life*:

'A test of a disease presents a rate of 5 per cent false positives. The disease strikes 1/1000 of the population. People are tested at random, regardless of whether they are suspected of having the disease. A patient's test is positive. What is the probability of the patient being stricken with the disease?'

This was a real quiz given to doctors, most of whom answered 95 per cent. Their answer was based on the assumption that the test had a 95 per cent accuracy rate. But this assumption was wrong! The correct answer was close to 2 per cent. Consider the following ratio:

Number of afflicted persons (1 out of 1000)

Number of true and false positives (1 true positive and 50 false positives).

He points out that a person who tests positive in this hypothetical scenario has a 1 in 51 chance of having the disease (assuming no false negatives). Explaining this to doctors no doubt took some time; explaining it to their patients presumably takes longer (unless they read the *Financial Times*, which featured this little gem). According to Hewison, the costs of providing information, counselling and support 'have usually been overlooked in economic analyses of prenatal screening programmes. The economists tend to include the cost of counselling for the women who are screen-positive but not the cost of giving information to the much larger numbers to whom the screening was offered originally.' (Hewison, in Fitzpatrick, 2000, p. 45). This suggests that the economic case for screening generally may be miscalculated, and that informed consent is being sacrificed as well.

HIV screening: a case in point?

In 1999, the Department of Health issued new antenatal HIV targets (HSC, 1999) as follows:

'All health authorities should ensure that arrangements are in place by December 2000 at the latest for:
  – all pregnant women to be offered *and recommended* an HIV test as an integral part of their ante-natal care (not including women arriving in labour or too late for ante-natal care, who should be offered and recommended a test after delivery)
  – an increased uptake of antenatal HIV testing to a *minimum of 50 per cent to be achieved*
  – health authorities that have effective monitoring systems in place and are already achieving 50 per cent or more *to increase uptake by a further 15 per cent.*

All health authorities should ensure that *arrangements are in place to achieve the following* by 31 December 2002:
  – an increase *in uptake* of antenatal testing to 90 per cent

- that nationally 80 per cent of HIV-infected pregnant women are identified during antenatal care.

These targets should result in an 80 per cent or so reduction in the number of children born with HIV.' (HSC, 1999)

Apart from the medical interventions offered to a pregnant woman who is HIV positive, there are other social consequences which need to be taken into account, for example, possible social stigma; the impact on her partner and immediate family; the consequences for her at work; problems if she wishes to obtain insurance, a mortgage or a pension in future; and problems with immigration and travel.

The DoH in March 1996 issued its own guidelines for pre-test discussion on HIV testing. This stresses the need for 'appropriate' pre-test discussion so that individuals decide whether to have the HIV test in a 'properly informed' way (p. 3). The DoH set out five main components of pre-test discussion. These were:

'1. Ensuring the individual understands the nature of HIV infection, provision of information about HIV transmission and risk reduction.

2. A discussion of risk activities the individual may have been involved in with respect to HIV infection including the date of the last risk activity and the perception of the need for a test.

3. Discussion of the benefits and difficulties to the individual, his or her family and associates of having the test and knowing the result whether positive or negative.

4. Providing details of the test and how the result will be provided.

5. Obtaining an informed decision about *whether or not* to proceed with the test.' (p. 6) [emphasis added]

These DoH guidelines addressed the situation in antenatal care as follows:

'... certain additional factors should be mentioned. These are:
- knowing her HIV status permits the women [sic] to make informed choices about the management of her pregnancy;
- advice on the avoidance of breastfeeding may be given as transmission of HIV from mother to child frequently takes place via breast milk;
- plan and arrange for early monitoring of the baby's health;
- prophylactic treatment for the mother and child (if HIV positive) may be given earlier which may prevent development of severe opportunistic infections, and
- here is an opportunity for clinicians to discuss the use of AZT (Zidovudine) as a treatment to significantly reduce the risk of transmission to the foetus.'

It went on: 'Where ante-natal testing is not routinely offered in ante-natal care i.e. in low prevalence areas, more time may be needed to be allotted to assessment of risk and the need for a test.' (p. 12)

The joint DoH and RCM leaflet *Information for Midwives* issued in November 1998 introduced itself with the slogan: 'helping women choose. ... It is time for midwives to give UK women the chance to make a choice.' It summarised the things midwives need to give pregnant women information about, as follows:

- what HIV is, and why we offer testing;
- routes of transmission, including mother to child;
- potential advantages and disadvantages of diagnosis;
- how the test is carried out, how long the results take, and what they might mean;
- confidentiality;
- *the woman's rights to take time considering her decision, to seek further advice before reaching her decision, and to refuse testing;*
- further sources of advice and support. [emphasis added]

There then followed a series of Questions and Answers. In answer to the question, How are we going to find the time to fit this into a busy booking visit?, the DoH and RCM replied: 'Effective pre-test discussion need only take a few minutes'! This is an extraordinary answer, in the light of the shopping list of topics just listed. For instance, how could any woman take time considering her decision, and even seek further advice before reaching her decision, in the space of just a few minutes? Furthermore, there could be no scope for individual advice, if everyone was allocated only a few minutes.

It is also not clear what is meant by 'effective' in this context: perhaps 'effective' meant that consent to testing was obtained? A pilot study by Chrystie *et al.* in 1993–4 found that booking visits in one antenatal clinic lengthened on average by 21 minutes, when discussions on HIV were built in (Chrystie, 1995). By contrast, Harrison and Corbett cite a study which showed that only 1.7 minutes was spent discussing HIV infection, in a consultation that lasted a mean of 33.1 minutes (Harrison and Corbett, 1999b). They comment: 'hardly a circumstance in which a midwife could obtain relevant information or the pregnant woman could make an informed choice over a complex issue' (p. 34, n.13). Judging by the DoH/RCM advice, already quoted, it appears that in practice midwives were expected to allocate only a token amount of time to deal with this topic, and that pregnant women were not expected to refuse. In other words, informed consent went out of the window.

What prompted this worrying development? One explanation (though not a justification) is, presumably, cost. In their pilot study, Chrystie *et al.* referred to earlier 1992 and 1994 DoH guidelines on HIV testing in antenatal care, and commented: 'to follow the Department of Health Guidelines, which require women to give explicit consent after appropriate counselling, is extremely costly (£150,000–200,000 for a population of 4000 woman a year)' (Chrystie *et al.*, p. 930). If, however, procuring consent is merely a rubber-stamping exercise, such costs can be avoided.

Furthermore, the DoH/RCM's claim that consent could be obtained in only a few minutes wilfully ignored the fact that, in order to obtain properly informed consent, midwives must allocate sufficient time to cover *not only* the five components which the DoH said were required in pre-test discussions, *but also* the additional factors which specifically apply to pregnant women. It is important to bear in mind that a failure to provide proper pre-test discussion may give rise to adverse legal consequences. A legal case, which settled, concerned this very issue (Thompson, 1999).

The facts were that the plaintiff was going abroad in 1992 and was told by his GP that he needed an HIV test (which was incorrect: an HIV test was *not* an immigration requirement). The plaintiff was asked if he were homosexual, or an intravenous drug user, and replied that he was not. He then saw a nurse, who gave him an out-of-date leaflet to read. She asked him if he had read it, and understood the implications of an HIV test. He said 'Yes', and was then tested. Later his GP told him over the telephone that the plaintiff appeared to be HIV positive, before the testing procedure was complete. At this stage, the lab had returned two positive results, and was awaiting the result of third. The third was negative. But by this time, the plaintiff had suffered a terrible shock. He suffered an acute stress reaction with suicidal ideas, an adjustment disorder with mixed emotional features of depression and anxiety, dermatitis and exacerbation of psoriatic tendencies. He sued and, amongst other things, alleged a failure to obtain his informed consent to HIV testing.

The plaintiff's experts were agreed that adequate pre-test counselling could not be provided by the mere provision of an information leaflet. Moreover, the questions which the plaintiff had been asked by the practice nurse were closed questions, requiring a 'yes' or 'no' answer merely, and in the opinion of his experts could not possibly constitute adequate pre-test counselling. The lesson to be learnt from this case is that a failure to provide adequate pre-test counselling and information will result in a failure to obtain informed consent, and this may lead to in a negligence action by someone who suffers as a result. Cursory or 'routine' testing procedures, which involve a few quick questions and giving a leaflet to someone, will not withstand hostile legal scrutiny.

The Terrence Higgins Trust (1999) states that life insurance companies will not generally insure anyone who has HIV. This is not therefore a potential disadvantage of HIV-positive diagnosis; it is an actual one. The same publication says:

'It is important to talk to an experienced counsellor or health adviser before you make your decision about taking an HIV test.' (p. 4)

'There is no good reason for having an HIV test *if you have not been at risk*.' (p.10) [emphasis added]

'If you test HIV positive, the news can be devastating.' (p. 11)

Can it be said that pregnant women as a class are 'at risk' of HIV infection? This cannot be right. The DoH stated that 300 women out of 600,000 giving birth are HIV positive (Nicol, Steele, Mortimer, 1999). This is a tiny percentage of the pregnant population: 0.05 per cent. Even in areas of high seroprevalence, such as London, high risk groups fall into specific categories, such as sub-Saharan Africans; or IV drug users. Presumably, if a pregnant woman in London is not from one of these high-risk groups, she is just as much 'low risk', as if she came from a low seroprevalence area. Yet the DoH aims to test 300,000 women by the end of 2000, and 540,000 women by the end of 2002. Both the DoH and the RCM had advised midwives that they need spend only a 'few minutes' in pre-test discussion. One is forced reluctantly to the conclusion that neither the DoH or the RCM intended that pregnant women should give properly informed consent to HIV screening. This is tantamount to being a compulsory scheme, the legality of which must be doubtful.

The pregnant woman and the foetus

It is axiomatic that duties cannot be owed to non-existent entities, and UK law has always adopted the position that a foetus is not a person until it is born (*Paton* v. *BPAS Trustees*, 1979; *Burton* v. *Islington HA*, 1993). Prenatally, the professional's duty of care is owed to the pregnant woman. If a baby is born injured, as a result of prenatal negligence, it then acquires a right to sue, based on the breach of duty to its mother. Equally, if the injury is caused by a refusal by the woman to accept advice or treatment, the baby has no independent right to sue. This may seem harsh, but is generally thought to be the only pragmatic solution (Congenital Disabilities Act 1976).

Pregnant women have, however, been involved in a series of exceptional court cases in which their refusals of treatment have been challenged by hospital authorities. Initially, these cases were conducted and decided in a decidedly eccentric fashion, with the women not being heard or represented on some occasions: an elementary denial of justice. In the famous St George's case (*St George's Healthcare NHS Trust* v. *S*, 1999), decided in 1998, the Court of Appeal considered the legality of a court order authorising an unwanted Caesarean section on a pregnant woman (S), who had been detained under the Mental Health Act 1983. S suffered from pre-eclampsia and had been detained, after she told her GP that she wanted a home birth. After S was taken to a maternity hospital, she continued to refuse offers of intervention, including drugs to reduce her high blood pressure. The order was obtained in her absence; the justification was that her own life and that of her baby were at serious risk unless surgical intervention was permitted. S was very angry and rejected the baby after she was born. Her legal battle attracted widespread attention. The hospital's arguments that it was acting to save life, and that S's pregnancy put her into a category of patient whose refusals could be overridden, were both rejected.

The Court of Appeal reiterated that adults are free to decide their own destiny. The fact S was detained under the Mental Health Act did not mean that she could not take decisions for herself. Her capacity had never been in issue. It also rejected the argument that pregnant women should be deprived of their autonomy for the sake of their foetuses. The Court decided that, if a pregnant woman could be subjugated to save her own life or that of her foetus, this would annihilate the principle of autonomy:

> how can a forced invasion of a competent adult's body against her will even for the most laudable of motives (the preservation of life) be ordered *without irremediably damaging the principle of self-determination?* When human life is at stake the pressure to provide an affirmative answer authorising unwanted medical intervention is very powerful. Nevertheless the autonomy of each individual requires continuing protection even, perhaps particularly, when the motive for interfering with it is readily understandable, and indeed to many would appear commendable: hence the importance of remembering Lord Reid's warning against making 'even minor concessions'. [emphasis added]

The Court pointed out that, if this principle were breached, then logically any adult might be forced to undergo bodily invasion to save a child:

> If it has not already done so medical science will no doubt one day advance to the stage when a very minor procedure undergone by an adult would save the life of his or her child, or perhaps the life of a child of a complete stranger. The refusal would rightly be described as unreasonable, the benefit to another human life would be beyond value, and the motives of the doctors admirable. If, however, the adult were compelled to agree, or rendered helpless to resist, *the principle of autonomy would be extinguished.* [emphasis added]

This is important because it can be tempting to argue that foetuses are uniquely vulnerable. But such an argument leads to the unattractive conclusion, as one American case points out, that foetuses have superior rights to those of people who have already been born (*Re AC*, 1990).

There is no legal basis on which an adult can be forced to undergo bodily invasion to save another – for example, by a bone marrow transplant, a kidney or a blood donation. As the case above shows, our law recognises no duty to rescue another (McIvor, 2000). The example given in law lectures is that you may see a small child drowning in a shallow pond, and walk by regardless. In other words, no one can be required to act to confer a benefit on someone else. Such 'Good Samaritan' actions are purely voluntary. The Court of Appeal in the St George's case considered an American case where the plaintiff suffered from a rare bone marrow disease, and desperately required a bone marrow transplant from a compatible donor (*McFall* v. *Shimp*, 1978). The defendant, his cousin, refused to submit to treatment to save the plaintiff's life, and was supported by the judge. Although the judge acknowledged that the defendant's conduct was morally indefensible, he refused to intervene, pointing out that coercion would defeat the sanctity of the individual.

Pregnant drug-users: the US experience

Scares about 'crack moms' in the US have led to much more brutal state intervention: an estimated 200 women addicted to drugs while pregnant have been arrested in over 30 US states, on theories of fetal abuse (Paltrow, 1999). The women were frequently also victims of racial and social prejudice. In South Carolina and California, addicted pregnant women attending antenatal clinics have been arrested and prosecuted, instead of being offered treatment. In 2001, the US Supreme Court allowed an appeal by ten women arrested while seeking maternity care at the MUSC hospital in Charleston, South Carolina. The women were covertly tested for drugs, and tested positive for cocaine (*Ferguson* v. *City of Charleston*, 2001). They were reported to the police, and arrested. All but one of the 30 women were African-American. One was kept shackled for two days during labour and delivery. Others were arrested after giving birth, and removed to prison. The US Supreme Court ruled that testing pregnant women for law enforcement purposes, without their consent and without a warrant, was unconstitutional.

Only one court in the States has decided that a foetus is a legal person in the context of these fetal abuse cases: South Carolina's Supreme Court, in 1997 (Paltrow, 1999, pp. 1029–35). The case concerned a black woman, Cornelia Whitner, convicted of criminal child neglect, for allegedly failing to provide proper medical care for her unborn child. He was born healthy, but a test indicated pre-natal exposure to cocaine. There were no in-patient residential drug programmes for pregnant drug users, when she was charged in 1992. No treatment was offered to her. She had a court-appointed trial attorney, who met her on the day of her trial. She pleaded guilty and was sentenced to eight years in prison. She appealed. The majority of the South Carolina Supreme Court declared that viable foetuses are persons protected by child abuse laws. (*Whitner* v. *South Carolina*, 1997) They accepted that, as a result of their ruling, such laws could be used to punish pregnant women who drank or smoked.

Two dissenting judges, including the Chief Justice, heavily criticised the majority decision. His co-dissenter complained: 'the impact of today's decision is to render a pregnant woman potentially criminally liable for myriad acts which the legislature has not seen fit to criminalize.' (*Whitner* v. *South Carolina*, p. 788) Thus, being overweight, failing to take exercise, taking too much exercise, and even drinking coffee might all potentially expose pregnant women to criminal sanctions. In Wisconsin, judges have rejected the argument that a pregnant woman could be taken into protective custody for the sake of her foetus (*State of Wisconsin ex rel. Angela MW* v. *Kruzicki*, 1997). But the Wisconsin legislature retaliated by passing a law that permits the authorities to detain a woman suspected of harming her foetus by 'habitual lack of self-control in the use' of alcohol, and other drugs. Some commentators believe that such initiatives are part of a concerted backdoor attack on abortion rights (Paltrow, 1999; and Schroedel, 2000).

In the UK, the legal experience has been far less dramatic. There have no comparable attempts to criminalise women for their conduct while pregnant. There was one attempt to detain a pregnant woman for a hospital birth in 1988 (*Re F*, 1988). The London Borough of Bromley claimed that she had a hippy lifestyle, and suffered from mental health problems. It tried to make her foetus a ward of court. It sought a court order for her arrest, to force her into hospital for the remainder of her pregnancy. Bromley's goal was to take the baby into care, when it was born. The court hearing was conducted in the woman's absence. The judge refused to make the order sought. Bromley appealed to the Court of Appeal, which also refused to intervene.

The Court of Appeal explained why English law should uphold a woman's autonomy. Firstly, English case law does not recognize foetuses as separate legal entities until they were born. Therefore, foetuses could not be made wards of court. Secondly, the question whether pregnant women's civil liberties ought to be curtailed in this way, is a matter for Parliament, and not for judges. Thirdly, the judges thought that if foetuses could be made wards of court, this would create a most undesirable conflict in cases involving pregnant women. Ordinarily, in wardship cases, the welfare of the child is paramount. How could the welfare principle be reconciled with a pregnant woman's autonomy? *Re F (in utero)* has been followed in Canada. The Canadian Supreme Court rejected an attempt to take a pregnant glue-sniffer into protective custody for the sake of her foetus (*Winnipeg Child and Family Services* v. *G*, 1997).

Human Rights Act 1998

This Act incorporates key provisions of the European Convention on Human Rights. So far there has been little litigation in the medical arena based on the Act, and it seems unlikely that the Act will make a significant difference to the way in which maternity services are provided (though the Act certainly helps to underpin the rights discussed in this chapter).

Article 2 of the Convention (which protects the right to life) has not so far been interpreted to include protection of fetal life (*Paton* v. *United Kingdom*, 1980). Article 3 prohibits torture and degrading treatment or punishment absolutely; but it requires a high threshold of maltreatment – the deliberate infliction of pain and suffering, which is most unlikely to arise in a therapeutic context. Article 8 of the Convention is perhaps the most important in this context. It guarantees the right to respect for one's private and family life. This Article encompasses the right to physical and moral integrity (*X & Y* v. *Netherlands*, 1986); the right to refuse medical treatment (*Peters* v. *Netherlands*, 1994); and also the right to medical confidentiality (*MS* v. *Sweden*, 1999). Nevertheless, Article 8 may be subject to interference by the state on a number of specified grounds:

'There shall be no interference by a public authority with the exercise of this right
except such as is in accordance with the law and is necessary in a democratic society in
the interests of national security, public safety or the economic well-being of the country, for the prevention of disorder or crime, for the protection of health or morals, or
for the protection of the rights and freedoms of others.'

Thus, it may be open to the state to justify a policy of universal vaccination,
on public health grounds (*Acmanne* v. *Belgium*, 1984).

When child protection issues are raised in the context of a child about to
be born, which a local authority plans to put on the At Risk Register at
birth, it is worth noting that the European Court of Human Rights in
Strasbourg has twice found that taking a newborn away from its mother in
hospital, under an emergency care order, violated Article 8: *K & T* v.
Finland (Judgement of the Grand Chamber, 12 July 2001); *P, C & S* v.
United Kingdom (Judgement of the Second Chamber, 16 July 2002). In
the latter case, it stated: 'the removal of a baby from its mother at birth
requires exceptional justification. It is a step which is traumatic for the
mother and places her own physical and mental health under a strain, and it
deprives the new-born baby of close contact with its birth mother and ... of
the advantages of breastfeeding' (para. 131).

In the light of the discussion of informed consent above, Article 10 may be
relevant: this guarantees the right to give and to receive information, especially
when taken together with Article 14 (the right not to be discriminated against,
in the enjoyment of one's Convention rights). So, for example, state measures
which involve giving pregnant women less information, and consequently less
choice, than other categories of patient (such as the universal HIV-testing policy
mentioned earlier) might be vulnerable to a human rights challenge.

The medicalisation of everyday life and experience – including pregnancy and
birth – coupled with the politicisation of medicine has serious implications for
individual autonomy. The temptation to treat pregnant women as a class which
is even less deserving of rights than everyone else, and which is expected to take
up certain types of care as routine, ostensibly in the name of public health, is
one which must constantly be guarded against, and challenged at all times.

References

Airedale NHS Trust v. *Bland* [1993] AC 789 at 864.
Acmanne v. *Belgium* (1984) 40 DR 251.
Atkins, K. (2000) Autonomy and the subjective character of experience. *Journal of Applied
    Philosophy*, **17**(1): 71–9.
Brett, P. *et al.* (1999) Correspondence in *The Practising Midwife*, **2**(8): 38–9.
Burton v. *Islington HA* [1993] QB 204.
Centre for Reproductive Medicine v. *Mrs U* (2002) 1 FLR 927.
Chrystie, I.L. *et al.* (1995) Voluntary, named testing for HIV in a community based ante-natal
    clinic: a pilot study. *British Medical Journal*, **311**: 928, 930.

Chrystie, I.L. *et al.* (1999) Correspondence in *The Practising Midwife*, **2(8)**: 38–9.

Collins v. *Wilcock* (1984) 3 All ER 374.

Congenital Disabilities (Civil Liability Act) 1976. Section 1, following the Law Commission's report No. 60: *Report on Injuries to Unborn Children* (1974).

Department of Health (1993) *Changing Childbirth: Report of the Expert Maternity Group*, Part I, para. 2.6.1. London: HMSO.

Department of Health (1996) *Guidelines for Pre-test Discussion on HIV Testing*. London: DoH.

Department of Health (2002) *Draft Standards for Antenatal Screening*. London: HMSO.

Family Law Reform Act 1969 section 8.

Ferguson v. *City of Charleston* (21 March 2001) 532 U.S 67

Fitzpatrick, M. (2000) *The Tyranny of Health: Doctors and the Regulation of Lifestyle*. London: Routledge.

Gillick v. *West Norfolk & Wisbech AHA* [1986] AC 112.

GMC (November 1998) *Seeking Patients' Consent: The Ethical Considerations*. www.gmc-uk.org/standards

Harrison, R. and Corbett, K. (1999a) Screening pregnant women for HIV: the case against. *The Practising Midwife*, **2(7)**: 24–9.

Harrison, R. and Corbett, K. (1999b) Authors' reply: *The Practising Midwife*, **2(9)**: 34–5.

HSC (1999) 183 *Reducing mother to baby transmission of HIV*.

Irish Times (15 June 2001) *Brain-dead woman was kept alive because of pregnancy*.

Irish Times (16 June 2001) *Attorney General refused to take part in case of brain-dead woman*.

Irish Times (4 July 2001) *Guidelines sought over pregnant woman declared brain-dead*.

Irish Times (13 August 2001) *Health: doctors respond*.

K & TV v. *Finland* (2001) 36 EHRR 257.

    Judgement of the Grand Chamber (12 July 2001).

Law Commission (1995) *Mental Incapacity* (para. 5.25). London: HMSO.

Law Society/BMA (2004) *Assessment of Mental Capacity*. London: BMJ.

McFall v. *Shimp* (1978) 127 Pitts, L.J. 14

McGlynn, A.G. (2002) *Caesarean Conference Report: from Audit to Action*, RCM Midwives' Journal, 3rd Rising Caesarean Rate Conference, 31 January 2002.

McIvor, C. (2000) Expelling the myth of the parental duty to rescue. *Family Law Quarterly*, **12(3)**: 220.

Midwives Act 1936 Section 1 (1).

MIDIRS Informed Choice Leaflet for Professionals, No. 10: *Place of Birth*.

MIDIRS News (24 August 2001) *Informed Choice – An Informed Future*.

Mill, J.S. (1975) *On Liberty: Three Essays*. Oxford: Oxford University Press.

Ms B v. *An NHS Trust* [2002] 2 All ER 449.

MS v. *Sweden* (1999) 28 EHRR 313.

National Health Service Act 1946, Section 23(1).

National Health Service Act 1977, Sections 1, 3.

Nicol, A. Steele, R. and Mortimer, P. (1999) Pregnant women and testing for HIV. *The Practising Midwife*, **2(8)**: 34–7.

North Western Health Board v. *H.W.* [2001] 3 IR 622, 747, 757.

Observer (2002) *Caesareans linked to risk of infertility*, 21 April.

O'Connor, M. *The Dublin Experience: Managing Mothers, Midwives and Markets* (submission to the Competition Authority), para 57, 46–71, 64.

Paintin, D. (1997) *Introduction to Antenatal Screening and Abortion for Fetal Abnormality*, BCT 5.

Paltrow, L.M. (1999) Pregnant drug users, fetal persons, and the threat to Roe v Wade. *Albany Law Review*. **62(3)**: 999, 1002. 1029–35.

P, C & S v. *United Kingdom* (2002) 25 EHRR 1075.

Paton v. *BPAS Trustees* [1979] QB 726.

Paton v. *United Kingdom* (1980) 3 EHRR CD 408.

Pearce v. *United Bristol Health Care NHS Trust* (1999) PIQR 53, 48.

Peters v. *Netherlands* (1994) No 21132/93, 77–A DR.

Rand v. *East Dorset HA* [2000] L R Med 181.

Re AC [1990] 573 A.2d 1235 at 1244.

Re C (Adult: Refusal of Treatment) [1994] 1 WLR 290.

Re F in utero [1988] Fam 122.

Re F (Mental Patient: Sterilization) [1990] 2 AC 1.

Re MB (Medical Treatment) [1997] 2 FCR 541

Re T [1993] Fam 95.

Reg. v. *North and East Devon Health Authority Ex parte Coughlan* [2000] 2 W.L.R. 622, 633–4.

Royal College of Midwives and Department of Health (November 1998) *Information for Midwives: HIV testing in pregnancy – helping women choose.*

S v. *McC* [1972] AC 24.

St George's Healthcare NHS Trust v. *S* [1999] Fam 26 at 46–7.

Schloendorff v. *Society of New York Hospital* [1914] NY 125.

Schroedel, J.R. (2000) *Is the Fetus a Person?* New York: Cornell University Press.

Seymour, J. (2000) *Childbirth and the Law.* Oxford: Oxford University Press.

Sidaway v. *Board of Governors of the Bethlem Royal Hospital and the Maudsley Hospital* [1985] A.C. 871, 904–5.

Stewart, G. (1999) Correspondence in *The Practising Midwife*, **2(9)**: 33.

State of Wisconsin ex rel. Angela MW v. *Kruzicki* [1997] 561 N W 2d 729.

Taleb, N.N. (2001) *Fooled by Randomness: The Hidden Role of Chance in the Markets and in Life.* London: Texere. 159–60, quoting material from Bennet D. J., (1988) *Randomness.* Cambridge, MA: Harvard University Press.

Terrence Higgins Trust (1999) *Testing Issues: A booklet for people thinking of having an HIV test.*

Thompson, A. (1999) A case study of some medico-legal issues in HIV testing. *Journal of Personal Injury Law* **1(99)**: 51.

Whitner v. *South Carolina* [SC 1997] 492 S E 2d 777, 788.

Winnipeg Child and Family Services v. *G* [1997] 3 BHRC 611.

X & Y v. *Netherlands* [1986] 8 EHRR 235.

Z v. *Finland* [1998] 25 EHRR 371.

CHAPTER 3

How Midwives Used Protective Steering to Facilitate Informed Choice in Pregnancy

VALERIE LEVY

Chapter Contents

- Introduction
- Outline of the study
- Controlling the agenda
- Protective gatekeeping
- Maintaining the hierarchy
- Trust
- Summary

Introduction

It has long been advocated that women should be enabled to make informed choices about their care during pregnancy and childbirth. For example, according to the '*Changing Childbirth*' document

> '[The woman] should be able to feel that she is in control of what is happening to her and able to make decisions about her care, based on her needs, having discussed matters fully with the professionals involved.' (DoH, 1993)

This often quoted statement contains several assumptions: for example, that the woman's needs can and will be identified, and that professionals are able and willing to 'discuss matters fully' with her. Facilitating informed choice is, in fact, a highly complex and skilled process involving many pragmatic and personal issues. The purpose of this chapter is to identify and discuss some of these issues.

Outline of the study

The chapter is based upon research carried out in England during the mid 1990s, comprising a grounded theory study of the processes involved when midwives facilitate and women make informed choices during pregnancy (Levy, 1997). Participants initially comprised a convenience sample of 12 pregnant women attending 'booking clinics' at about 16 weeks of pregnancy, and the midwives carrying out these 'booking' interviews, recruited from the antenatal clinics of two Consultant Units and one GP Unit in the East Midlands, England. 'Booking' interviews between these women and midwives were observed and tape-recorded, and transcripts written. Booking clinics were chosen because they were likely to involve the sharing of information between midwife and woman, leading to the making of choices. The midwives and pregnant women were then interviewed separately by the author, using extracts from the transcripts to trigger comments about what they thought was happening at various points. Theoretical sampling was employed to provide variability in the sample and to enable emerging categories to be more fully described. For example, a midwife/woman 'pair' from a progressively run midwife-led practice in an inner-city area was studied in the same way as described above, and community midwives and women in their care were also recruited. Occasions other than 'booking' interviews were studied at this time; for example, home visits in later pregnancy were included and these produced rich data when information was exchanged and discussions ensued influencing choices. These midwives and women were followed up in the same way as before and invited to describe their perceptions of the interaction; these interviews were also tape-recorded and transcribed as above, and, together with the other transcripts, provided the data for the study. A total of 17 midwife/woman 'pairs' were included and 48 transcripts produced.

Data were analysed using a grounded theory approach. Categories were identified that formed two theoretical frameworks describing the processes of facilitating and making informed choices during pregnancy, from the midwives' and pregnant women's perspectives respectively.

The purpose of this chapter is to discuss issues arising from the data relating to the midwives' perspectives. Further details of the research protocol have been published elsewhere (Levy, 1997; Levy, 1999 a,b,c). The categories emerging from the data have also been described elsewhere and they will not be discussed in any detail; rather the issues arising from them.

During observations of interactions and from the 'follow-up' interviews it was apparent that the midwives largely controlled the agenda of what was discussed. Their choice of topics was guided firstly by the institution's policies of what should be included, secondly, their own personal and professional views, and thirdly, by the woman's personal needs, either expressed or as perceived by the midwife. The process of actually providing information and guiding discussion was influenced by several factors, including constraints of time and place, the midwife's personal views about the topic, and the need to give the appropriate amount and level of information. At times midwives were constrained by the necessity of giving permissable information – in other words, information approved by those in authority. Midwives also needed to feel able to trust women with information. These are the issues that will be discussed in this chapter, illustrated with examples taken from observation of interactions between midwives and women in their care, and follow-up depth interviews with midwives (pseudonyms have been used).

Controlling the agenda

Particularly during 'booking clinics', midwives had an agenda to work through in a limited period of time, and they tended to retain control of this agenda. For example, Linda prioritised breastfeeding as a topic, whereas Lily (in early pregnancy and recently arrived from Malaysia and unaccustomed to Western food) wished to discuss her diet:

> Linda: 'Are you going to breastfeed? – Sorry, were you going to say something?'
> Lily: 'Yes. I'm just wondering is it all right to drink coffee and tea and things like that?'
> Linda: 'Yes, and a nice normal diet, yes, of course (laughs). Breastfeeding – you're going to do it again?'
> Lily: 'Yes, I enjoyed it.'

Linda then talked about breastfeeding for the next few minutes; the topic of diet was not returned to during the interaction, although information about diet would probably have been more useful to Lily. Mishler (1986, p. 54) pointed out that medical questioning tends to focus upon certain topics, whilst selectively ignoring others. Freire (1970) calls the process 'naming the world', whereby the health professional, by pursuing certain topics and ignoring others, constructs and prescribes what is relevant for both the professional and the client.

The agenda was also influenced by what choices existed. Midwives saw no point in discussing options if they were not available; not only would this waste time but it may also raise false expectations in the woman and reflect badly on the unit for not providing that facility. For example, Doreen said she would not inform a woman about, for example, water birth unless the woman initiated the topic, as that facility was not available at her unit at the time.

Midwives often worked under time constraints and it could be difficult to give the depth and breadth of information they thought women should have. As Shirley said:

'I think we need the time to do it … to translate it, if you like. We act as translators. Women get bombarded with information … we can try to pull it all together so they can make choices.'

Women were encouraged (or permitted) to raise their own concerns. Hilary said she would try to discuss adequately topics initiated by the woman, but was constrained by time:

'I was constantly aware of time, you see, and if I had a whole hour then perhaps we would have explored more topics. Everything she said I tried to pick up on, but maybe I could have given her an opportunity of more things, I don't know.'

Midwives were, however, reluctant to appear to be short of time. They did not wish to appear to be hurrying the woman along as this could negatively affect building a relationship with the woman. Despite the shortage of time that appeared to constrain many interactions (particularly in hospitals) midwives felt some topics were far too important to be neglected. For example, midwives spent relatively long periods of time raising women's awareness about 'routine' fetal screening tests. Women were often given printed information regarding these, which they were expected to read and think about before their appointment with the midwife. This was intended to save time whilst giving the woman an opportunity to consider issues before discussion. Midwives would often reiterate the information, however, as they were not convinced the woman had understood it, or because they doubted that she had read it at all.

Paula [talking about the triple test]:'I go right the way through from the beginning, I think you have to … because the Community midwife just says it's a screening test but they don't actually go through it … the booklet and leaflets that we give ladies, they do read through it but not always.'

Katherine said that she would offer to answer any questions the woman might have about the triple test as a strategy to avoid 'going through the whole information sheet again', but (as can be seen below) she deflected Laura from asking questions. Soon Katherine returned to the topic afresh with an offer to summarise the information:

Katherine:'Did you have the triple test last time?'
Laura:'Yes'
Katherine:'Would you like to ask me any questions about it? Oh, by the way, the Hepatitis C survey is finished. '
Laura:'Oh, right. I must admit, with all the problems I've had this pregnancy … I thought, oh no, not another one. '
Katherine:'Would you like me to go over the triple test again? '
She then spent several minutes explaining the triple test and its implications.

Some issues would be discussed at parentcraft classes, but not every woman attended all of them (some women did not attend any), and midwives were aware that these issues would also need to be addressed. Leaflets could be given, but they were seen as 'second best' to an explanation from the midwife. It appeared that midwives considered some topics too important to be dealt with by leaflets (or even trusted to professional colleagues) and preferred to risk duplicating the information, and thus wasting time, rather than risk omitting the information.

Protective gatekeeping

Midwives sometimes felt constrained when giving information by their desire to protect women from both physical and emotional harm. If the level of information was not appropriate the woman would either have insufficient or excessive information. Thus, midwives acted as gatekeepers of information, controlling its release in order to achieve a balance of providing enough information to permit safe informed choices to be made whilst avoiding excessive information that might confuse or frighten the woman. Women needed to understand and contextualise (in other words, assimilate) information. Assimilation was perceived by midwives as appropriate if women indicated they had

- understood the facts contained within the information.
- contextualised the information, that is, personalised it appropriately to themselves.

Midwives often held strong views on what was safe or potentially dangerous or undesirable, and these views affected the direction in which midwives steered women when helping them make informed choices. For example, Evelyn did not think home births were safe, and said she would try to steer women away from home births. There were some scenarios that midwives found personally unacceptable and this could lead to the midwife withdrawing choice from the woman as the following illustrates. Judy said she would not give a woman in her care the opportunity to be delivered in a bath or pool:

> 'I would not go along with that. Also, I do not think I should be expected to do that either. I do not like, you will have to excuse me, I cannot cope with faecal matter ... you will never see me have a delivery where there is faecal matter all over the place ... the anus does dilate a lot and if they are in water I do feel it will circulate round and whatever gauntlet gloves you have got they do not come up to your armpits so it also means it will be flowing round my arms and I do not want that.'

In this example, the midwife had the power to impose her wishes upon the woman by withholding the information that water birth might be available (or by refusing to carry out the water birth had the woman requested it). At the time the research was carried out it is likely that some women did not know about the possibility of water birth and would not therefore have asked about it; unless women know what questions to ask they may not receive useful information.

Some midwives claimed they would not try to lead or influence women, but this was not always borne out by analysis of their interactions. For example, midwives often said they did not want to frighten women. It appeared, however, that if the midwife felt strongly about the importance of a particular issue in regard to the woman's health (or the baby's), she would risk frightening the woman, or might even intentionally scare her into following the course of action she deemed correct. For example, Joan cited a list of dangers to the baby when trying to persuade a woman to stop smoking cigarettes:

'It is important, not only for your own health, but you're much more likely to miscarry, you're more at risk of the baby not growing well, you're more at risk of going into labour earlier than usual, and after the baby's born you're more at risk of the baby having ear infections, chest infections, that sort of thing, and also from cot death. ...There's also some recent research about miscarriages that if you're expecting a girl child her fertility may be affected too, and she will be more likely to miscarry if her mother smokes.'

Joan [to the author, later]: 'I'm not sure that I actually gave her a choice – I just wanted her to stop smoking – I am very anti-smoking, I know that, so anybody I come across who smokes I will always advise them of all the disadvantages.'

Joan added that her own young son had just started smoking cigarettes, much to her dismay, and so smoking was very much on her mind and she had very strong feelings against it. The dangers to health of smoking are well known (for example, Gritz, 1980; Plant, 1990, p. 82) and there is no intention to further discuss them here, but rather to point out that strong views held by midwives may sometimes influence the verbal force with which the midwife attempts to steer the woman's behaviour. Joan made it clear that if the woman continued to smoke her baby would be more likely to experience a whole range of problems. Women during pregnancy are often extremely vulnerable to suggestion, particularly regarding the well-being of their babies, and rarely knowingly carry out actions likely to harm them; indeed, they may well be frightened if such a prospect is suggested. The midwife released the information in a way she thought would influence the woman to take the course of action she (the midwife) felt was 'right'. The midwife may not feel so strongly about other issues known to be damaging to the mother and child, however, and may not use similar tactics, or may even exclude them from the agenda of what is to be discussed. For example, Joan, when asked about the importance she gave to diet in pregnancy, said she had no strong feelings about it, but would merely ask the woman if she had read and understood the advice given in the handouts.

'It's a personal thing, so I probably don't spend as much time talking about it (diet) as smoking. I can't remember with this particular lady whether we talked about diet ... I always mention it, but I don't go on about it.'

It could be argued that advice about diet was at least as important as advice against smoking (Spedding *et al.*, 1995), but the midwife steered the conversation towards the topic about which she felt strongly, largely ignoring an issue in which she had little interest.

In contrast with Joan's intentions, Evelyn, although recognising the dangers of smoking, was concerned not to frighten women by the advice she gave. She wished to avoid scaring the woman into changing her behaviour, preferring an approach that stopped short of that by 'picking her line' and choosing her words carefully.

'You just say to the mothers it's a good idea to stop smoking – but again, you could say, are you going to frighten them [laughs] by saying something awful could happen! But you've got to sort of pick your line.'

'Picking your line' was a difficult activity, demanding sensitivity and perception on the part of the midwife. Midwives wanted to be realistic, preparing women for events that might (but would probably not) occur. There were certain issues that midwives considered ethically important to address in as much detail as possible. For example, Linda said she always gave a full explanation about fetal screening tests and their implications:

' ... because if they had a child with Down's syndrome and then said that no one explained it properly to them I couldn't carry that on my conscience.'

A balance needed to be struck; sufficient factual information was required to enable choices to be made but if too much information was given there was a danger that the woman would not successfully assimilate it, misunderstand or inappropriately personalise it with consequent worry or fright. The greater the perceived ability of the woman to assimilate information, the further into detail and hypothetical realms the midwife would be prepared to go. Women who were able to assimilate knowledge were considered to able to deal with hypothetical information, and not inappropriately personalise it. For example, Barbara justified her detailed account of fetal screening tests:

'Actually, she was quite an intelligent woman, wasn't she? [Laughs.] She did understand, it was a lot of information to give someone, wasn't it, but she did understand.'

Women who were already well informed were thought to be less at risk of being frightened because they could more readily contextualise the information.

Although they tended to understand information, however, the way in which they operationalised the information could be perceived by midwives as problematic

> Midwife Francis [talking about schoolteachers]: 'They get terribly upset if they do not do so well as they think they ought to be ... we have to be very firm with these ladies ... they write a lot, they want to know a lot, they need a lot of support because their expectations are so high.'

Midwives assessed ability to assimilate information by means of feedback from the woman:

> Evelyn: 'I get a response from the mother, that she is interested, she's listening to me and picking up various points or asking questions about them, and you're aware then that she's listened and is aware of what you've said, and can make her own mind up about the choices that are available to her.'

A balance also needed to be struck between protection and overprotection. For example, Fiona said:

> 'I sometimes think that I must not be patronising or condescending, those again are not entirely the right words, sometimes I cannot find the right words, but do you understand what I am saying? I must make sure that no matter what they are like I must put myself on a level with them, and not sort of be as if they are my chicks if you like, do you see what I mean?'

Midwives tended to limit information more if they were doubtful of the woman's ability to understand, either because she was perceived as not being bright enough, or as having language problems. On other occasions, midwives were concerned that women would take actions not thinking of the possible personal consequences. This applied particularly to fetal screening tests. Several midwives commented that women often had the tests never considering that they might reveal a potential problem; women underwent the tests to confirm normality, not to suggest abnormality:

> Janet [talking about the triple test]: 'They read the information – or not – they listen, but do not understand sometimes. They don't have it (the test) in order to find out if something is wrong, they have it thinking it is going to reassure them that everything is all right ... I don't think it really hits home to some these women until the phone rings and they find they are at high risk.'

Alternatively, although aware of the danger of worrying women unnecessarily, midwives would often wish to empower women to cope with events that may occur in the future by providing accurate and realistic information. For example, whereas Doreen said:

'It's very difficult to talk about screening tests because we are talking about abnormalities and miscarriage and women don't want to think about that at sixteen weeks.'

Evelyn commented:

'I think it's better to be informed than to suddenly have it thrust upon you by a phone call that the test has come back abnormal.'

Midwives tried to protect women from emotional distress by steering them through potential 'minefields' within the health care system without alarming them. Fiona had concerns about the implications for women of taking part in a study of Hepatitis C, and attempted to protect women by, whenever possible, guiding them away from participating.

'I think that there are implications in this for later in life if they are found to be carriers of this virus. Implications for their own health, their own life, when they get older … What I do is I say to them, have you read the letter [explaining the study]? Do you want to take part in the research? If they say no, I say fine and I not do anything to dissuade them. If they say yes, I normally say to them I think you ought to phone up this person whose name and phone number is on the bottom of your letter if you are not certain about the implications of it. I know that's passing the buck … it's got to do with liver cancer, liver sclerosis, liver failure when people reach their 50s. I think that is something I am not prepared to start talking to them about.'

Not only did midwives wish to protect the women in their care, they also were aware of the need to protect themselves. They defined and located themselves as practitioners working within hierarchy in terms of their power and knowledge and areas of practice. Constraints were perceived as being imposed either externally by the structure within which they worked, or internally when they were self-imposed. When defining their territory, midwives steered between, and balanced, these constraints demarcating their territory from that of other professionals such as obstetricians and general practitioners.

Maintaining the hierarchy

Midwives in this study tended towards subservience to hierarchical controls imposed over their practice by medical and organisational models. Medical power was referred to frequently as a factor guiding what information midwives could give; even though they felt competent to take or advise certain courses of action, midwives often acceded to policies made by those seen as more powerful, such as GPs. At the same time, however, they often used various strategies to circumvent medical dominance.

Policies and procedures are set by the senior staff of hospitals and other medical institutions, and midwives are required to know what these policies are (UKCC, 1994). Some midwives felt themselves bound not only to know the policies, but also to follow them, feeling powerless to make autonomous decisions. This depended to some extent upon the personal confidence of the midwife, and the perceived 'ownership' of the area of the decision. Evelyn was a newly qualified midwife who saw herself as relatively inexperienced and powerless. At antenatal booking visits she wanted to discuss with women the administration of intramuscular Konakion to the baby at birth to prevent haemorrhagic disease of the newborn, but felt that she could not initiate such a discussion because this was not hospital policy.

Other midwives chose not to follow the policies and procedures, adapting their practice as they perceived it safe and reasonable to do so; these tended to be more senior (and therefore, presumably, more experienced and confident) midwives who appropriated the power to self-direct their practice. Linda had worked in the unit for several years and was sufficiently confident to refuse to follow a procedure set by consultants and senior midwife managers that made little sense to her; namely, asking the woman she was 'booking' how long she would like to stay in hospital after the birth. This, however, concerned a relatively minor issue which was unlikely to affect the more powerful others directly. Morriss (1987, pp. 32–34) differentiates between 'power to' effect outcomes and 'power over' other individuals to persuade or coerce them to take a certain course of action. This midwife was accorded the 'power to' adapt the procedure since she was not assuming 'power over' the more dominant individual, that is, the obstetrician. Linda went on to describe another situation when she had tried to make life easier for a woman due to be admitted for elective Caesarean section:

> 'the woman had said, can I put the children to bed, and I said of course, you can come in a bit later to the ward. There was a big rumpus about it, this woman had missed the anaesthetist and they blamed me ... So there are some things I am bound by till they change and it is the anaesthetists really that we have got to get round now.'

Changing the time of admission would have allowed Linda to assume 'power over' the anaesthetist, requiring him or her to change the time of their ward visit, and this was strongly resisted. Linda spoke in terms of 'getting round' the anaesthetist in order to achieve her goal which would, in her view, improve care. This implies a more covert, less challenging approach than that originally used, reflecting Stein's (1978) description of the strategies used by nurses when interacting with doctors, and Tannen's (1992) observations of how women may use indirect methods of communicating what they want from more powerful others, rather than asking or acting outright.

Midwives often remarked that they felt constrained when giving advice, if the consequences of that advice had implications for their more powerful colleagues. An example of this was home birth. Alison had previously worked as a community midwife, and she had felt quite confident recommending home birth. Now, working in the hospital clinic, she was wary of *'stepping on toes'*.

Alison: 'We know that the GPs don't want [home births] ... you can cause an awful lot of trouble by mentioning it to women when you know that the people who will be looking after them don't want to take that responsibility ... I mean, you can imagine, if a woman said "I hadn't thought of a home delivery until I went to the hospital and the midwife that booked me suggested that I could have my baby at home, and I thought oh, that's a good idea", it would be like horrendous.'

Alison went on to say that complaints would probably be made, as it was not for her as a hospital midwife to suggest something that, if taken up by the woman, would cause work to the community staff. If this happened, she said, community staff would be committed to caring for the woman during her home delivery, and would be thereby inconvenienced and possibly annoyed by her (the midwife's) actions. Complaints may be made by more powerful others (GPs) to those in power over the midwife (Consultants), and her power and professionalism would be diminished in the eyes of the woman, and possibly others. Paradoxically, committing community staff to areas of care other than intrapartum were not seen as problematic. For example, Alison said that following birth it would be the hospital's (and presumably the woman's) decision when she and her baby were transferred home to the care of the community staff.

'I don't think it should have anything to do with the community as to (when) they accept them back again ... you might say, well discuss it with your community midwife but I don't think that comes into it, personally.'

'Hierarchies of work' may be one explanation of this apparent paradox. Labour is a subject of intense public interest (which Foucault (1977) termed the 'gaze') as evidenced by the number of articles about labour published in newspapers and journals, whereas postnatal care is rarely accorded the same degree of public attention. It is possible that, because of the intensity of this interest, the work of caring for a woman during labour and delivery is considered as being of higher order work than that of postnatal care, which is not subjected to the same degree of public surveillance. In this example, Alison said that she would not tread upon the toes of the community staff by suggesting to a woman that she should consider a home birth, but would not hesitate to transfer the woman home early to be cared for by community staff. I would suggest that there is a hierarchy of work in midwifery. The attention accorded to labour by the media confers, by the intensity of the media 'gaze', an importance that exceeds other aspects of care in childbirth, such as postnatal care. These observations arise from Alison's comments that if a woman was delivered in hospital, the hospital staff (together with the woman) could specify to the community staff when she would be returning home for postnatal care, but yet Alison felt unable to commit the community staff to the 'work' of caring for the woman in labour. It appeared that whoever did the 'higher order work' – that is, delivering the woman, had the right to prescribe where the 'lower order work' of postnatal care should take place. This perception may be influenced by the preponderance of technology surrounding intrapartum care, compared with that in postnatal care, or – and more likely – it is the 'gaze' that reflects the interest in intrapartum events that has led to the technological control.

Trust

The final issue discussed here is that of trust. In order to promote the exchange of information, not only did women need to trust the midwife, but the midwife needed to trust the woman with the information that would enable her to make decisions. For example, Marion (a member of a team of midwives working in an inner city area) said that she went to considerable lengths to help women make informed choices, giving as much information as she could, but she trusted the woman in her care to act sensibly if things went wrong, and to trust her judgement. This was borne out by the observation of the interaction between Marion and Anne, which lasted well over an hour in Anne's home. Issues such as the administration of Syntometrine and Konakion were discussed. Anne eventually decided not to have Syntometrine during her home birth, unless Marion (or whoever of the team midwives was with her) thought it necessary. Marion later told the author that she would not give Syntometrine if the third stage of labour was normal, but trusted Anne to agree to the administration of Syntometrine if she, Marion, thought it necessary. In other words, she trusted Anne to trust her, and trusted her not to take a foolish course of action that would harm Anne, and possibly Marion, putting her in a professionally and ethically dangerous situation.

Marion and Anne knew each other well; they had built up a relationship during Anne's pregnancy. Conversely Pauline, working in a hospital antenatal clinic, seldom saw women more than once or twice during pregnancy, and those interactions tended to be brief, perhaps lasting fifteen to twenty minutes. She commented that she felt unable to trust the women in her care; she would not rely upon them to follow sensible courses of action. Indeed, she felt it likely that without a lot of advice and guidance that they would act unwisely compromising themselves, and possibly herself; she might be blamed for their actions.

The woman, by virtue of the midwife being a member of a profession which is generally considered as trustworthy, has a stereotype upon which to base initial trust. Several studies concerning trust in health care relationships emphasise the importance of this trust by the patient/client towards the nurse. As argued above, it is probably equally important for the midwife (or nurse) to trust the woman (or patient). The midwife has a limited range of stereotypes (such as social class, ethnicity) upon which to judge how far she can trust a woman she does not know with information. Until the relationship, and trust, develops beyond that based upon stereotype, it is difficult for the midwife to 'open the gates' for fear of what the woman might do with that information (Levy, 2000). Continuity of care, either by means of care by an individual or by a group of known midwives, is likely to facilitate the growth of mutual trust.

It was also necessary for the midwife to trust the organisation within which she worked. Johns (1996) pointed out the importance of this. Marion worked within a system where she said she felt well supported by her manager. She felt that her manager shared her ideals about midwifery practice and sharing information, and trusted her to support her if conflicts arose with other powerful figures who did not share those ideals.

Summary

Midwives regarded facilitating informed choice as an essential part of their job. Facilitating choice was seen mainly as providing information, and making women aware of what choices were available. When facilitating informed choice, however, midwives 'walked a tightrope' in attempting to meet the wishes of women, steering their way through several dilemmas. For example, midwives were anxious to meet the wishes of women and to appear unbiased in their advice, but acknowledged their own strong feelings regarding certain issues. Midwives also had to strike other balances, for instance between giving enough information for the woman to make a choice but not giving too much information and frightening the woman, particularly when talking about, for example, screening tests for fetal abnormality.

Facilitating informed choice involved making the woman aware what options were, and were not, open to her. Midwives recognised that many women had strong feelings regarding their care, but whether they did or not, women often needed the opportunity to talk through the issues involved with a midwife who would provide facts and information tailored to the individual woman's circumstances and wishes. This required both time and knowledge on the part of the midwife, which were not always perceived by the midwife as adequate. Time in particular was often at a premium and the midwife needed to limit the amount of time she could spend with a woman, whilst trying to appear not to do so. The midwife needed to feel able to trust the woman to use the information to make 'sensible' decisions that would not compromise the woman or the midwife, and also she needed to have confidence that people within the organisation for which she worked would provide support and back-up.

In conclusion, midwives tried constantly to strike the right balance and this was difficult, especially if women were not well known to them. Often, particularly at the hospital booking clinics, they were meeting each other for the first time and the midwife had little to guide her, only her initial impression of the woman and the stereotype this may have triggered. Midwives were constantly looking for clues to indicate what information was needed, and to what depth it could be assimilated. This in turn had to be considered in relation to employer's policies, the midwife's place in the hierarchy, constraints of time and, possibly, knowledge, and the midwife's own views and opinions. If the 'right line' was not 'picked' highly undesirable outcomes could result. The woman could be frightened, feel patronised, or lack accurate information to make an informed choice, colleagues could be upset, unrealistic expectations could be encouraged, and the woman's (and the midwife's) well-being and safety compromised.

Facilitating informed choice is a highly complex activity, demanding of the midwife great sensitivity and personal awareness, as well as highly developed professional skills and knowledge.

References

Department of Health (1993) *Changing Childbirth: Report of the Expert Maternity Group*. London: HMSO.

Foucault, M. (1977) *Discipline and Punish: The Birth of the Prison* (translated by A. Sheridan). London: Penguin.

Freire, P. (1971) *Pedagogy of the Oppressed*. New York: Herder & Herder.

Gritz, E.R. (1980) Problems related to the use of tobacco by women. In O.J. Kalant (ed.), *Alcohol and Drug Problems in Women: Research Advances in Alcohol and Drug Problems*, Vol. 5, pp. 487–543. London: Plenum Press.

Johns, J.L. (1996) A concept analysis of trust. *Journal of Advanced Nursing*, **24**: 76–83.

Levy, V. (1997) Facilitating and Making Informed Choices During Pregnancy: A Study of Midwives and Pregnant Women. PhD thesis, University of Sheffield.

Levy, V. (1999a) Protective steering: a grounded theory study of the processes involved when midwives facilitate informed choices during pregnancy. *Journal of Advanced Nursing*, **29(1)**: 104–12.

Levy, V. (1999b) Maintaining equilibrium: a grounded theory of the processes involved when women make informed choices during pregnancy. *Midwifery*, **15**: 109–19.

Levy, V. (1999c) Midwives, informed choice and power: Part 1. *British Journal of Midwifery*, **7(9)**: 583–6.

Levy, V. (2000) Making and facilitating informed choices during pregnancy: the importance of trust. Proceedings of 25th Triennial Congress of the International Confederation of Midwives, Manila, Philippines: 332–4.

Mishler, E.G. (1986) *Research Interviewing: Context and Narrative*. Harvard, MA: Harvard University Press.

Morriss, P. (1987) *Power: A Philosophical Analysis*. Manchester: Manchester University Press.

Plant, M. (1990) Maternal alcohol and tobacco use in pregnancy in J. Alexander, V. Levy and S. Roch (eds), *Midwifery Practice: A Research-Based Approach; Antenatal Care* (pp. 73–87). London: Macmillan.

Spedding, S., Wilson, J., Wright S. and Jackson, A. (1995) Nutrition for pregnancy and lactation, in J. Alexander, V. Levy and S. Roch (eds). *Aspects of Midwifery Practice: A Research Based Approach*. Basingstoke: Macmillan.

Stein, L. (1978) The doctor-nurse game in R. Dingwall and J. McIntosh (eds), *Readings in the Sociology of Nursing* (pp. 108–117). Edinburgh: Churchill Livingstone.

Tannen, D. (1992) *You Just Don't Understand*. London: Virago Press.

United Kingdom Central Council (1994) *The Midwife's Code of Practice*. London: UKCC.

CHAPTER 4

Can Leaflets Deliver Informed Choice?

ALICIA O'CATHAIN

Chapter Contents

■ The MIDIRS *Informed Choice* leaflets

■ Evaluating the leaflets

■ Measuring informed choice

■ Were the leaflets used?

■ Did any of the leaflets deliver informed choice?

■ What does this say about leaflets?

■ Is maternity care different from other health care settings?

■ Is this just about leaflets – what about other media?

■ Conclusion

Leaflets are commonly used in health care to communicate information about the prevention and treatment of health problems. Their aim is often to improve consumers' knowledge levels – that is, act as information aids – and indeed they have been shown to be effective for this purpose (Little *et al.*, 1998; O'Neill *et al.*, 1996). Evidence of their effect beyond improving knowledge is mixed. For example, they have been shown to reduce re-consultations for respiratory problems in primary care (Macfarlane *et al.*, 1997) but have not helped people to adhere to drug treatment (Peveler *et al.*, 1999). There is often conflicting evidence, for example information prior to colposcopy has been shown both to reduce (Marteau *et al.*, 1996) or have no effect on women's anxiety levels (Howells *et al.*, 1999).

Leaflets can be developed as decision aids rather than simply information aids, with the purpose of helping people to make decisions about their individual health care. Decision aids provide information on the treatment

71

options available, alongside research evidence on their effects, to help people to make specific and deliberative choices (O'Connor *et al.*, 1999). They come in formats other than leaflets, including decision boards, videotapes, computer programs, booklets and interactive multimedia (Murray *et al.*, 2001). They tend to have a range of objectives such as improving knowledge, satisfaction, participation in decision-making and reducing decisional conflict. They have been shown to improve knowledge and reduce decisional conflict when tested with small numbers of patients (O'Connor *et al.*, 1999; Molenaar *et al.*, 2000; Estabrooks *et al.*, 2001). However, they have rarely been put to the test with large groups of patients in everyday practice.

A study of a set of decision aids in maternity care, in leaflet format, offered the opportunity to address whether leaflets can help consumers to make decisions in everyday health care (Kirkham and Stapleton, 2000). In this chapter I discuss these leaflets and their aim, describe the study used to evaluate them, present some findings about specific leaflets in maternity care, and discuss whether leaflets can actually deliver informed choice.

The MIDIRS *Informed Choice* leaflets

An addition to the small pool of available decision aids is the set of ten *Informed Choice* leaflets produced by MIDIRS (Midwives Information and Resource Service) and the NHS Centre for Reviews and Dissemination. The leaflets summarise research evidence on ten decisions which women face in pregnancy and childbirth, in order to promote informed choice. The titles of the leaflets are displayed in Box 4.1. They come in pairs – a simple version for women and a more complex one for health professionals which includes the references to research upon which they are based. They were designed to be given to women by health professionals as an integral part of the care process, rather than simply displayed on leaflet racks. They present the options available to women, the pros and cons of those options, and give some help in how women can make choices by asking women to think about the questions they need to ask health professionals and the issues they value. They are 'simple' decision aids because they offer women guidance in their decision-making rather than provide an explicit process for making a decision.

Information and decision aids can differ in quality. The MIDIRS *Informed Choice* leaflets meet the quality criteria developed for such supports to patients' involvement in decision-making by containing research-based data in a form acceptable to patients, giving a balanced view of the effectiveness of different treatments, presenting uncertainties, taking a non-patronising tone, and being developed and tested with multi-disciplinary groups including people for whom they are developed (Coulter *et al.*, 1999). They were based on systematic reviews of the research literature, peer-reviewed by international experts, the text in the women's version was

---

Box 4.1 MIDIRS *Informed Choice* **leaflets**

	Women's version	Professionals' version
1	Support *in* labour	Support *in labour*
2	*Listening to your baby's* heartbeat *during labour*	Fetal *heartrate* monitoring *in* labour
3	Ultrasound scans – *should you have one?*	Ultrasound screening in the first half of pregnancy: *is it useful for everyone?*
4	Alcohol *and pregnancy*	Alcohol *and pregnancy*
5	Positions *in labour and delivery*	Positions *in* labour *and* delivery
6	Epidurals *for pain relief in labour*	Epidural pain relief *during labour*
7	*Feeding your baby –* breast *or* bottle?	Breastfeeding *or* bottle feeding: *Helping women to choose*
8	*Looking for* Down's syndrome *and* spina bifida *in pregnancy*	Antenatal screening for congenital abnormalities: *helping women to choose*
9	Breech baby: *What are your choices?*	Breech presentation – *options for care*
10	*Where will you have your baby –* hospital or home?	Place *of* birth

---

drafted by a journalist, they received a Plain English kite mark, and they were tested among focus groups of women and health professionals (Entwistle *et al.*, 1998).

Evaluating the leaflets

The NHS Centre of Reviews and Dissemination commissioned researchers at the Universities of Sheffield and Glamorgan to determine whether using this set of ten MIDIRS *Informed Choice* leaflets would promote informed choice in maternity care. A randomised controlled trial of the use of the leaflets in everyday practice was undertaken as part of a wider study of the leaflets (Kirkham and Stapleton, 2001). The trial involved giving the leaflets to some maternity units and not to others, which then acted as controls. The conclusions were that, overall, the MIDIRS *Informed Choice* leaflets did not promote informed choice (O'Cathain *et al.*, 2002). However, changes occurred in *some* of the maternity units receiving the MIDIRS *Informed Choice* leaflets and in *some* of the maternity units in the control arm of the trial. These control maternity units had introduced their own leaflets on some of the topics covered by the MIDIRS *Informed Choice* leaflets during the course of our study. This offered the opportunity to undertake a more detailed exploration of the data collected, to understand more about the role of different types of leaflets in delivering informed choice.

The study was a pragmatic cluster randomised controlled trial with maternity units as clusters. The methods have been described elsewhere and are merely summarised here (O'Cathain *et al.*, 2002). Thirteen maternity units, where the MIDIRS *Informed Choice* leaflets were not in use, were grouped into ten clusters because some shared management or clinicians. Five clusters were randomised to the intervention arm of the trial and five to usual care. Two samples of users of these maternity units were identified. The first sample was all women reaching 28 weeks gestation during a six-week period who were receiving antenatal care in any setting (antenatal sample). The second sample was all women who had delivered during a six week period in any setting (postnatal sample). An antenatal sample and a postnatal sample were identified before the introduction of the leaflets, and again some months after they had started to be used. Outcomes were assessed using a postal questionnaire to these four different samples of women. Antenatal samples received the questionnaire at 28 weeks gestation and postnatal samples received the questionnaire eight weeks after delivering their babies.

Measuring informed choice

The key outcome for the evaluation was the change in the proportion of women exercising informed choice. The hypothesis was that this would increase in maternity units using the MIDIRS *Informed Choice* leaflets and remain the same in maternity units in the control arm of the trial. Yet how is informed choice best measured? Although some validated measures of involvement in decision-making and decisional conflict exist (Degner and Sloan, 1992; O'Connor, 1995), doubt has been cast on the validity of some of these measures for all health care encounters (Entwistle *et al.*, 2001) and some researchers have recently developed other measures in recognition of the dearth of appropriate measures (Marteau *et al.*, 2001). The outcome measure used in the evaluation of the MIDIRS *Informed Choice* leaflets was developed specifically for this study, based on other validated measures and developed and tested with women attending antenatal clinics and childbirth classes. The measure identified women's perceptions of whether they had exercised informed choice and was the proportion of women saying 'yes' to the question, 'Have you had enough information and discussion with midwives or doctors to make a choice together about all the things that happened during maternity care', with the options 'yes', 'partly', 'no', 'there was no choice', 'did not apply'. This question was asked for eight of the ten topics covered by the MIDIRS *Informed Choice* leaflets, as well as about 'all the things that happened' in maternity care.

Other outcomes measured were knowledge, satisfaction with information, satisfaction with how choices had been made, and whether women felt they had had sufficient discussion with health professionals. Knowledge was measured using ten multiple choice questions about each of the topics covered by the leaflets (Kirkham and Stapleton, 2001). Each woman completed knowledge questions on two randomly chosen topics.

Were the leaflets used?

Each maternity unit in the intervention arm of the trial was given a set of professionals' leaflets for each midwife, and enough women's leaflets so that every woman delivering in an eight month period could receive a full set of leaflets. Since the leaflets were designed to be given to women by midwives, and the trial was of their use in everyday practice, the process of offering the leaflets to women was left to the discretion of each maternity unit.

Women were asked to report whether a midwife or doctor had given them each of the MIDIRS *Informed Choice* leaflets. The names of each of the leaflets were given, including the 'tick' symbol which is part of the MIDIRS *Informed Choice* logo, and women were given the option of saying they were not sure whether or not they had received those leaflets. Nonetheless, approximately 40 per cent of the women reported being given at least one of the MIDIRS *Informed Choice* leaflets prior to the start of the study, in both the intervention and control maternity units, when they were not available. This was explained by the qualitative study which ran alongside the trial – women could not distinguish the MIDIRS *Informed Choice* leaflets from the many other leaflets available in maternity care (Stapleton *et al.*, 2002).

Comparison of leaflet use before and after the MIDIRS *Informed Choice* leaflets were made available showed considerable increases in the proportion of women reporting that they had been given each of the MIDIRS *Informed Choice* leaflets in each of the maternity units in the intervention arm of the trial (Table 4.1). One of the maternity units was reluctant to use the leaflets on ultrasound scanning, screening for Down's syndrome and spina bifida, and epidurals because they had limited availability of these services. Thus they had smaller increases in use of these leaflets than the other maternity units in the intervention arm.

Table 4.1 Percentage point change in the proportion of women reporting that they received a MIDIRS *Informed Choice* leaflet

Leaflet *		Alcohol	Ultrasound scans	Screening	Place of birth	Support	Positions	Epidurals	Monitoring	Feeding	No. of women#
Intervention	1	**20**	**30**	**36**	**21**	**22**	**22**	**30**	**16**	**21**	222
	2	**29**	**16**	**14**	**19**	**39**	**28**	**33**	**28**	**39**	548
	3	**20**	**22**	**23**	**18**	**31**	**27**	**30**	**28**	**28**	272
	4	**45**	**47**	**44**	**35**	**34**	**25**	**40**	**25**	**29**	222
	5	**27**	**43**	**38**	**25**	**21**	**20**	**26**	**24**	**30**	150
Control	1	2	9	−8	0	−3	−3	4	−2	1	239
	2	0	3	17	5	4	3	1	5	4	425
	3	2	4	27	2	4	3	9	0	12	336
	4	−2	0	−8	1	8	8	10	8	7	173
	5	−3	**36**	15	3	6	−7	1	5	−6	155

Notes:

Bold indicates statistically significant change at 1 per cent level

* Leaflet about breech babies not included because relevant to small numbers of women only

minimum number of women in each time period.

Surprisingly, there were increases in leaflet use in maternity units in the control arm of the trial of a similar order to those seen in the intervention arm. On investigation, the qualitative researchers from the wider study found that control unit 3 had introduced a 21-page A5 leaflet on screening tests for Down's syndrome and spina bifida and had started to use it during the trial. This leaflet was produced by the health authority with considerable input from staff at control unit 3 during its development. The leaflet clearly stated that testing was optional and gave some information about risks and benefits. Control unit 5 introduced a sheet of A4 on ultrasound scans, which had been constructed by an ultrasonographer, midwives and obstetric staff at that unit. It clearly stated that ultrasound scans were optional and that they might identify problems as well as date the baby. Neither of these leaflets could be described as decision aids because they did not present detailed risks and benefits of different options and made no attempt to help women to make decisions. However, they were more than simple sources of information because they introduced the concept of choice to women. As well as this, one of the two maternity units in control unit 2 introduced the MIDIRS *Informed Choice* leaflet on screening tests for Down's syndrome and spina bifida.

Did any of the leaflets deliver informed choice?

The unexpected introduction of leaflets about ultrasound scans and screening tests for Down's syndrome and spina bifida in control maternity units during the study presented an opportunity to explore the effect of different leaflets for these two decision points in maternity care, and to explore whether leaflets about one decision point could affect women's perceptions of informed choice overall in their maternity care. However, prior to exploring these issues it is worthwhile considering the limitations of the analysis.

A cautionary note

Any analysis of changes which occurred in individual maternity units is limited by a lack of statistical power. The trial was designed to have an 80 per cent chance of detecting an increase from 50 per cent to 60 per cent in the proportion of women reporting that they made informed choices in the intervention units compared with no change in the control units, at a two-tailed significance level of 5 per cent. To find a minimum 10 percentage point increase in informed choice in one of the maternity units would require 390 women in that maternity unit in each time period. Since the sampling technique used was to take a six week cohort of users in each maternity unit, larger samples were taken from larger maternity units and only two units had samples large enough to detect this difference. In fact the analysis below has the power to detect minimum differences of 15 percentage points in each of the maternity units. A second problem is the use of multiple statistical tests, where so many tests are undertaken that differences are found where none exist. Because of these limitations it is best to use the results reported below to identify hypotheses for further testing rather than for drawing firm conclusions.

Ultrasound scans

The introduction of the MIDIRS *Informed Choice* leaflet on ultrasound scans was associated with small increases in women's knowledge levels, informed choice, satisfaction with information, satisfaction with how choices were made, and whether they had had enough discussion with health professionals, in some of the maternity units only. Further, the size of the increases in knowledge, informed choice etc. was not associated with the size of the increase in leaflet use. Decision aids have been shown to increase knowledge by an average of 1.6 out of 10 points for simpler aids (O'Connor *et al.*, 1999). Given that there was approximately a 30 percentage point increase in the use of leaflets, we would expect to see a half point increase in knowledge in the intervention units. Only two of the maternity units managed an increase of this size.

Two units reached the threshold of a 10 percentage point change in the primary outcome of whether women felt that they had exercised informed

Table 4.2 Percentage point change in the proportion of women reporting different outcomes about ultrasound scans

Maternity unit		Received leaflet	Knowledge	Informed choice	Satisfied with information	Satisfied with way choices made	Enough discussion	Minimum number of women
Intervention	1	**30**	0.71	4	7	10	9	224
	2	**16**	0.20	8	**10**	1	7	552
	3	**22**	−0.18	3	6	6	0	275
	4	**47**	0.26	**13**	9	2	**15**	220
	5	**43**	0.73	−7	0	−3	−5	150
Control	1	9	0.37	9	3	3	4	242
	2	3	0.00	8	2	0	1	424
	3	4	0.04	−4	−3	1	−5	342
	4	0	0.00	5	4	−2	5	174
	5	**36**	−0.28	**28**	**18**	**20**	12	159

Note:
Bold indicates statistically significant change at 5 per cent level.

choice – one of the five intervention units and the control unit which had introduced their own leaflet. The size of effect was considerably larger for the control unit than any of the intervention units, as were the increases in the other outcomes.

Screening for Down's syndrome and spina bifida

No maternity unit reached the minimum 10 percentage point change in the proportion of women reporting that they had exercised informed choice, including the control unit which introduced their own leaflet (Table 4.3). The changes in other outcomes were small.

Informed choice overall

It is possible that each of the MIDIRS *Informed Choice* leaflets had a small effect individually, but combined had a large effect on women's views of informed choice overall in their maternity care. It is also possible that introducing a leaflet on one topic can affect views of informed choice overall. These issues are

Table 4.3 Percentage point change in the proportion of women reporting different outcomes about screening for Down's syndrome and spina bifida

Maternity unit		Received leaflet	Knowledge	Informed choice	Satisfied with information	Satisfied with way choices made	Enough discussion	Minimum number of women
Intervention	1	**36**	0.08	–2	**13**	–2	9	223
	2	14	0.40	**8**	6	3	6	553
	3	**23**	–0.22	6	–1	6	1	273
	4	**44**	0.17	–3	3	1	2	220
	5	**38**	0.37	–8	–4	–10	–2	152
Control	1	–8	–0.16	8	6	3	4	242
	2	**17**	0.46	6	1	–3	3	423
	3	**27**	–0.20	1	–3	3	–2	341
	4	–8	0.35	4	0	0	1	174
	5	15	0.18	6	**11**	**15**	2	159

Note:
Bold indicates statistically significant change at 5 per cent level.

explored by looking at women's views of informed choice for all the things that happened in their care (Table 4.4). Focusing on the intervention maternity units, two of the five intervention maternity units had the minimum 10 percentage point increase in informed choice overall in their maternity care, and three of them in total had evidence of increases in many of the outcome measures. Again, the size of increases in informed choice were not related to the size of increases in use of the MIDIRS *Informed Choice* leaflets.

Two of the control maternity units showed changes in informed choice larger than the minimum 10 percentage point change. Both were units which had introduced their own leaflets on one topic. Control unit 5, with the introduction of a leaflet on ultrasound scans, had an improvement overall in informed choice of twice the order seen for any intervention unit and increases also occurred for many of the other outcomes. Control unit 3, with the introduction of a leaflet on screening for Down's syndrome and spina bifida, had a reduction in informed choice and discussion.

What does this say about leaflets?

Changes in informed choice occurred in some maternity units that introduced leaflets on choice within maternity care. Therefore it seems that leaflets *can* have

Table 4.4 Percentage point change in the proportion of women reporting different outcomes overall in antenatal care

Maternity unit		Received leaflet	Knowledge	Informed choice	Satisfied with information	Satisfied with way choices made	Enough discussion	Minimum number of women
Intervention	1	**30**	−0.06	10	7	7	9	221
	2	**23**	**0.37**	**10**	**8**	**9**	**11**	549
	3	**27**	−0.12	1	10	2	5	270
	4	**41**	**0.50**	8	10	**11**	10	221
	5	**45**	0.38	−5	−3	−7	−3	147
Control	1	−7	0.25	3	5	6	5	239
	2	**12**	0.05	6	3	−1	4	418
	3	**21**	−0.27	**−13**	−3	−4	**−12**	337
	4	−2	−0.31	3	−1	0	0	171
	5	**19**	**−0.58**	**19**	10	**13**	**13**	158

Note:
Bold indicates statistically significant change at 5 per cent level.

an effect on informed choice, as found elsewhere (O'Connor *et al.*, 1999; Molenaar, 2000; Estabrooks *et al.*, 2001). However, application of Bradford Hill's conditions necessary to identify leaflets as a *cause* of promoting informed choice were not present (Bradford Hill, 1965). A strong relationship between changes in leaflet use and informed choice was present in one maternity unit only, and there was no evidence of a dose-response gradient between changes in leaflet use and informed choice. Overall, leaflets did not deliver informed choice in this study. This lack of effect was not specific to the MIDIRS *Informed Choice* leaflets because another leaflet on Down's syndrome had a similar lack of effect on informed choice for that specific decision.

Other important points to emerge from the above analysis is that improving informed choice for one decision point can affect views about informed choice overall. On a less positive note, it is possible for the use of one leaflet on one topic to have a negative effect on informed choice overall. This may be due to the fact that time is a fixed resource in health care and promoting informed choice for one decision point may mean that there is less time for discussion on other decision points. Finally, there is an issue about the quality of leaflets used. The leaflet which had the largest impact in the above study did not meet the quality criteria met by the MIDIRS *Informed Choice* leaflets.

Informed choice – a difficult objective

Information can be a powerful tool, for example it can change the uptake of prenatal screening (Thornton *et al.*, 1995). Leaflets are tools for imparting information, and although information is necessary to attain informed choice, it is not sufficient. Informed choice is 'not a simple concept that can easily be implemented, particularly in national/public health care systems' (Entwistle *et al.*, 1998b, p. 223). Information and education are relatively ineffective ways of facilitating this complex objective, compared with the context and social influences (Bekker *et al.*, 1999). Thus it is more likely that what happened *alongside* the leaflets in the study outlined above facilitated or hindered their effectiveness. Barriers to the use of the MIDIRS *Informed Choice* leaflets and to the promotion of informed choice in maternity care are now well documented (Stapleton *et al.*, 2002). The influence of the health professional in resisting the use of leaflets (Oliver *et al.*, 1996) and in influencing the decisions made – the uptake of antenatal HIV testing differed between 15 per cent and 48 per cent depending on midwife seen (Simpson *et al.*, 1998) – has been highlighted. This has led to a call for more time available within consultations, improved ways of communicating risk to patients, and an acquisition of new communication skills rather than for more decision aids (Elwyn *et al.*, 1999). The success of the 'home-grown' leaflet on ultrasound scans in the study detailed above may have resulted from changes in health professionals' approaches to choice rather than the leaflet itself. This is pure speculation because there is no information available on what actually happened in that maternity unit. However, perhaps it is time to turn our attention from the barriers to informed choice towards understanding what positively contributes to the promotion of informed choice in health care everyday practice.

Is maternity care different from other health care settings?

The complexities of involving people in decision-making about their care is common to many health settings. Maternity care may be different from other health settings because women are making decisions about another person as well as themselves, and they are usually healthy throughout the process of health care. In addition, leaflets are commonly used in maternity care for some issues, especially breastfeeding, and if we continue to use this medium for decision aids in maternity care then it will be important to ensure that these leaflets are distinguished from the many others available. Perhaps the most striking difference between maternity care and other settings is the sheer number of decisions that need to be made. Taking hormone replacement therapy may involve many decisions such as whether to do so, which type to take, when to start and when to stop taking it. A decision aid about taking hormone replacement therapy focuses on whether or not women should take it (O'Connor *et al.*, 1998). Women in maternity care have many of these 'whether or not' decisions to make and this is why there are ten MIDIRS *Informed Choice* leaflets rather than one. This makes it difficult to know whether it is best to address informed choice overall in maternity care or focus attention on one decision point only. It is likely that both approaches are needed because there are some generic issues concerning the delivery of informed choice in maternity care (Stapleton *et al.*, 2002) but each decision point may face different pressures (Oliver *et al.*, 1996).

Is this just about leaflets – what about other media?

It could be argued that a leaflet is a static throwaway medium associated with information giving, and ubiquitous in maternity care. Perhaps another medium might be more successful? A comparison of a leaflet about prenatal tests, with a touch screen information system in an antenatal clinic setting, resulted in the same understanding of the purpose of the test, although the information system resulted in increased uptakes of anomaly scans (Graham *et al.*, 2000). A comparison of a video with a simple leaflet and an expanded leaflet about screening test for Down's syndrome showed that they performed the same in terms of knowledge, decision-making process and test uptake (Michie *et al.*, 1997). Thus the medium may not be the important issue.

Indeed, the conclusions from a study on birth plans read similarly to the conclusions of the evaluation of the MIDIRS *Informed Choice* leaflets:

> It is clear from the existing literature on birth plans that context and setting play a critical role. The degree to which hospital staff are involved in developing and implementing birth plans devised by women themselves or adapted from other settings, are likely to have powerful effects. How birth plans affect practice, and how well they achieve the purpose of promoting communication between women and care-givers cannot be separated from existing hospital policies and cultures, the extent of support for evidence-based practice, degree of continuity of care, and commitment to involving women and their partners in decision-making. (Brown and Lumley, 1998, p. 114).

Conclusion

The title of this chapter poses the question 'can leaflets deliver informed choice?' The conclusion is that it seems unlikely that they can *deliver* informed choice in maternity care but possible that they may *help* to deliver it. That is, they might perform better when employed as part of initiatives to promote informed choice rather than the driver of such initiatives. There are barriers to informed choice which go beyond the mere presentation of evidence-based information and decision-making strategies, and these must be addressed before leaflets and other decision aids can make their mark in the complex world of health care.

References

Bekker, H., Thornton, J.G., Airey, C.M., Connelly, J.B., Hewison, J., Robinson, M.B. *et al.* (1999) Informed decision making: an annotated bibliography and systematic review. *Health Technology Assessment*, **3**(1).

Bradford Hill, A. (1965) The environment and disease: association or causation? *Proc. Roy. Soc. Med.*, **58**: 295–300.

Brown, S.J. and Lumley, J. (1998) Communication and decision-making in labour: do birth plans make a difference? *Health Expectations*, **1**: 106–16.

Coulter, A., Entwistle, V. and Gilbert, D. (1999) Sharing decision with patients: is the information good enough? *British Medical Journal*, **318**: 318–22.

Degner, L.F. and Sloan, J.A. (1992) Decision-making during serious illness; what role do patients really want to play? *Journal of Clinical Epidemiology*, **45**: 941–50.

Elwyn, G., Edwards, A. and Kinnersley, P. (1999) Shared decision-making in primary care: the neglected second half of the consultation. *British Journal of General Practice*, **49**: 477–82.

Entwistle, V.A., Watt, I.S. and Davis, H., *et al.* (1998a) Developing information materials to present the findings of technology assessment to consumers. *International Journal of Technology Assessment in Health Care*, **14**: 47–70.

Entwistle, V.A., Sheldon, T.A., Sowden A. and Watt I.S (1998b) Evidence-informed patient choice. Practical issues of involving patients in decisions about health care technologies. *International Journal of Technology Assessment in Health Care*, **14**: 212–25.

Entwistle, V.A., Skea, Z.C. and O'Donnell, M.T. (2001) Decisions about treatment: interpretations of two measures of control by women having a hysterectomy. *Social Science in Medicine*, **53**: 721–32.

Estabrooks, C., Goel, V., Thiel, E., Pinfold, P., Sawka, C. and Williams, I. (2001) Decision aids: are they worth it? A systematic review. *Journal of Health Services Research and Policy*, **6**: 170–82.

Graham, W., Smith, P., Kamal, A., Fitzmaurice, A., Smith, N., Hamilton, N. (2000) Randomised controlled trial comparing effectiveness of touch screen system with leaflet for providing women with information on prenatal tests. *British Medical Journal*, **320**: 155–9.

Howells, R.E., Dunn, P.D., Isasi, T., *et al.* (1999) Is the provision of information leaflets before colposcopy beneficial? A prospective randomised study. *British Journal of Obstetrics and Gynaecology*, **106**: 528–34.

Kirkham, M. and Stapleton H. (2001) *Informed choice in maternity care: an evaluation of evidence-based leaflets.* York: University of York.

Little, P., Griffin, S., Kelly, J., Dickson, N. and Sadler, C. (1998) Effect of educational leaflets and questions on knowledge of contraception in women taking the combined contraceptive pill: randomised controlled trial. *British Medical Journal*, **316**: 1948–52.

Macfarlane, J.T., Holmes, W.F. and Macfarlane, R.M. (1997) Reducing reconsultations for acute lower respiratory tract illness with an information leaflet: a randomised controlled study of patients in primary care. *British Journal of General Practice*, **47**: 719–22.

Marteau, T.M., Kidd, J. and Cuddeford, L. (1996) Reducing anxiety in women referred for colposcopy using an information booklet. *British Journal of Health Psychology*, **1**: 181–9.

Marteau, T.M., Dormandy, E. and Michie, S. (2001) A measure of informed choice. *Health Expectations*, **4**: 99–108.

Michie, S., Smith, D., McClennan, A. and Marteau, T.M. (1997) Patient decision-making: an evaluation of two different methods of presenting information about a screening test. *British Journal of Health Psychology*, **2**: 317–26.

Molenaar, S., Sprangers, M.A.G., Postma-Schuit, F.C.E., Rutgers, E.J.T., Noorlander, J., Hendriks, J. and De Haes, H.C.J.M. (2000) Feasibility and effects of decision aids. *Medical Decision Making*, **20**: 112–127.

Murray, E., Davis, H., See Tai, S., Coulter, A., Gray, A. and Haines, A. (2001) Randomised controlled trial of an interactive multimedia decision aid on benign prostatic hypertrophy in primary care. *British Medical Journal*, **323**: 493–6.

O'Cathain, A., Walters, S.J., Nicholl, J.P., Thomas, K.J. and Kirkham, M. (2002) Use of evidence based leaflets to promote informed choice in maternity care: randomised controlled trial in everyday practice. *British Medical Journal*, **324**: 643–6.

O'Connor, A.M. (1995) Validation of a decisional conflict scale. *Medical Decision Making*, **15**: 25–30.

O'Connor, A.M., Rostom, A., Fiset, V., Tetroe, J., Entwistle, V., Llewellyn-Thomas, H. *et al.* (1999) Decision aids for patients facing health treatment or screening decisions: systematic review. *British Medical Journal*, **319**: 713–4.

O'Connor, A.M., Tugwell, P., Wells, G.A., Elmsie, T., Jolly, E., Hollingworth, G. *et al.* (1998) Randomised trial of a portable, self-administered decision aid for postmenopausal women considering long-term preventive hormone therapy. *Medical Decision Making*, **18**: 295–303.

Oliver, S., Rajan, L., Turner, H., Oakley, A., Entwistle, V., Watt, I. *et al.* (1996) Informed choice for users of health services: views on ultrasonography leaflets of women in early pregnancy, midwives, and ultrasonographers. *British Medical Journal*, **313**: 1251–5.

O'Neill, P., Humpris, G.M. and Field, E.A. (1996) The use of an information leaflet for patients undergoing wisdom tooth removal. *British Journal of Oral and Maxillofacial Surgery,* **34**: 331–4.

Peveler, R., George, C., Kinmonth, A.L. *et al.* (1999) Effect of antidepressant drug counselling and information leaflets on adherence to drug treatment in primary care: randomised controlled trial. *British Medical Journal,* **319**: 612–5.

Simpson, W.M., Johnstone, F.D., Boyd, F.M., Goldberg, D.J., Hart, G.J. and Prescott, R.J. (1998) Uptake and acceptability of antenatal HIV testing: randomised controlled trial of different methods of offering the test. *British Medical Journal,* **316**: 262–7.

Stapleton, H., Kirkham, M. and Thomas, G. (2002) Qualitative study of evidence-based leaflets in maternity care. *British Medical Journal,* **324**: 639–43.

Thornton, J.G., Hewison, J., Lilford, R.J. and Vail, A. (1995) A randomised trial of three methods of giving information about prenatal testing. *British Medical Journal,* **311**: 1127–30.

CHAPTER 5

Is There a Difference Between a Free Gift and a Planned Purchase? The Use of Evidence-based Leaflets in Maternity Care

HELEN STAPLETON

Chapter Contents

- Background to the *Informed Choice* study
- Research design and methods
- Background to the phase one study of the ethnographic units
- Funding arrangements for purchasing the *Informed Choice* leaflets
- The *Informed Choice* leaflets in everyday practice
- Different understandings of the concept of 'informed choice'
- Informed choice, equity and consumerist values
- Choice, inequality and stereotyping
- The evidence imperative, informed choice and professional accountancy
- The overall significance of the *Informed Choice* leaflets
- Conclusion

The material in this chapter is derived from a Department of Health (DoH) funded evaluation (Kirkham and Stapleton, 2001) of the MIDIRS (Midwives Information and Resource Service) *Informed Choice* leaflets. The aim of the chapter is to describe the main findings from the first phase of this research, which entailed an ethnographic study of three maternity units where the leaflets had been purchased and used for some time. Selected themes from the analysis of this qualitative data are discussed in conjunction with findings from the second phase of the study, where qualitative data was collected alongside a randomised controlled trial (RCT) (see Chapter 4).

Background to the *Informed Choice* study

In 1993, the (then) government policy document, *Changing Childbirth* (DoH, 1993) charged providers of maternity care to work towards making the service more woman-focused. Although patient-centredness is not exactly a new idea (Balint, 1957), *Changing Childbirth* modernised and expanded the concept by emphasising the need for childbearing women to have access to good quality information in order to make more informed choices about their care.

Our evaluation examined the use of the *Informed Choice* leaflets in maternity units which had independently purchased the leaflets and, subsequently, within the context of an RCT in which intervention units received the leaflets as a 'free gift'. The research aimed to assess the effectiveness of the leaflets in promoting informed choice. The relationship between leaflet use and evidence-based practice was not a primary focus of this research. Midwives' use of individual leaflets in clinical practice has, however, been described elsewhere (Stapleton, 2000).

The timing of our research acknowledged a shift of emphasis and philosophy in the NHS agenda. In recent years, UK government directives have moved on from stressing the importance of patient informed consent to treatment, to rather more complex notions of incorporating evidence-based care, informed choice and patient partnership (NHS Executive, 1996; DoH, 1997). The imperative for NHS trusts to deliver a service in accordance with predetermined quality indicators, which include the aforementioned concepts, has since become a legal requirement (DoH, 1999) and the present government has continued to push the need to improve the quality of patients experiences (Secretary of State for Health, 2002). Public inquiries into the performance of NHS doctors and nurses (for example, Bristol Royal Infirmary, Royal Liverpool Children's Hospital, Clothier Report, Shipman Inquiry) have also emphasised the need for a more responsive and accountable service with built-in safeguards to protect patients. The means by which this 'fine rhetoric' (Coulter, 2002) is turned into reality has not, however, been addressed although an expanding body of midwifery research has identified cultural and organisational impediments to change (Hunt and Symonds, 1995; Kirkham, 1999; Kirkham and Stapleton, 2001; Hughes *et al.*, 2002).

The development and publication of the MIDIRS Informed Choice leaflets

In 1994 the Department of Health made funding available for MIDIRS and the NHS Centre for Reviews and Dissemination to collaboratively produce evidence-based information for maternity service users in an accessible and useable form. This resulted in the production of the MIDIRS *Informed Choice* leaflets (see Chapter 4, Box 4.1). The joint expertise of MIDIRS and the NHS Centre for Reviews and Dissemination ensured that the initial ten leaflets would be based on the best available research evidence, utilising the Cochrane Database of Systematic Reviews. They were intended to provide research-based information to inform choice in accordance with women's individual needs. The leaflets, the production of which is now funded solely by MIDIRS, were last updated in 2003 and are available in electronic format: http://www.infochoice.org

Research design and methods

The research was undertaken in two phases. The first phase comprised an ethnographic study of three maternity units in England and Wales. This phase informed the second phase of the research, in which an RCT was carried out alongside qualitative research. The intervention for the RCT consisted of the full set[1] of ten MIDIRS IC leaflets and training in their use. The five intervention units were supplied with one set of leaflets for every woman delivering in an eight-month period; one set of professional's leaflets was also supplied for each midwife (see Chapter 4).

The qualitative research, undertaken in women's homes, community and hospital-based NHS antenatal and ultrasound clinics, included non-participant observation of clinical practice, in-depth interviews with women and health professionals, and focus groups with women. Participants included childbearing women and health professionals providing maternity care. The sample of maternity service users included multiparous and primiparous women covering the social class spectrum and the age range for childbearing; they were at all gestational stages. The postnatal sample included women who had given birth within the previous six months. The sample of health professionals included midwives, doctors (including general practitioners, obstetricians and obstetric anaesthetists at registrar level and above), and ultrasound practitioners (including medically and non-medically trained).

The majority of those observed and interviewed were midwives and maternity service users. The focus on midwives was deliberate as they are currently designated the lead professionals where normal pregnancy and birth are concerned and they were almost exclusively responsible for ensuring the transfer of *Informed Choice* leaflets to childbearing women. During phase two of the study, the researchers' observed 886 antenatal consultations and undertook 383 interviews (see Table 5.1). A substantial number of interviews followed on from an episode of observation. Observational work and interviews allowed the researchers to access participant's views on the *Informed Choice* leaflets; it also provided opportunities to examine women's and health professionals' attitudes to broader concepts such as evidence-based information, informed choice, and decision-making in maternity care.

Table 5.1 Summary of the qualitative methods used in phase two
of the study

Respondents	Episodes of observation	Interviews
Childbearing women	All observations concerned childbearing women; n=886	163: 85 antenatal : 78 postnatal
Midwives	653	177
Obstetricians	167	28
Obstetric ultrasonographers	66	12
Obstetric anaesthetists	n/a – observation of women in labour was not undertaken	3
Total	**886**	**383** of which 17 were conducted in Welsh

An ethnographic approach to the qualitative data collection was adopted during both phases of the study in order that the researchers might observe the use of the *Informed Choice* leaflets in a 'natural' setting. The phrase 'ethnographic approach' is used deliberately in order to convey that this was a partial, rather than complete, ethnography with the focus of data collection limited to aspects of pregnancy and childbearing and not the wider dimensions of participants' lives. In its broadest sense, ethnography is a description of a people and the cultural basis of their peoplehood (Peacock, 1986); 'doing' ethnography then, is a complex and time-consuming enterprise which involves negotiating access, establishing rapport, selecting and interviewing participants, mapping fields, keeping a diary, transcribing texts (Geertz, 1973). The ethnographer strives to observe and record events without censoring or filtering phenomena and to leave the field with 'thick' (contextual) descriptions. It is taken for granted in qualitative research that the observations and detailed fieldnotes made by the ethnographer are inevitably shaped by the 'personal biography of the gendered researcher who speaks from a particular class, racial, cultural and ethnic community perspective' (Denzin and Lincoln, 1994). The researchers' fieldnotes were included in the data analysis.

The four qualitative researchers, all of whom were midwives (including the author, HS), and one of whom was a Welsh-speaker, each spent between seven and eighteen working days in each of the study sites. As the majority of sites were previously unknown to the researchers, it was necessary to undertake a rapid assessment exercise about the way in which maternity care was accessed and delivered. The assessment exercise consisted of reading literature such as existing audits of the maternity service, scanning patient information booklets and other in-house literature, noting information displayed on notice boards, attending departmental and other meetings and, all the while, observing and listening to interactions amongst staff and between themselves and the childbearing women in their care. During this time the researchers also spent time informally chatting to both service providers and users wherever they congregated: in waiting rooms, canteens, foyers and wards and in staff sitting rooms, offices and kitchens. Such intensive networking, with both NHS and non-NHS service providers and users, enabled the researchers to identify a number of key participants and initial lines of enquiry at an early stage of the fieldwork.

Qualitative and quantitative research: combining methodological approaches

The various qualitative methods enabled us to examine the same issue from a range of different perspectives and to explore beyond health professionals' and childbearing women's 'official' accounts of choice and decision-making.

The combination of qualitative and quantitative methods in the study design, data collection and analysis reflected the changing priorities in health services research (Murphy *et al.*, 1998). Undertaking qualitative research alongside the RCT subsequently proved invaluable in aiding our understanding of the evaluation findings. Indeed, the combination of methods facilitated the pragmatic approach adopted in this study and enabled us to explore issues arising throughout the study period which were often of a multidimensional and multidisciplinary nature. An additional advantage, noted by other researchers (Ronka *et al.*, 2002), was that it enabled us to target qualitative interviews to 'get at' issues identified by the quantitative data, and to move in the reverse direction. The spectrum of methodologies employed was thus mutually supportive and permitted a detailed illumination of the complex processes underlying change and continuity (Laub and Sampson, 1998). This approach also assisted us in generating and testing hypotheses directly from observation of clinical practice. The findings from the qualitative research illustrated the complexity of the environment in which the intervention was applied and suggested reasons why the *Informed Choice* leaflets did not promote informed decision-making (O'Cathain *et al.*, 2002; Stapleton *et al.*, 2002).

Data analysis

A grounded theory (Glaser and Strauss, 1967) approach to data collection and analysis was adopted in all qualitative phases of the research. The software package QSR NUD*IST (Non-numerical Data Information Systems and Technology) was used to organise and interrogate the complex data sets.

Ethics and consent

Ethics committee approval was obtained for both phases of the study. Written consent was obtained from all participants prior to interview. Difficulties were occasionally experienced in obtaining verbal consent from maternity service users for some of the observation episodes because staff assumed consent to observation alongside clinical care (see Kirkham and Stapleton, 2001, Chapter 11).

Confidentiality

In order to protect the identity of participants, generic terms such maternity service user, midwife, GP, ultrasound practitioner, obstetric anaesthetist, obstetrician are used throughout this chapter. The 'signature' of an individual participant is qualified in some instances by the insertion of descriptors such as *community* midwife, *caseload* midwife, *Head of Midwifery* (HoM), midwifery *manager* or *consultant* obstetrician.

Notations used in the text

Quotations from phase one and phase two participants are differentiated as follows:

Phase one participants carry the inscription: Site 1, 2 or 3 to indicate in which of three maternity units they were based.

Phase two participants are distinguished between those working on 'intervention' sites, which received the MIDIRS *Informed Choice* leaflets, and those working on 'control' sites.

The inscription 'small maternity unit' is used to indicate participants working in maternity units in which the annual birth rate was less than 500.

The term 'service user' is used interchangeably with 'childbearing woman'.

Background to the phase one study of the ethnographic units

This phase of the research was crucial to the design and development of the questionnaire tool used in the RCT; it also served to alert the qualitative researchers, early on in the study, to a number of key themes.

Two of the three maternity units in the ethnographic study were in England and one was in Wales. The sites were very different geographically, in the clientele they served, and in the organisation of maternity care. The annual delivery rates for the units ranged from approximately 1500 to 4500; the latter served as a regional referral unit for women from local and surrounding areas with high-risk pregnancies. One of the units served an inner city, multi-ethnic population; the remaining two units served smaller, mainly white, working-class populations.

Throughout this chapter, reference is made to 'leaflets'. These are the MIDIRS *Informed Choice* leaflets unless otherwise stated.

Funding arrangements for purchasing the *Informed Choice* leaflets

The ethnographic units varied in funding arrangements for their initial purchases of the leaflets. In one unit the Head of Midwifery (HoM) used the leverage of risk management to persuade her employing trust:

> 'As soon as I saw them I thought they were a really good thing. I presented them as evidence to the trust hospital negligence scheme and got money to fund the purchase immediately. The trust here are very hot on risk management and we've got a very efficient complaints system here so anything that might play a part in reducing complaints and dealing with high-risk situations gets a hearing.' (HoM, site 1.1)

The health promotion unit on another site agreed to fund the leaflet on alcohol:

> 'The health promotion unit isn't trust based so they're a bit more independent with what they can do. They had a bit of money so they bought the alcohol leaflets for us.' Midwifery manager, site 1.3

Midwives in the third unit, including the HoM who was not in post at the time the leaflets had originally been purchased, did not know how the leaflets had been funded.

None of the units appeared to have any strategy in place for re-ordering leaflets when current stocks eventually ran out. The following comment, made by an HoM but echoed by participants all three sites, suggested that hospital departments would be expected to become increasingly self-sufficient in producing written literature for their own client groups:

> 'Trust policy is now for all clinical fields to develop the production of their own in-house materials ... the MIDIRS leaflets will be a great help.' (HoM, site 1.2)

Very few health professionals, however, indicated that they had any awareness of the enormous amount of research and preparatory work which had preceded the launch of the *Informed Choice* leaflets and none mentioned possible infringement of intellectual property rights in the event that information contained in the leaflets was replicated.

Maternity service managers, especially those who were not practising clinicians, expressed only positive sentiments about the leaflets. The majority valued the opportunity to be seen to be 'doing the right thing' by addressing risk management concerns that service users be adequately informed and that the information they received from health professionals was based on good clinical evidence. A more cynical view is that the purchase of the *Informed Choice* leaflets constituted little more than a public relations exercise which ensured that, if things did go wrong, the hospital trust would not be seen as culpable.

The *Informed Choice* leaflets in everyday practice

The leaflets were used almost exclusively by midwives on all three sites and they were used in a similar manner during both phases of the study. To summarise: leaflets were often disguised by being 'wrapped' with other pregnancy-related information (including advertising materials) or inserted into Bounty packs[2]; leaflets were often given to women without any discussion; the timing of leaflets did not always synchronise with women's requirements; once leaflets were given, there was generally no further reference to the leaflet topic(s); women were given leaflets in 'batches' and at fixed points in pregnancy rather than having them individually 'prescribed' according to need; midwives were selective in which leaflets they gave to women; women of lower social class tended to be given fewer leaflets.

Unsurprisingly perhaps, the way in which the *Informed Choice* leaflets were transferred to women seemed to play a crucial role in whether the contents were subsequently read and/or acted upon. Very few midwives were observed spending time discussing the contents of the leaflets with women and even fewer were observed to 'prescribe' the leaflets in response to a specific situation. For different reasons perhaps, both staff and childbearing women seemed to place more value on the 'tried and tested' knowledge they had already acquired, than on that which was provided by the *Informed Choice* leaflets. This is not to suggest that staff were already conversant with the information contained in the leaflets and had changed their practice in line with the evidence stated therein. Sadly, clinical practice which reflected the evidence base of the leaflets was rarely encountered in this study. Many clinicians did not appreciate the evidence base of the *Informed Choice* leaflets, possibly because the health professionals', fully referenced version, was rarely seen on any of the sites. Indeed, many participants in both phases of the study did not know that a professionals' version existed.

The leaflets (and/or the presence of the researchers) often appeared to threaten staff and many reacted defensively and aggressively when invited to explain their initial response to using the leaflets in practice. Many midwives presumed that the researchers had been involved in the leaflet production and publication processes and hence we were often subjected to a diatribe on the various shortcomings of individual leaflets.

It was customary practice across all three ethnographic sites for a selection of the *Informed Choice* leaflets to be routinely inserted into the woman's hand-held notes, or the Bounty pack, together with a variable range of other routine information, including advertising materials. This package was then given to all women at the booking consultation. Sometimes the leaflets remained bundled up with the other information for the duration of the pregnancy, following which the *Informed Choice* leaflets, in pristine condition, were occasionally retrieved from the woman's notes for recycling. Midwives' 'wrapping' of the leaflets in this way thus rendered their contents invisible. It required childbearing women to exercise considerable initiative and discrimination if they were to appreciate the significance of the (well disguised) leaflet contents. It appeared that very few women achieved this.

A considerable number of health professionals were of the opinion that the *Informed Choice* leaflets should not be given to maternity service users if they contained information which contradicted local policies. This was especially so if the leaflets contained information which staff thought might potentially create a demand for services which were not locally available. A small number of women, who accessed information which was neither locally available, nor contained in the *Informed Choice* leaflets, reported frustrating experiences when they invited comments from staff:

> 'I downloaded information off the net about this [the pros and cons of neural tube screening over chorionic villus sampling] because they didn't seem to have anything. They wouldn't even look at it. I couldn't believe it. They just refused to discuss it. ... They acted like the Internet was some kind of adult movie...like it was censored or something. ... It was really good quality information but they didn't even want the address of the site.' (Service user, intervention site)

When health professionals were 'put on the spot' in this way by service users, they were commonly observed to dismiss either the source, and/or the quality, of the information. It was as if they were only comfortable when able to exert control over the flow of information and it is possible that the *Informed Choice* leaflets undermined their position in this respect. It is also likely that the choices offered in the leaflets served to (painfully) remind midwives of their powerlessness in effecting change.

Many women were often given leaflets inappropriately. For instance, women in the third trimester were observed being offered leaflets on ultrasound scanning and screening for fetal abnormalities long after these decisions had been made (albeit sometimes by default). With respect to the leaflet on alcohol, women who had clearly stated that they did not drink alcohol, or that they had stopped because of pregnancy, were nonetheless given this leaflet without the midwife ascertaining whether it was wanted. Midwives generally did not discuss the information contained within specific leaflets, for example that a small amount of alcohol in pregnancy was probably all right, and neither did many midwives give women the option of refusing leaflets. The vast majority of midwives were observed documenting in the woman's maternity record, however, that the leaflets had been dispensed.

Women were usually given the *Informed Choice* leaflets with a vague recommendation from the midwife 'to go away and read them'. The following extract, taken from fieldnotes, illustrates a typical interaction between a community midwife and a pregnant woman during a routine antenatal consultation.

Midwife: '*There are some leaflets here about some of the things we've discussed, so if you have a read of them and then you can ask me if you have any questions.*'

As she stands up, the community midwife hands the woman her notes, plus a bundle of information including three *Informed Choice* leaflets: alcohol, ultrasound and place of birth. This woman is 22 weeks pregnant and has already received three ultrasound scans (two 'mini', and one anomaly scan) and has said that she does not drink alcohol. There has been no suggestion during the consultation that she might exercise any choice in where she has her baby nor in questioning the need for further 'mini' scans (which are routinely used by some obstetricians in this unit to listen to the fetal heart during abdominal palpation). Antenatal clinic, site 1.3

It was customary practice for some community midwives to discuss birthplans with women in their caseloads when they were around 35–7 weeks pregnant. This was often the time when the *Informed Choice* leaflets describing labour-related decisions, such as positions, support, epidurals and monitoring were handed out to women. The birthplan consultation was also the occasion where a degree of variation in practice was observed in that a very small number of midwives were seen to open leaflets and initiate discussion of the contents with the woman concerned. This was much more likely to occur if the midwife already had an established relationship with the woman and if she expected to be looking after her when in labour.

Parentcraft classes were also used as access points for disseminating leaflets to women, often as supplementary reading to topics which had been presented in the class. Typically, the leaflets were handed to the woman sitting closest to the midwife teaching the class, with the instruction for her to take one and to pass the remainder on; in this way the *Informed Choice* leaflets were distributed. The majority of women removed leaflets from the bundles as instructed. They put them straight into their handbags, laid them on their laps or flicked through the contents whilst the midwife continued talking. Women were rarely invited by the midwife to read the leaflets during the class but were typically requested to 'read them at home', 'show them to your partners' and to 'come back with any questions'. The researchers did not observe one parentcraft class when specific reference was made by the midwife to any of the *Informed Choice* leaflets previously given to women.

Very occasionally, midwives removed an individual leaflet from the pre-packed bundle during the antenatal consultation. When midwives enquired about alcohol intake or infant feeding, for example, the cover of the leaflet referred to might be shown to the pregnant woman. Mostly, however, the leaflets were simply referred to in passing. Maternity service users were not heard to have the differences between the *Informed Choice* leaflets, and any other sources of information explained to them, and this may have acted to render the leaflets even more invisible. These and related issues were also observed throughout the second phase of the study.

Written information and quality issues

In addition to the *Informed Choice* leaflets, midwives often gave childbearing women written information produced 'in house'. A number of women were critical of both the quality and content of this material:

> 'Take the information they gave us about Vitamin K. First of all it was so badly photo-copied it was almost unreadable. And the information was so biased. For instance they didn't say it had been linked with childhood cancers. They didn't mention that research at all, which is a bit stupid of them really, because it's so widely available.' (Service user, control site)

The researchers scrutinised a selection of maternity-related literature that had been produced in-house across all the research sites. Most of it was undated, photocopying was often of such poor quality as to make reading difficult, errors in spelling and punctuation were common and evidence to support the claims made was generally lacking. The topics covered by these in-house materials frequently duplicated those covered by the *Informed Choice* leaflets although there were often substantial differences in content and 'tone', with the former being more directive, alarmist, and describing only the options which were locally available. With reference to the preceding quotation, the vast majority of babies on all study sites were given Vitamin K. The 'choice' which the researchers heard midwives offering to women was between oral and subcutaneous administration; opting out altogether did not appear to be a choice. As has been explained elsewhere (Stapleton *et al.*, 2002), women's trust in health professionals' recommendations ensured their compliance with professionally defined 'right' choices and only very rarely were women observed asking questions or making alternative requests. Hierarchical power structures resulted in senior doctors defining the norms of clinical practice and hence which choices were possible. This reinforced notions of 'right' and 'wrong' choices rather than 'informed' choices.

A small number of midwives suggested that the MIDIRS *Informed Choice* leaflets had provided them with an important measure of quality against which to critique the in-house information produced by their own employing trust. The quality of the leaflets was also commented on by a small number of (middle-class) women who were surprised and excited to see such an initiative within an NHS context:

Researcher: 'Did you appreciate they [*Informed Choice* leaflets] were all based on research?
Maternity service user: 'Oh yes, it's obvious… Yes I did appreciate that. You can see that a lot of effort has gone into producing these … a lot of people have been involved. That's what gave me so much confidence when I read them … it's very exciting to think leaflets of this quality will be available to people using the NHS.'

One such service user, an expert in the use of information technology systems, suggested, however, that education would be necessary before information based on research evidence could bring about change:

'The main downfall is always that people aren't briefed properly on how to handle this kind of information [*Informed Choice* leaflets]… You might as well just not bother with it. It's just a complete waste of paper.'

Sadly, our research findings support the opinion of this service user. Despite their impressive and scientific credentials, there was no evidence that the *Informed Choice* leaflets were effective in increasing the proportion of women who reported having exercised informed choice. The lack of a coherent strategy, including educational reform, was identified as a significant factor.

Withholding leaflets; maintaining power

A number of midwives were observed withholding certain *Informed Choice* leaflets because they contradicted their personal philosophy, their customary clinical practice or because the leaflets conveyed 'a negative image'. Initially, the leaflets pertaining to epidural, place of birth, ultrasound scans and breech presentation appeared particularly troublesome but, as the study proceeded, almost all the leaflets, with the possible exceptions of alcohol and infant feeding, were problematic for health professionals in this respect. Indeed, the negative opinions of medical staff on one intervention site carried such weight that three of the leaflets (epidural, ultrasound scans and antenatal screening) were withheld for the duration of the RCT. When asked about these issues during follow-up interviews, a number of midwives on all intervention sites admitted that they were 'more selective' with information which contradicted local policies and which might thus provoke confrontation with medical colleagues. More than any other group, obstetricians voiced concerns about 'bias' in the leaflets and the potential for harm to women if they were given information, which 'pointed out the downside of everything'. A worrying number of obstetricians appeared, however, to view any information which described the disadvantages of obstetric interventions as 'biased'. It is perhaps worth stating that, as with midwives, a significant number of obstetricians did not appear to have read the *Informed Choice* leaflets and even towards the close of phase two of the study, some did not know that the unit in which they were working had been allocated to the intervention arm of the RCT.

Doctors exercised considerable power over the information given to women and, therefore, over the options which midwives subsequently made available to them. For example, one consultant obstetrician would not allow the *Informed Choice* leaflet on breech presentation to be used because she disagreed with women being offered any choice in the mode of delivery; she was of the opinion that all women with a breech presentation should undergo an elective Caesarean section (CS). Another consultant obstetrician refused to allow women booked with him to have access to the *Informed Choice* leaflet on antenatal screening because he considered the current tests to be insufficiently accurate. A community midwife did not offer women the leaflet on place of birth because of GP opposition to home birth.

Midwives largely colluded with doctors in withholding leaflets from women and thus with the reduction in the choices they made available. Some midwives voiced their disquiet about this during the course of an in-depth interview:

> 'I wasn't directly involved with her but I still feel awful about not having said anything. Watching her go through a [Caesarean] section [for a breech presentation] and knowing that she'd had two perfectly normal vaginal births before. What upset me most was that she wasn't given any choice about it. She wasn't given any options. She was just told in the clinic to come in the next day for a section. I felt awful about not having said anything, knowing that if that woman had been a patient of consultant X, she'd have been offered ECV and if she'd wanted to, a try at a vaginal birth.' (Midwife, site 1.3)

The researchers observed a number of occasions when women were not informed that alternative options were available and nor were women routinely informed about the possible outcomes of certain choices. Withholding such information was problematic when, as in the case described in the above quotation, referral to a different consultant, skilled in ECV and vaginal breech delivery, might have avoided an operative delivery. In this study the researchers frequently observed information being 'framed' (Marteau, 1989) in such a way as to 'steer' (Elwyn *et al.*, 1999; Levy, 1999) or 'sway' (Freeman and Sweeney, 2001) women towards making decisions which reflected the point of view advanced by the health professional.

Different understandings of the concept of 'informed choice'

The researchers invited participants on all sites to explain what they understood by the phrase 'informed choice'. The variety of responses elicited a broad range of concerns and suggested that many participants had reservations about the potential of one utility (such as the *Informed Choice* leaflets) to achieve something as complex as informed choice. Some of the themes identified during the first phase of the study, such as power relations, economic and time pressures, educational and skill deficits and inequality of service provision, were also identified as key themes in the data collection during the RCT phase of the study.

The following quotations reveal what a selection of participants understood by the term 'informed choice':

'Informed choice should only be offered when the service is well prepared and can meet the extra needs this will create. If we [health professionals] are not given information about what exactly is meant by informed choice, then we cannot be expected to provide it ... informed choice is more than providing information.' (GP, site 1.2)

'Well, for a start, there's a lot more to informed choice than spending a few hundred quid on some leaflets. It seems to me that informed choice is only available for the women who've already got libraries of books and more than enough information. They're the ones getting the informed choices.' (Midwife, site 1.1)

'Frankly I don't think they [childbearing women] get much choice at all ... they're told what's on offer and that's that, really ... and it's the same with the information we give them, I think a lot of it is not very impartial. It's what we think is the right thing to do ... so we're advising them what we think is right rather than giving them impartial information and letting them choose ... I think informed choice is an issue we've ducked out of really.' (GP, site 1.1)

'What I understand by informed choice is that I'll have all the information I need to make decisions ... that the information will come from a respected source ... that I won't be pressured into doing something I really don't want to do.' (Maternity service user, site 1.3)

'Where the idea of informed choice falls down for me is where primips choose to have a home birth or where women want to have water births, or they don't want to be monitored ... or don't want to have scans ... I have great difficulty in understanding those decisions, but I also accept that they are probably making informed choices because in order to go against the tide, they need to be well informed.' (Consultant obstetrician, site 1.2)

'Informed choice is really about women using their initiative to find out what's not available, rather than what is.' (Midwife, site 1.2)

'Informed choice is about women asking for choice ... it's about them asking for it ... the women who ask for home birth or ECV for turning breech babies are well informed, but no-one's going to tell them about these things ... No-one's going to tell them what their options are – they have to find out for themselves.' (Midwife, site 1.1)

In 'finding out for oneself' or 'asking for it', however, the onus of responsibility for ensuring that choices are made available is on the service user, not the service provider.

Information seeking requires a command of English and a level of personal assurance which many service users may not posses; it also emphasises the imbalances in power relationships between women and their care providers. The following quotation graphically illustrates the difficulties women, especially those pregnant for the first time, experienced when they attempted to 'find out for themselves':

> 'The GP doesn't seem to trust the midwife and the midwife doesn't seem to have any real authority and the consultant just acts like he's god… It's exhausting. It's also very easy to offend them if you say the wrong thing to the wrong person. … You're stumbling around in the dark and none of them help you to find out who's who or how the system works. They leave it all up to you to find out.' (Service user, control site)

As choice is also related to 'categories of contingency' (Pope, 2002) about which women are not routinely informed, for example staff preferences, and the availability of equipment and services, it seemed unlikely that the leaflets alone could promote informed decision-making. With particular regard to antenatal screening, it has been suggested (Press and Browner, 1997) that the act of offering a test may, in itself, be interpreted as a recommendation to have the test, which compromises the very notion of a free, and informed, choice. One commentator on this subject (Robins, 2002) has recently proposed that 'a fully informed choice is not possible in the antenatal setting' because 'an offer that is made under conditions that take advantage of a woman's vulnerabilities … does not respect her voluntariness' (ibid.).

The choices offered to women then, inevitably reflected the policies of the local unit, the normative standards of local clinical practice and the decisions of powerholders such as obstetricians. This reiterates what has been described elsewhere: 'For many patients, what happens to them depends more on locally accepted practice than rigorous clinical evidence'; hence the phrase 'geography is destiny' (Farrell and Gilbert, 1996, p. 21). The choices health professionals offered to women conformed to accepted societal and behavioural norms, perhaps because:

> 'the strength of the normative standard is so powerful that our society is constrained to go to extraordinary lengths to perpetuate a clear distinction between what is considered normal and acceptable and what is considered abnormal and intolerable.' (Shildrik, 2002, p. 68)

In this study, for example, many midwives working in the small maternity units facilitated labour without recourse to pharmaceutical pain relief. This was locally perceived as a normative practice and was much valued by local childbearing women. Staff working in neighbouring consultant obstetric units, however, tended to discount these midwifery skills, perhaps because epidural use in labour is now so common as to be widely accepted as 'the' normative standard for pain relief in labour.

Verbal information and non-verbal cues: sowing seeds (of doubt)

Midwives and women sometimes used metaphorical language such as 'seeds', 'sowing' and/or 'planting' when describing the way in which non-verbal information was conveyed. Midwives often stressed the importance of 'getting off to a good start' with women in their care and this included laying the foundations for a relationship of trust to be established at the first consultation:

> 'The first impression the women get of the maternity service and of us midwives is really, really important. If you let the woman see any seeds of doubt at that stage, before she's got any trust going with us, then you're sunk really. You can't pick it up so easily later on.' (Community midwife, control site)

In the following quotation, a woman interviewed late in her second pregnancy, recounts how the suggestion of a repeat Caesarean section was 'planted' in her mind by an obstetrician at her first hospital appointment. In her first pregnancy, two years previously, she had undergone an emergency Caesarean in early labour for a previously undiagnosed breech presentation.

> 'The doctor planted the seed right at the beginning. He asked me at my first appointment if I'd thought about a Caesarean section. I hadn't. I'd just thought I'd have it naturally unless anything went wrong again and then I'd have to have another Caesarean. That's what I'd thought but then he planted the seed. He said he could book me in so then there wouldn't have to be any emergency, no panic sort of thing. I suppose if he hadn't said anything, I'd be sitting here waiting for labour to start instead of packing my bag to go hospital.' (Service user, intervention site)

Women's faith in health professionals almost always resulted in their unquestioning acceptance of the options they suggested.

Many midwives reported practising under considerable time pressures and whilst some said they would have preferred to give women individualised, and appropriately timed, information, this was rarely possible. Midwives often complained that the booking visit was especially problematic and many felt that they 'bombarded' women with questions and information at this time. This was particularly the case where the information midwives were asking women to impart, or that which they were conveying to them, was of a sensitive nature. The widespread lack of continuity of both care, and of carer, observed throughout this study, only served to increase the sense of pressure midwives widely reported feeling in their interactions with women. Some midwives reported occasionally acting prematurely on cues they picked up from women during their first encounters because the organisational priorities were such that they knew they would have little further contact with them.

Sometimes, women reported that health professionals preempted their readiness to receive information. This was often the case when the health professional adduced the notion of risk. In the following quotation, a woman with a breech presentation at 37 weeks describes how staff seriously undermined her belief in her capacity to deliver her baby vaginally:

> 'Now whether it was for them to sow the seed in my mind first before I found out about what options I had myself I don't know. They obviously thought that this [elective CS for breech presentation] was going to be better for me but it was the first time I had heard that mentioned. I didn't know anybody who'd had a Caesarean section before. I'd only had two straightforward home births before. They planted a seed of doubt in my mind and it stuck there. ... I did have a normal [vaginal breech] delivery in the end but I never stopped worrying that the head would get stuck because that was the seed of doubt they sowed in my mind. That was the risk they said I'd be taking. It was very hard not to imagine that happening. The baby's head getting stuck inside me. It was horrible.' (Service user, five weeks postnatal)

Many health professionals were observed to inflate clinical risk by recounting 'horror stories' to women as a means of securing their compliance with the suggestions they made. Women who opted for a different course of action were commonly labelled as 'difficult'. The woman in the preceding quotation went on to give birth vaginally but, as this excerpt demonstrates, her memory of the (mis)information she was given at a critical time in her pregnancy did not assist her in assessing her situation, nor did it help her to make an informed decision with which she felt comfortable. Five weeks after her baby's birth she still appears to be troubled by the imagery 'planted' in her mind by her care providers. Little is known about the longer-term affects on women's mental health when unwanted mental imagery is created which they find difficult to eradicate subsequently.

Lack of information about a common intervention: Caesarean section

Given the privileging of technocracy in modern obstetrics, and the increasing frequency with which Caesarean section is performed (Thomas and Paranjothy, 2001; DoH, 2001) it was surprising to hear women on the majority of the research sites complaining about the paucity of information they received about this 'mother of all interventions'.

The quotations selected to illustrate this part of the chapter are all from women who underwent an elective CS. The majority reported that they had accessed information of relevance to them from sources other than health professionals.

> 'You'd think with this mother of all interventions that they'd at least be able to give you some decent information. After all, that's what they're supposed to be good at isn't it?

I got nothing that was of any use. They didn't even tell me I wouldn't be able to pick up my baby… I wouldn't be able to drive for six weeks … Like it was nothing for them.' (Service user, small unit, CS for pre-existing hypertensive disease)

'I'd had two normal deliveries and you're on a bit of a high after delivery. You really think you've achieved something when you give birth. There's none of that after a Caesarean. I felt very miserable on some days.' (Service user, site 1.2, CS for suspected fetal growth restriction)

'Nobody had ever said to me that if you have a Caesarean that you might need a general anaesthetic if the epidural doesn't work … I knew that obviously it's a medical operation and I knew that the recovery time was a lot longer than a normal birth. But that was about all I knew. I'd only had normal births before… It wasn't as if they didn't know I needed a Caesarean. They knew that from early on … But as I say it was all at the last minute. Things were being thrown at me.' (Service user, intervention site, CS as the placenta was partially occluding the Os)

'I did feel cheated actually afterwards because I'd sort of gone into hospital pregnant and come out having had an operation and there was this baby in a sort of little fish tank at the side of the bed that I just didn't feel … Well I knew she was mine but it didn't feel as though I'd had anything to do with her birth … No-one told you what to expect afterwards.' (Service user, control site, elective CS for breech presentation)

The main issues which women in this research wanted more information about *in advance of* a CS included:

- *The need for help afterwards.* Some women had to pay for extra household help or ask friends or relatives who were sometimes in poor health themselves and/or lived some distance away.
- *Restrictions on driving, lifting and carrying.* Some women living in rural areas gave birth during lambing season and the additional burden on partners having to drive children to school, as well as shop and clean, placed an enormous stress on a relationship already stressed in accommodating a new baby. These restrictions also created breastfeeding problems when women could not easily lift, nor lie down, with their babies to feed.
- *Lack of emotional affect*
- *Loss of independence*
- *Pain* – particularly for women who had only previously experienced uncomplicated birth
- *Complications afterwards:* wounds that failed to heal and antibiotic resistant thrush were frequently mentioned.
- *Post-operative physiotherapy:* 'Nobody taught me to cough before my Caesarean…'
- *Unfamiliarity of a hospital environment:* This was especially problematic for women who had not previously been an in-patient as an adult and for

women who had previously given birth only at home. This lack of experience in dealing with a medical environment made it difficult for women to formulate questions as they didn't know what 'the rules' were.

The vulnerability of women living in rural or remote areas was greatly increased by the impact of surgery which severely restricted their mobility. Not knowing 'what to expect afterwards' was frequently mentioned by this group and this seemed to exaggerate their sense of disbelief and dislocation in the early postnatal period. The agitation and distress which was evident when women articulated this sense of 'not knowing' also seemed to preoccupy their focus of attention, moving this away from their newborn baby.

It was something of a paradox that women who wanted the fewest interventions very often amassed the most information (usually as a result of their own efforts and often in anticipation of having to defend their decision to a health professional) whilst those undergoing the extreme end of the intervention continuum were given very little information by health professionals and what they did receive was often neither helpful nor relevant to their lives as new mothers.

Informed choice, equity and consumerist values

The way in which informed choice was described by some health professionals gave credence to the myth that pregnancy affords all women choices whereas, especially within the context of a welfare system, choice is very limited for disadvantaged women. The following quotations are illustrative:

> 'Women who are undemanding of the service may lose out on being well informed and they're certainly far less likely to make decisions which are right for them.' (GP, site 1.3)

> 'Informed choice is a nonsense for women who cannot access and use written information ... they are likely to remain powerless and helpless because there are no resources being invested in them ... Take these leaflets, they're useless for most of my women because they're only available in English [and not in the Asian languages spoken by most of the women in this midwife's caseload].' (Midwife, site 1.2)

These views suggest that some health professionals recognised that women on the receiving end of the maternity services are not all equal and that effecting change will require strategic planning and investment on a number of levels. It is extremely doubtful, however, whether informed choice can be presented as a viable option to either women or health professionals until the issue of inequality is acknowledged and strategies are put in place which make it easier for disadvantaged women to access the full range of maternity services.

Informed choice has become something of a fashionable concept in recent years and this is reflected not only in NHS directives but is also evident in the terminology of advertising and commerce. In a welfare state, healthcare is rationed and choices for health service users are set by government priorities, with some flexibility for manoeuvring at a local level. Given the variability in maternity service provision throughout the UK, however, the information contained in the *Informed Choice* leaflets will undoubtedly continue to contradict local norms of practice and this will make it particularly difficult for women who are disadvantaged, and/or who are unassertive, to achieve informed choice in their maternity care.

Choice, inequality and stereotyping

A number of community midwives considered the leaflets to be inappropriate for particular women in their caseloads. Midwives' dealt with this issue in varying ways but the end result was that certain women were stereotyped.

'I've had many women in this area refuse the *Informed Choice* leaflets because they look too complicated … I think they're a bit too posh for some of these girls around here … a lot of the girls I look after don't read … their reading matter is probably limited to the newspaper around the fish and chip package.' (Midwife, site 1.3)

'There are a lot of women in my caseload I wouldn't dream of giving the leaflets to … like I wouldn't give some of them certain information because I don't want them having certain choices … like not having a scan or having the baby at home for instance … it would be a complete waste of time giving them leaflets to read … anyway, they can't read, a lot of them and I don't want them feeling even worse about that than they do already.' (Midwife, site 1.2)

As has been previously described (Kirkham *et al.*, 2002), midwives sometimes made incorrect judgements about women's abilities, capacities and their desire to participate in their maternity care and, as a consequence, women were negatively stereotyped, for example, as 'demanding' and/or as 'unco-operative'. Midwives often formulated opinions about their clients on the basis of circumstances over which childbearing women exercised little control. Unfortunately, once pregnant women were 'typecast' in this way by health professionals, they usually remained so for the remainder of their pregnancy and, occasionally, these same descriptions resurfaced in a subsequent pregnancy.

The following quotation is unusual in that it demonstrates a midwife's sensitive and creative approach to presenting information to women with different needs:

'There's a lot of women around here who may not want *Informed Choice* leaflets because they can't read … but one of the important aspects of informed choice is about finding out what people are good at so you know how to help them to get what they want …

if they can't read for instance, then you draw or tell them stories about how other women did it, so they get the ideas in a different ways.' (Midwife, site 1.3)

Such flexible and individualised care, whilst undoubtedly of great value to childbearing women, creates problems for midwives working within the time constraints of contemporary NHS, where lack of staff time has been identified as a major obstacle in making services more patient-centred (Dunn, 2002). (See Chapter 6.)

A number of midwives correctly implied that management decisions to purchase the leaflets were driven not so much by a commitment to informed choice, but by concerns about quality assurance indicators and risk management strategies. Thus, a range of other concerns militated against the leaflets being used to promote informed decision-making by service users. These issues also jeopardised the professional–client relationship and served to worsen the inequity of maternity care provision as is illustrated by the following quotation:

'I don't want to use the leaflets ... they make me angry because they make the inequality issue a lot worse ... especially with the way we've been told to use the leaflets. We've been given strict instructions about that. We were told that because of finance, we were only getting a limited supply and that we had to make them last us, so we're only to give them to those who would really benefit from them and who would look after them so that when they were given back, they would be in good condition.' (Midwife, site 1.1)

The quotations in this section all serve to illustrate the dilemmas midwives faced in clinical practice. In trying to do best by the women in their care many midwives assumed decision-making responsibility on their behalf and this tended to increase the likelihood of stereotyping. This seemed more likely to happen when women were materially disadvantaged. It is suggested that such responses may have encouraged midwives and other health professionals to accept, rather than challenge, sweeping judgements as accurate reflections ('women in this area can't, or don't read...') which are then held to be true for all women, in that geographical patch, for all time.

The evidence imperative, informed choice and professional accountability

Participants valued many different sorts of evidence which emanated from a wide variety of sources. From the analysis of the research findings it seemed that the 'evidence' offered to defend, or support the many, and often conflicting, views was not only extremely varied, but often did not appear to have any rational basis. Given the privileging of rationality in biomedicine this was somewhat surprising, at least insofar as the health professional participants were concerned. The lack of a rational evidence base influenced the information health professionals conveyed to childbearing women and affected the decisions made by both parties.

The evidence cited by participants often appeared to be underpinned by a moral judgement (good/bad; right/wrong) and this sometimes made the research enquiry a delicate undertaking, perhaps because of the emotional investment in the belief underpinning the evidence. The 'mixed bag' of evidence from which respondents drew, ranged from the verbally disseminated 'wisdom of our grannies' to the meta-evidence of RCT's (as illustrated by the MIDIRS *Informed Choice* leaflets).

Conflicts arose when 'evidence' was positively or negatively weighted by those in positions of authority and power, especially when this was without reference to the possible interests and concerns of other parties. Perhaps because of the long established power imbalances within the paternalistic, and technology driven, maternity services, powerholders on all sites tended to make unilateral decisions; it was relatively easy to suppress, or discount, the 'anecdotal' evidence from powerless others (including midwives and childbearing women).

For some staff, only evidence from 'approved' sources, such as an RCT or a systematic review, was admissible for the purpose of clinical decision-making. As the following quotation demonstrates, however, this created problems where the woman's decision was informed by other evidence, such as her successful past experiences of childbearing.

> 'I have had a recent incident which has made me think about informed choice from the professional's point of view. We've had a complaint against a fairly junior midwife. She seems to have decided that evidence-based practice is more important than the woman's choice ... the husband was writing on her behalf ... his wife [who was Asian] had wanted to lie flat on her back to give birth because this was what she had done before with the other births and it had worked fine so she wanted to do it again. ... But it seems that the midwife did not want this and kept telling her that it was better for her, and better for the baby, if she was upright ... The husband said he had to keep helping his wife to lie down, while the midwife kept trying to help her up again... I can see the midwife's dilemma but informed choice is not for midwives to be forcing on women.' (Midwifery manager, site 1.2)

Providing decisions emanated from sources considered legitimate by the health professional, they were usually seen as 'right' decisions. Many staff appeared to experience difficulty in dealing with alternative models of decision-making. Many health professionals seemed unable to acknowledge women's agency in the decision-making process and reacted with expressions of hurt and rejection when women disregarded their recommendations and advice:

> 'It's disappointing when women are given the information and they don't make the choices you want them to or, when you try to give women information, they refuse it and say that they're not bothered or they're not interested.' (Midwife, site 1.3)

When women made decisions which were disapproved of, staff often appeared uneasy. Some health professionals adopted an adversarial stance whilst others anticipated feelings of blame, from which they sometimes attempted to protect themselves by shifting the blame back to women:

> 'Some women are never satisfied with the information or the explanations you give them…it doesn't matter how evidence based it is…but if they then make choices that are not based on good evidence, whose problem is it?' (Midwife, site 1.2)

> 'They tend to blame me rather than themselves.' (Consultant obstetrician, site 1.2)

> 'Women … shouldn't put the blame on us when we try to tell them the other side of the story … like the *Informed Choice* leaflets … you tell them that it's all evidence-based and that it can give them ammunition to argue a case for themselves but a lot of them just don't want to know.' (Midwife, site 1.1)

This last quotation is somewhat ironic given the ambivalence displayed by the majority of midwives towards the (evidence-based) information contained in the *Informed Choice* leaflets and their own reluctance to use them as 'ammunition' in confronting medical staff about the absence of research evidence for many of the 'choices' offered to women. The quotations in this section also attest to the very real tensions many health professionals felt to exist between the concepts of evidence, informed choice and accountability.

The evidence informing women's decisions

Considerable numbers of women drew upon their embodied 'evidence' of previous childbearing experiences when they made decisions about their maternity care. This 'know how' often gave women with the necessary confidence to 'do it differently' in the current pregnancy. For many women, decisions were often contingent upon domestic arrangements and the potential impact on other family members. The following quotation illustrates this with respect to a woman expecting her third baby who has decided to take up the offer of antenatal screening, which she had declined in her two previous pregnancies:

> 'With each pregnancy it's a tougher decision because of the effect on the other kids. We both know from the work we do [in the field of disability] that having a first child with a major disability is one thing but I think the decision isn't so difficult with the first child as it is with the second and third. They're much tougher decisions because of the effect on the family as a whole. It's not a simple case of whether you think you, as an individual, have the capacity to handle it. What you can't predict is the effect on the family as a whole. But they never talk about that in the arguments they put for and against having screening tests.' (Service user, intervention site)

The preceding quotation highlights the hierarchy of the factors considered important in this woman's decision-making process. Interestingly, she does not mention her increasing age (37 years), which would almost certainly be ascribed considerable significance by midwives and obstetricians.

In the following quotation, a young woman cites the evidence of her mother's successful bottle-feeding and antipathy to breastfeeding, together with the economic advantage of not having to buy equipment, as motivating forces in her decision to bottle-feed her baby:

> 'No, I don't think I'll be breastfeeding, my mum's dead against it. I live at home so it would be difficult to go against her. She fed us all with the bottle, so I think that's what I'll do to. My sister has just finished using all the stuff [equipment for bottle-feeding] for her baby so I can have it all after it's born.' (Maternity service user, site 1.1)

Many women reported that the decisions that they made in pregnancy were simply 'repeats' of what had worked previously. In the following quotation a woman describes her surprise at the reactions she met following her previous vaginal breech birth. As this was perceived to be a normal labour, she states her intention to do the same again:

> 'Afterwards, everyone asked me why I'd had a normal labour with a breech baby but he [consultant obstetrician] told me it were normal. I didn't know it were any different. I just thought that's how babies were born. I'd do the same again.' (Service user, intervention site)

Female health professionals and their experiences of choice in the maternity services

Despite their expert knowledge and 'insider' status, when health professionals became pregnant they often experienced similar struggles in having their voices heard, and their views respected, as any other childbearing woman. In both of the following quotations, different midwives describe their difficulties in securing their preferred type of care:

> 'I have no risk factors. I've had two normal births so I thought I'd be an ideal candidate for the new midwife-led team they've just started up here. ... I wanted to be looked after by the team midwives of this unit, but I didn't want to have to book under a consultant. But basically here you can't do that. You cannot have midwifery-led care without actually booking under a consultant. And you have to be seen by that consultant regularly during your pregnancy. That's how they see midwifery-led care here and it's all the same if you're a midwife or whoever you are.'

> 'I couldn't have midwifery-led care unless I had a dating scan. I don't believe in dating scans. I know when I had my last period so I know when my baby is roughly due. I just wanted an anomaly scan but then I found I couldn't have that unless I'd had a dating scan. In the end I had both. I just didn't want the hassle.'

As these excerpts reveal, manipulating the maternity system to achieve the care which these midwives had identified as best suited to their individual needs was an arduous undertaking which required sophisticated, 'insider' knowledge. Even so, considerable compromise on their original choices was required.

The final quotation in this section is from a consultant obstetrician who reflects back on the birth of her first child five years earlier when she was a senior registrar. Her poignant account demonstrates the enduring, and corrosive, sense of regret when important decisions about maternity care are subsequently identified as erroneous. It is not known whether health professionals, with their 'expert' knowledge base, suffer post-decision regret more, or less, than any other childbearing woman.

> 'At the time I'd been very much the good little girl. I took the advice of the senior consultant and I've lived to regret it. I simply hadn't anticipated that the decision [to have an elective CS] would mean so much to me. I suffered with post-natal depression after the birth and eventually I went back to that consultant and told him that the decision had been wrong for me. The next baby I had with a midwife I knew and trusted. It has changed me. It really matters to me that women are helped to make decisions which are right for them, not for the medical profession. I get very angry when I hear women saying things like "Oh well, it doesn't matter, as long as the baby is all right." because I know from my own experience that it matters very much. Sometimes long after the birth it's still mattering.'

The value of health professionals' personal childbearing experiences was often a powerful stimulus in changing their professional behaviour. A number of these participants reported that 'feeling what it's like from the other side' increased their ability to empathise with their clients and improved their facilitation skills in providing choice.

The overall significance of the *Informed Choice* leaflets

At the time the fieldwork was undertaken, none of the units had instituted any on-going training in the use of the leaflets and neither had any unit implemented systems for evaluating their use. This is in marked contrast to what Jill Demilew has described in Chapter 8. This lack of vision may explain why participants in this research appeared largely unable to comment on the long-term strategies for leaflet use or to reflect on possible changes in outcome measures which might have been expected if the information contained within the leaflets was applied to clinical practice. This absence of vision; of forward thinking and long-term planning, did not appear to be particularly unusual in the maternity services. Rather, the introduction of the *Informed Choice* leaflets was simply another change which a compliant workforce absorbed. Such an attitude of resignation and acquiescence may be a contributing factor in the process whereby any innovation rapidly becomes 'routinised'. Hence, the leaflets were gradually assimilated into the existing model of care, rather than being seen as a vehicle to facilitate and promote choice for pregnant women. They certainly were not generally perceived as a vehicle for change.

It was perhaps understandable then, that the majority of the midwives who were observed dispensed the *Informed Choice* leaflets in the same manner as all other information was issued to pregnant women. The fact that midwives were not heard discussing the contents of the leaflets and were not themselves heard asking questions about the anticipated purpose, or function of the leaflets, suggests that the leaflets were not particularly valued. Observational work confirmed that the leaflets did not in any way challenge the power of the institution to direct the choices of service users, in part because midwives tended to maintain the status quo.

Conclusion

Regardless of whether participants in this study had access to the *Informed Choice* leaflets in the form of a 'free gift' during the RCT or as a 'planned purchase' provided by managers, the outcome was the same. The majority of health professionals observed did not use written information in such a way as to suggest that service users could do other than 'go with the flow' of local obstetric custom and practice. These findings support existing research suggesting that written materials alone do not appear to effect change in the behaviour of health professionals (Bekker *et al.*, 1999; Freemantle *et al.*, 1996). Service users also largely conformed to what was expected of them and remained passive recipients of maternity care rather than as 'partners or coproducers' (Tudor Hart, 1998) in that care.

This outcome was somewhat unexpected given that one of the primary motivations underpinning the production of the *Informed Choice* leaflets was that they would increase (evidence-based) knowledge and that this, in turn, would enable staff to facilitate informed choice with childbearing women. In other words, the leaflets would challenge, rather than reinforce, behavioural norms. The acquisition of knowledge, however, may have been privileged over other factors known to negatively affect informed choice, such as power imbalances, inadequate resources and the exclusion of key players in the planning and debates which precede the implementation of new technologies (Williams *et al.*, 2002). In this study, the clinical midwives who were responsible for dispensing the leaflets did not appear to have been involved in discussions or decisions at any stage of the *Informed Choice* initiative, either in advance of leaflet purchase in the ethnographic sites, or participation in the RCT. Decision-making was thus appropriated on behalf of midwives' and this paralled the way in which they made decisions on behalf of women in their care. Neither were significant attempts were made on any of the research sites to include doctors in the *Informed Choice* initiative. If the evidence base of leaflets had been applied to clinical practice, it would have revealed that many of the cherished beliefs held by obstetricians could not be substantiated. Sadly, however, staff, policies, and the maternity care system, remained largely unchanged.

Over the past decade, a number of factors have altered the status quo with respect to the relationship between midwives and their clients. University-based education has resulted in midwives entering the profession with a substantially different knowledge base and personal skills inventory; midwives are less accepting of their traditional (low) position in the institutional hierarchy; difficulties in recruiting and retaining midwives (Ball *et al.*, 2002) have been exacerbated by a 'declining altruism' (Jones, 2002) amongst health professionals in training; consumers have become powerful advocates in their own health care (Bastian, 1998) and are less reliant on health professionals for information; 'advances' in reproductive technologies and a growing awareness of ethical and legal issues require that consumers are well informed and actively involved in decision-making.

Health-related information is no longer the exclusive province of health professionals, and whilst pregnant women are unlikely to completely eschew pregnancy information from staff providing maternity care, they are likely to become far more critical. At the time this research was undertaken, the concepts of evidence-based information and informed choice did not appear to have entered the consumer discourse and thus the majority of service users were not well placed to challenge the information they received from health professionals, nor indeed the decisions they made on their behalf. It is anticipated that promoting consumers' demands for evidence-based medicine (Domenighetti *et al.*, 1998) will lead to a greater degree of 'healthy skepticism' (ibid.) with respect to orthodox medicine and will eventually result in a public who are better informed and who expect to share decision-making processes. But information is only one component in the decision-making process. In this study, lack of continuity, work pressures and social contexts served to distance health professionals from childbearing women and these factors impeded women's ability to make informed choices and to translate these into preferred actions or inactions. It is these aspects of the maternity service culture which we need to change.

Notes

1 The 'full set' of MIDIRS *Informed Choice* leaflets consisted of ten leaflets, on ten discrete topics of maternity care, arranged as pairs of leaflets. One leaflet was designed to be used by the pregnant woman and the other, fully referenced leaflet, for the health professional. In the event of women wanting more information it was intended that they be given the professional's version.

2 The Bounty pack comprised a pack of free samples and advertising materials routinely given to pregnant women at the booking visit.

References

Balint, M. (1957) *The Doctor, His Patient and the Illness*. London: Tavistock.

Ball, L., Curtis, P. and Kirkham, M. (2002) *Why do Midwives Leave?* London: Royal College of Midwives.

Bastian, H. (1998) Speaking up for ourselves: the evolution of consumer advocacy in health care. *International Journal of Technology Assessment in Health Care*, **14(1)**: 3–23.

Bekker, H., Thornton, J.G., Airey, C.M., Connelly, J.B., Hewison, J., Robinson, M.B. *et al.* (1999) Informed decision-making: an annotated bibliography and systematic review. *Health Technology Assessment*, **3(1)**.

Bristol Royal Infirmary Inquiry (2001) *Learning from Bristol: The Report of the Public Inquiry into Children's Heart Surgery at the Bristol Royal Infirmary 1984–1995*. London: Stationery Office. www.bristol-inquiry.org.uk

Clothier report following an investigation into the deaths and injuries caused by Beverley Allitt: http://www.iodclothier.co.uk

Coulter, A. (2002) After Bristol: putting patients at the center. *British Medical Journal*, **324**: 648–51.

Denzin, N.K. and Lincoln, Y.S. (1994) Introduction: Entering the Field of Qualitative Research. In N.K. Denzin, and Y.S. Lincoln (eds), *Handbook of Qualitative Research*. London: Sage.

Department of Health (1993) *Changing Childbirth: Report of the Expert Maternity Group*. London: HMSO.

Department of Health (1997) *The New NHS: Modern, Dependable*. London: HMSO.

Department of Health (1999) *Clinical Governance: Quality in the New NHS*. London: HMSO.

Department of Health (2001) *Government Statistical Service: NHS Maternity Statistics, England 1995–96 to 1997–98*. London: Department of Health.

Domenighetti, G., Grilli, R. and Liberati, A. (1998) Promoting consumers' demands for evidence-based medicine. *International Journal of Technology Assessment in Health Care*, **14(1)**: 97–105.

Dunn, N. (2002) Commentary: Patient centred care: timely, but is it practical? *British Medical Journal*, **324**: 651.

Elwyn, G., Edwards, A., Gwyn, R. and Grol, R. (1999) Towards a feasible model for shared decision-making: focus group study with general practice registrars. *British Medical Journal*, **319**: 753–6.

Farrell, C. and Gilbert, H. (1996) *Health Care Partnerships*. London: King's Fund.

Freeman, A.C. and Sweeney, K. (2001) Why general practitioners do not implement evidence: qualitative study. *British Medical Journal*, **323**: 1100–02

Freemantle, N., Harvey, E.L., Grinshaw, J.M. *et al.* (1996) The effectiveness of printed educational materials in changing the behaviour of healthcare professionals. In *The Cochrane Database of Systematic Reviews*, Issue 3 [updated 6 September 1996] Oxford: Update Software.

Geertz, C. (1973) *The Interpretation of Cultures: Selected Essays*. New York: Basic Books.

Glaser, B. and Strauss, A. (1967) *The Discovery of Grounded Theory*. New York: Aldine.

Hughes, D., Deery, R. and Lovatt, A. (2002) A critical ethnographic approach to facilitiating cultural shift in midwifery. *Midwifery*, **18**: 43–52.

Hunt, S. and Symonds, A. (1995) *The Social Meaning of Midwifery*. Basingstoke: Macmillan.

Jones, R. (2002) Declining altruism in medicine. *British Medical Journal*, **324**: 624–5

Kirkham, M.J. (1999) The culture of midwifery in the NHS in England. *Journal of Advanced Nursing*, **30(3)**: 732–9.

Kirkham, M.J. and Stapleton, H. (eds) (2001) *Informed Choice in Maternity Care: An*

Evaluation of Evidence-based Leaflets. University of York: NHS Centre for Reviews and Dissemination.

Kirkham, M.J., Stapleton, H., Thomas, G. and Curtis, P. (2002) Stereotyping as a professional defence mechanism. *British Journal of Midwifery.*

Laub, J.H. and Sampson, R.J. (1998) Integrating quantitative and qualitative data. In J.Z. Giele and G.H. Elder (eds), *Methods of Life Course Research: Qualitative and Quantitative Approaches.* Thousand Oaks, CA: Sage.

Levy, V. (1999) Protective steering: a grounded theory study of the processes involved when midwives facilitate informed choice in pregnancy. *Journal of Advance Nursing,* **29**(1): 104–12.

Marteau, T.M. (1989) Framing of information: its influence upon decisions of doctors and patients. *British Journal of Social Psychology,* **28**: 89–94

Murphy, E., Dingwall, R., Greatbatch, D., Parker, S. and Watson, P. (1998) Qualitative research methods in health technology assessment: a review of the literature. *Health Technology Assessment,* **2**(16).

O'Cathain, A. Can leaflets deliver informed choice? In: M. Kirkham (ed.) *Informed Choice in Maternity Care: An Evaluation of Evidence-based Leaflets.* York: NHS Centre for Reviews and Dissemination: University of York.

O'Cathain, A., Walters, S., Nicholl, J.P., Thomas, K.J. and Kirkham, M. (2002) Use of evidence-based leaflets to promote informed choice in maternity care: randomised controlled trial in everyday practice. *British Medical Journal,* **234**: 643–6.

Peacock, J.L. (1986) *The Anthropological Lens: Harsh Lights, Soft Focus.* Cambridge: Cambridge University Press.

Pope, C. (2002) Contingency in everyday surgical work. *Sociology of Health and Illness,* **24**(4): 369–84.

Press, N. and Browner, C. (1997) Why women say yes to prenatal diagnosis. *Social Science and Medicine,* **45**: 979–89.

Robins, J. (2002) Compliant behaviour in the antenatal setting. *British Medical Journal,* **324**: 7338, Letters, 19 March.

Ronka, A., Oravala, S. and Pulkkinen, L. (2002) 'I met this wife of mine and things got onto a better tack': Turning points in risk development. *Journal of Adolescence,* **25**(1): 47–63.

Royal Liverpool Children's Hospital at Alder Hey: http://www.rlcinquiry.org.uk

Secretary of State for Health (2002) *The NHS Plan.* London: Stationery Office.

Shildrick, M. (2002) *Embodying the Monster: Encounters with the Vulnerable Self.* London: Sage.

Shipman Inquiry (2002): www.shipman-inquiry.org.uk

Stapleton, H. (2000) The MIDIRS *Informed Choice* leaflets in clinical practice. *MIDIRS Midwifery Digest,* **10**(3): 388–92.

Stapleton, H., Kirkham, M. and Thomas, G. (2002) Qualitative study of evidence based leaflets in maternity care. *British Medical Journal,* **324**: 639–43.

Thomas, J. and Paranjothy, S. (2001) *The National Sentinel Caesarean Section Audit.* London: RCOG Press.

Tudor Hart, J. (1998) Expectations of health care: promoted, managed or shared? *Health Expectations,* **1**: 3–13.

Williams, C., Alderson, P. and Farsides, B. (2002) Too many choices? Hospital and community staff reflect on the future of prenatal screening. *Social Science and Medicine,* **55**: 743–53.

CHAPTER 6

The Culture of the Maternity Services in Wales and England as a Barrier to Informed Choice

MAVIS KIRKHAM AND HELEN STAPLETON

Chapter Contents

- Obstetric authority and its implications

- Fear and the technological imperative

- Midwives in the middle: balance and vulnerability

- Rhetoric and resistance

- Childbearing women's response to the maternity service

- Contrasts in scale and culture

- Conclusion

This chapter is drawn from the *Informed Choice in Maternity Care* study (Kirkham and Stapleton, 2001), as are Chapters 4 and 5. The aim here is to use the qualitative aspect of that study, together with the literature, to explore the culture of the NHS maternity services studied. The overall study was a randomised controlled trial of the MIDIRS *Informed Choice* leaflets (MIDIRS, 1996). The women's version of each leaflet carries the heading: *Informed Choice for Women. This leaflet is based on research to help you make your own choice.* This study therefore provides both an analysis of the culture of the maternity service and an opportunity to examine how that culture interacts with requirements for clients' informed choice in their care.

Obstetric authority and its implications

In the sites studied, which included the majority of the maternity units in Wales, doctors were held in high regard and their words carried authority. Clients and staff saw doctors as decision-makers.

> 'At the end of the day the patient looks up to the doctor as somebody who knows what they're doing ... who knows best ... who knows what's right for them. Doctors have the overview of the situation that the patient doesn't have.' (Registrar, intervention site)

Consultant obstetricians' words carried great, and ultimate, authority:

> '...it's a consultant-led service. You may disagree with what your consultant says but if you're working for that consultant that's what you've got to tell the patient. Whether you like it or not that's what you do, whether you totally disagree, you've got to do it.' (Registrar, intervention site)

Service users held doctors in high regard and expected them to make decisions:

> 'It was a case of the doctor telling me and he's got to be right ... He's obviously a doctor and he's qualified and done all his exams, and I just thought "OK then, whatever he's telling me must be right."' (Service user, intervention site)

Women sometimes indicated that they disagreed with doctors' views but the majority nonetheless withheld their criticism, maintained their silence and deferred to medical opinion:

> 'Even when you disagree with what they're saying, you tend not to say anything ... There's no point in arguing with them. Whatever you think, they'll do what they think is best.' (Service user, intervention site)

Authoritative knowledge was clearly vested with obstetricians. As Brigitte Jordan observed, 'The power of authoritative knowledge is not that it is correct but that it counts' (Jordan, 1997). The hierarchically organised maternity services studied fitted Rapp's description of authoritative knowledge as 'a way of organising power relations ... which makes them seem literally unthinkable in any other way' (Rapp, 1992).

These hierarchical structures were reinforced by economic imperatives and an NHS management culture of 'getting it right'. Staff justified their behaviour with reference to policies, procedures and guidelines, which tended to be treated as rules. Evidence-based practice was often equated with the clinical decisions with which senior obstetricians felt most comfortable.

In such a culture there was a locally defined 'right way' to behave in particular circumstances and a 'right choice' for each of the decision-making occasions addressed in the MIDIRS leaflets.

Manipulation,[1] blame and stereotyping

Accepting that doctors make the important decisions, some clients sought to achieve their aims in a manner widely documented for nurses and midwives (Stein, 1967; Stein, Watts and Howell, 1990; Kitzinger, Green and Coupland, 1990), by making the doctor think it was their idea. For a few women this extended to conveying a false clinical picture:

W, G5P4 and at term, is attending a routine antenatal appointment to see the consultant obstetrician. The researcher (R) engages in conversation:
W: *Had enough now...want to be induced. Don't want to be in over Easter (in 2 weeks' time).*
R: *So what do you hope to get out of today's appointment?*
W: *Talk the doctor round to inducing me. (Grins) Tell him it's not moving as much now.*

Since they accepted the obstetrician's authority, women sometimes blamed him in retrospect:

'I were bored and fed up so when the doctor offered me a date to come in I were really pleased … but I'd not do it again. I'd never go through that again. It were so intense … I regret it really. [If the doctor had not booked the induction] I'd still have been bored and fed up, but I'd have listened to him. You do, don't you, because they're the experts … you know … doctor knows best sort of thing. So if he'd said that I'd be better off waiting for it to come naturally, I'd have had to wait. I'd have had no choice would I?' (Service user, control site)

Such responses were common, especially from poor women who lacked control and choice in the rest of their lives. Nevertheless, this response created tensions for doctors, as is illustrated in the following quotation from a consultant obstetrician:

'One thing I have noticed is that I do get a bit angry when I've put a lot of time into explaining difficult and sensitive issues to women but when women don't understand or misinterpret what I've said, then they tend to blame me rather than themselves.'

Blame and manipulation by service users served to reinforce obstetricians' need for control of the service.

This climate of blame and obstetricians' need for control provided fertile ground for stereotyping of women who did not agree with the medically defined 'right' options. Many women also appeared to be stereotyped on the basis of circumstances (age, dwelling, parity, marital status or social class) over which they had little, or no, control.

'There's no amount of information that will enable them to see that they must [do what the obstetrician suggests]. Some of them lead problem lives but they're not the types to take the information in.' (Consultant obstetrician, control site)

'The most distressful thing is to have a client that you do your best to communicate information to and because of her own what I will call stubbornness, will like to take a risk, for example the grand multip I discussed with you earlier [who wanted a home birth] or a girl who is smoking heavily and has evidence of intrauterine growth retardation or a girl who has breech presentation who insists she must be delivered in her caravan. Such clients I think are really just being stubborn. They don't really want any information.' (Consultant obstetrician, intervention site)

Stereotyping always demonstrated the unreasonableness of women and their lack of attention to the reasoned, but often spuriously based, arguments of the health professional. Other factors influencing women's decision-making were not considered and certainly not allowed as evidence to support those decisions (see Chapter 5). On the rare occasions when obstetric authority failed to convince women, 'fear tactics' were used to inflate risk and thus dissuade women from making choices with which the health professional disapproved. One woman said of the obstetrician:

'He's a real Jekyll and Hyde that one. He was fine as long as he thought I was going to the hospital but as soon as I said I wanted to have the baby at home it was all about haemorrhage and the risks to the baby … if anything went wrong it would be my own fault. It would be on my head. It was horrible. I came home and cried.' (Service user, intervention site)

Thus, obstetricians' response to women who did not do as they wished was exactly the same as that of women when obstetricians' did not do as they wished: manipulation or blame. The power of obstetricians was greater but the parallel processes are clear in the actions of all involved. Sadly neither manipulation nor blame could improve the overall situation.

Fear and the technological imperative

Fear of litigation cast a dark shadow for health professionals working in the maternity services on all the study sites. Many volunteered that they worked 'with a lot of fear around' although very few were able to identify specific triggers for their fears, except for that of litigation. Some obstetricians were of the opinion that it was fear of litigation, rather than striving for standards of excellence, which was currently the primary motivation for change in the maternity services:

'I've been working since '91 and I can honestly say that the nature of people around is changing. There's now more and more stress on evidence-based medicine. You've got to be able to justify yourself. But it's not just because of the evidence-based medicine... You do things out of fear and litigation comes into it. So if you've done something you've got to be able to justify it. You can't just be strong-headed about it and say "that's what I always did and that's what I'll always do ...". I think that is hurting people more than the evidence-based.' (Senior registrar, control site)

Fear (of litigation), rather than security with evidence based information, was also reported to be a major factor influencing the way in which choices were presented to, or withheld from, service users:

'[I'm] saddened that obstetricians are forced to practise defensive obstetrics [because of] the fear of litigation. We let them [women] do what they want to do and then when things go wrong we get sued... We are now in a stage where are afraid to go against the women's wishes ... [But] you get very skilled at smelling a rat. We know now when trouble is approaching and that woman smells like trouble.' (Obstetrician, intervention site)

This particular obstetrician was observed striving to offer choice to service users, but nonetheless his words reflect an attitude of mistrust and fearfulness lest women he perceived as 'trouble' catch him unawares and unprotected. The qualitative research suggested that a number of health professionals maintained a similarly uneasy, if not adversarial, position with respect to women in their care and this made it difficult to foster alliances built on the principles of mutual respect and partnership. It has been suggested (De Ville, 1998) that the threat of malpractice has accelerated the trend towards a more conservative and defensive clinical practice not the least because health professionals tend to use technology as a 'prophylaxis' against being sued.

Decision-making around breech presentation illustrates this situation well.[2] There appeared to be very few obstetricians on any of the research sites who were sufficiently skilled in either external cephalic version (ECV), or in facilitating vaginal delivery, to offer women with a breech presentation any real choice in mode of delivery. Medical staff who did have such skills were most likely to have acquired them overseas and/or be too junior to cast much influence over senior (male) obstetricians. This was particularly the case if the junior doctor was female.

The following quotation is an extract from an interview with a registrar who had recently taken up post in one of the intervention units in which the policy for breech presentation was elective Caesarean section. During the interview the registrar disclosed that in her previous post the consultant obstetrician had 'allowed' her to make good use of her considerable expertise in ECV and vaginal breech delivery. She had assumed a similar approach would be condoned in her new job.

Researcher: 'Are you finding the same approach to the management of breech presentation here as you were used to in X [previous hospital]?'
Registrar: 'No. Here I've found you've got to work more as a team. Never mind what

your experience is, never mind the differences between yourselves as doctors, you don't air those in front of patients.'

Researcher: 'So you're not able to offer women the experience you have in ECV and vaginal breech birth?'

Registrar: 'No. The policy in this unit is Caesarean section for all breeches. ... At the end of the day the patient looks up to the doctor as somebody who knows what they're doing, who knows what's right and if you give the patient two different opinions, obviously the patient loses confidence in you.'

Very few women who were identified by the researchers' as having a breech presentation late in pregnancy indicated that they were aware of alternatives to routine elective Caesarean section or, indeed, that debates on this issue had been in progress for some time. They were not, therefore, well placed to challenge medical decision-making. The absence of a knowledgeable, and potentially critical, advocate in the consultation room was identified as a factor in the tendency for staff to conceal from women the real reasons for the some of the clinical decisions they made on their behalf but not always with their consent. The following extract, from the fieldnotes of one of the midwife researchers, illustrates this with regard to the obstetrician's 'failed' attempt at ECV and his decision to undertake an elective Caesarean section:

After the palpation W, G2P1 37/40, attempts to get up from the couch. The consultant obstetrician (O) stops her and begins a conversation. It appears, from what he says, that he has diagnosed the baby as being breech,

O: *I can offer you a choice of three things. I can try to turn it, you can try labour and see how you get on, or we could do a Caesarean section. Have you any preferences yourself?*

O does not wait for W to respond but returns his focus to her abdomen and begins to move his hands over her fundal area. I wonder idly what he is doing as I watch him bring, what I assume to be the baby's head, across to W's midline and then release it. He does this a couple of times before announcing: '*This baby is not for turning; some are and some aren't and this one isn't. It doesn't want to be turned so I think it's best we leave it alone.*' It is slowly dawning on me that I have just witnessed an attempt at an ECV.

O does not return to his earlier question about W's preferences but tells her to get dressed and wait outside whilst he organises her section. W duly leaves the room. O phones labour ward: 'Hello staff. We've got a lady coming in next Tuesday. I hope you can oblige us. It's a breech ...'

Of all the clinical scenarios in maternity care, antenatal screening and breech presentation appeared to generate attitudes of fear and blame in most obstetricians. Some reacted to these perceived threats by expressing a need to have the issue of accountability more clearly defined. Fear seriously impinged upon the development of trusting relationships and, as the following quotation reveals, when trust between women and their carers cannot be assumed, the language of risk and blame becomes foregrounded:

> 'I have a lot of experience with breeches … probably more than anyone in this unit so if it really matters to the woman then I will put myself on call for her. But then, I think well, why should I if she's going to turn round and sue me if something unpredictable happens … if it all goes wrong. I think if women want me to take these risks then they are going to have to accept the uncertainty involved. I'm very careful to assess the individual woman before I'll go on call. I want to know that they will really give it a go but that they'll also listen to me when I'm concerned. I don't want them to be telling me what to do when I'm seriously concerned about something. I don't panic easily but I do need to feel they can put their trust in me.' (Senior registrar, intervention site)

Little is known about the factors which assist or deter childbearing women from placing their trust in an obstetrician or a midwife and even less is known about the effect of trusting relationships on optimising clinical outcomes. This is especially the case where a degree of clinical risk has been identified.

The widespread belief that technological intervention would be viewed positively in the event of litigation, reinforced notions of 'right' and 'wrong' choices rather than 'informed' choices. Thus 'right' practice became that which was tried and tested and with which obstetricians felt skilled and secure. Informed choice was hence defined as making the locally defined 'right' choice.

Midwives in the middle: balance and vulnerability

Midwives' experiences held many parallels with that of obstetricians and childbearing women in their care. Like doctors and clients, midwives usually acted in conformity with local norms or took the options of manipulation or blame. The rigid observance of hierarchical norms hindered communication and midwives not infrequently found themselves 'caught in the crossfire' when they attempted to support women making decisions which went against unit policies and/or consultant preferences. One midwife described this position in the following way:

> 'You're a bit of a piggy in the middle … you're caught between trying to advocate for the women but you're also having to mediate for the consultant.'

Midwives appeared to expend considerable amounts of energy in trying to 'keep both sides happy' and many struggled to maintain an equilibrium (Levy,

1999), especially in situations where what women wanted was very different from what was considered appropriate, in terms of the local, medical agenda (see Chapter 3).

Going with the flow

The majority of midwives appeared to 'go with the flow' of obstetric opinion because 'it made life easier'. Adopting this stance could, however, have a divisive effect upon relationships between midwives:

> 'There is a lot of good will amongst the midwives here. Many of the midwives try and facilitate women and their choices but there are still a lot of midwives who are quite happy to follow obstetric procedure because in many ways it's easier for them ... because it doesn't make a fuss. So they tend to go with the flow. It's not so confrontational. So yes, they'll go along with what the obstetricians ask because it makes their life easier. You end up with an awful lot of aggression and back-biting between the midwives ... between the ones who go with the consultants and the ones who go with the women.' (Community midwife, intervention site)

Most midwives sought to avoid 'trouble' and therefore identified strongly with medical powerholders.

> 'You always come back to "this is what we normally do" and the women will just comply with it. If you look at Vitamin K, you've got to give the information and sometimes we slant it in a way that they would comply with us. We're very powerful and very able to do that. Not always, but when it suits us. When it doesn't, we manipulate the situation. We give them informed choice as long as they make the choice we want so we still hold the power. I think obstetricians have had a lot of power and I think midwives are taking on that power.' (Midwife, control site)

Midwives certainly ensured that the vast majority of women complied with medical authority in making what were seen locally as the 'right' choices. However, considerable numbers of midwives volunteered that it was only by resorting to tactics of 'doing good by stealth' (Stapleton *et al.*, 1998) that they were able to balance differing agendas and support women in making choices which they felt to be right for them. Many midwives complained that balancing conflicting loyalties, in addition to managing intense, and ever increasing, pressures upon their time made their working lives very stressful.

Going against the flow

Some excellent care was observed around the facilitation of informed choice but this was the work of individual midwives rather than the strategy in any particular unit. One characteristic of midwives who were prepared to challenge the medical hegemony was that, although they were often powerful agents for change within their local communities, they appeared to occupy a fragile position with respect to the institutional hierarchy, where they endeavoured to keep a low profile. A further distinguishing feature of these midwives was that they were very often union representatives or members of groups working to improve the maternity services. Thus their largely invisible, but highly political, work also benefited their midwifery colleagues as much as it did users of the maternity services.

The small number of midwives who did attempt to challenge the medical hegemony by openly confronting obstetric policies, sometimes confided during interviews that they lived in constant fear of reprisal, from both midwifery and obstetric colleagues. Their challenging actions were also potentially self-defeating because they risked effecting an increased scrutiny over the midwife's practice:

'I think you get looked at a lot more. I know that I've personally had things brought back to my attention a lot more than I've noticed with other midwives. Certain people see my name and will therefore look more closely at what's happened and what's been written and what's been done.' (Midwife, intervention site)

As is implied in the following quotation, making one's politics public, and working towards changing the local culture, was stressful and not without potential repercussions for the individual's personal health and well-being:

'You feel a bit out on a limb. It's very stressful ... but with any revolution, there are always the sacrificial lambs. That's how I see myself. But better me than the women ... I think midwives like me are a bit like those SAS hit-men. We should only be exposed on the front-line for short bursts and then we should be brought back to recuperate! You can't be on the front line all the time. But there isn't any choice. You have to keep going for the women.' (Community midwife, intervention site)

Midwifery managers varied in their ability and willingness to support midwives working 'on the front line'. Their allegiance to a woman-centred and/or a midwifery model of care could not necessarily be assumed:

'You do get support from some [midwifery managers] but you have to be careful. There is one in particular who will always go on the medical side. She'll always take the side of the medics over the midwives. So you just choose who you go to for support if you've got a woman who wants something they [consultants] disagree with.' (Midwife, intervention site)

Midwives who did prioritise women's expressed needs had a tendency to undervalue themselves and demean their own efforts. They frequently lacked support and were often kept at a distance by their peers who considered them to be 'a bit radical' or as 'offering women too much'. There was a strong sense of censorship in these comments, possibly because such modelling of practice threatened to expose and undermine the position of colleagues who preferred 'a quieter life'. But these were the midwives who were striving to facilitate informed choice for women in their care and, given the conservative nature of the maternity culture, this required that they constantly challenge the status quo. They did this at considerable personal cost.

> 'I'm shattered. I've been called out every night this week. Last night I was out all night for a home birth. I'm here doing the clinic today because there's no-one else to cover. I'm praying that one of my home birth women won't phone tonight … It's moments like this when I think my colleagues are right not to touch Dominos or home births because they do put a lot of extra stress on you. We get no support.' (Community midwife, intervention site)

In a recent paper (Davies, 2002) on organisational culture in the context of the NHS reforms, it was suggested that the continued emphasis on surface, or structural, change has been at the expense of the 'below surface', or more hidden, manifestations of culture which work against real change occurring. Our research concurs with the need to address these deeper levels, such as power imbalances, lack of resources and health professionals' perceived lack of support and fear of litigation, rather than continuing to update the rhetoric and jargon.

Hierarchical oppression and collusion

As mentioned earlier in this chapter, the hierarchical structure of the maternity service was evident and accepted at all levels. Many midwives (and some childbearing women) openly acknowledged their lowly status:

> 'You drop into the waiting-on mode before you've even realise you've done it. It's automatic to think they're [consultants] top and you're bottom.' (Midwife, intervention site)

> 'It's the pecking order thing, isn't it? You know who's boss as soon as you walk in there [consultation room].' (Service user, control unit)

The researchers observed midwives on all sites, especially in consultant antenatal clinics, undertaking 'waitressing' tasks on behalf of their medical colleagues. These included serving them refreshments, intercepting their (sometimes personal) phone calls and altering the seating in the consultation room to ensure their maximum comfort. Midwives were also observed undertaking many of the 'secretarial' aspects of the consultation such as placating women when consultants were late (or failed to arrive) for prearranged appointments, chasing laboratory results and (re)arranging appointments. On a number of sites midwives were also observed testing women's urine, recording their weights and measuring their blood pressures before ceremonially ushering them in to see the doctor, who was often at SHO grade.

Some midwives even used the term 'handmaiden', with varying degrees of irony or frustration, when describing their unequal relationship with medical colleagues:

> 'Everywhere there are medics and midwives working together there will always be the handmaidens. Some midwives just can't help falling into the role of being there for the doctors ... It's very hard to say no to doing something your colleague has always done for the doctor without making her feel like shit.'

A number of midwives divulged during interviews that they had been angered by a colleague who had conducted herself in an obsequious or demeaning manner with a medical colleague. Very few of these same midwives reported, however, that they had openly shared their feelings with the colleague concerned. A sense of professional loyalty, fear, and/or dislike of conflict were cited as the main reasons for midwives avoiding discussion of these issues. Midwives' reinforcement of one another's collusive patterns of behaviour thus maintained the status quo and they also contributed to their feelings of powerlessness and demoralisation.

Bullying

The bullying of midwives by those more powerful within the hierarchy was not uncommon, as described in an RCM report on industrial relations in Wales (Tinsley, 2000):

> Bullying and harassment of midwives is a serious concern within Wales. Despite a campaign in 1998, we return to this topic regularly in stewards' training. The incidence and severity of the bullying and the difference in treatment received by midwives compared to other members of staff have all been considered. Violence by obstetricians against midwives has occurred on more than one occasion, to the concern of both Trust management and the RCM. The Trusts agree that bullying cannot be tolerated, but difficulties have been experienced in applying the policies to all staff, irrespective of position.

Bullying by powerholders has been identified as a key issue with regard to decisions to leave nursing (Dobson, 2002) and midwifery (Ball, Curtis and Kirkham, 2002) and with regard to the lowered morale of many who remain in both those professions (Quine, 1999; Hadikin and O'Driscoll, 2000). This is a widespread problem which is certainly not confined to Wales. Bullying behaviour by powerholders often appeared to be accepted simply as a negative aspect of their role: as institutionalised oppression which, whilst constantly bemoaned in its individual manifestations, was rarely challenged in terms of its embodiment within NHS structures and cultures. Yet it works in opposition to the need to 'help NHS staff feel more valued', which is identified as key to achieving the 'good staff morale and motivation' – 'critical to achieving the government's ambitious plans for modernising the NHS' and which 'have positive impacts on patient care and outcomes' (Finlayson, 2002).

Horizontal violence

Some midwives described colleagues policing their practice to ensure conformity with local norms. This, together with much of the behaviour described above, fits the analysis of midwives as an oppressed group. 'Horizontal violence' is not just a description of inter-group conflict or various forms of 'bullying': it embodies an understanding of how oppressed groups direct their frustrations and dissatisfactions towards each other as a response to a system that has excluded them from power. In midwifery this manifests as:

> scapegoating, back-stabbing and negative criticism. The failure to respect privacy or keep confidences, non-verbal innuendo, undermining, lack of openness, unwillingness to help out, and lack of support have all been described as horizontal violence. (Leap, 1997, p. 689)

In the following quotation, a community midwife is reflecting on the inappropriate use of continuous electronic fetal heart monitoring in labour for low-risk women. She complains that introducing evidence-based practice, such as intermittent monitoring in labour for this group of women, is difficult to achieve because of the power and control exercised by midwifery colleagues holding permanent positions on central delivery suite:

> 'We don't trust each other enough. We're too quick to criticise instead of supporting each other a little bit more... Some of the G grades here are getting to be like the doctors: "Why haven't you done an ARM [artificial rupture of membranes]? Why isn't she monitored? Why haven't you done a VE [vaginal examination]?" [They're] often on your back.' (Community midwife, intervention site)

This respondent illustrates one of the many dilemmas midwives face in their attempts to foster trusting relationships when the imposed model of care was not one which all midwives held in equal regard, was rarely evidence-based, and, perhaps most importantly, was not woman-focused.

The caring, self-sacrificing culture of midwifery

As well as external pressures, it is important to consider the many pressures upon midwives from within their own culture. For a more detailed analysis of this culture see Stapleton *et al.*, 1998 and Kirkham, 1999. This is a female culture of caring expressed through service and sacrifice. This caring takes place within institutions with very different culturally coded values which depend upon, but do not acknowledge, the importance of such caring work

(Davies, 1995). Therefore, whilst midwives gave care, their role as professional carer discounted their need for personal and professional support. Yet NHS midwives' perceived lack of, and pressing need for, support has been acknowledged in several studies (e.g. Stapleton *et al.*, 1998; Kirkham and Stapleton, 2000), and this has also been identified as a key factor in midwives' decisions to leave midwifery (Ball, Curtis and Kirkham, 2002). This perceived lack of support is in stark contrast to the way in which changes in the maternity services have encouraged childbearing women to expect appropriate support as a right; it is somewhat ironic that the midwives caring for them did not perceive themselves as having parallel rights. As the following quotation illustrates, however, midwives tended to release their frustration in individual expressions of cynicism and despondency, rather than in collective, political activism or, indeed, in anger.

> 'The managers here aren't real midwives. They haven't practised in years. They don't give a fig about us shop floor midwives. All this place cares about is keeping the number of complaints down. We get feedback on how we're doing on that one every month [laughs]… What the women want is what the women get. That's the motto here. What the midwives want, well, who cares what the midwives want? That's not important is it?'
> (Midwife, control site)

In some cases, powerful role models of self-sacrifice reinforced the lack of support voiced by 'shop floor' midwives. Midwives often reported that they experienced a lack of mutual support as well as a lack of role models of support. Such a culture, with deeply internalised values of service and self-sacrifice, together with midwives' mutual pressures to conform, produced considerable guilt and blame. Self-blame was widespread and, whilst this may be a female characteristic in the wider culture surrounding midwifery, it had an undermining effect upon many midwives.

In such a context, looking after oneself was seen 'selfish'. This word, chosen by midwives seeking to address their own needs, was itself an indictment in the caring, self-sacrificing, client-centred culture. 'Selfish' resolutions were unlikely to be implemented because of the strong resistance within the prevailing culture. Lack of provision for their own needs and support enhanced the sense of midwives' vulnerability.

Pressures of time

Throughout this study staff spoke, often and at length, of the pressures on their time. A number of midwives in the first phase of the study reported that they had initially thought that the *Informed Choice* leaflets would save them time because the information they routinely conveyed verbally could now be dispensed as a written package. As the following quotation illustrates, however, the anticipated timesaving effect was rarely demonstrated in practice:

'When we first got the leaflets, I thought well, that's great. You just give them the leaflet on, say, screening which is so complicated to get across and you know then that they've got the information and it saves you a lot of time … Well that's what I thought, but it isn't like that, because you still have to explain what's written and with some of them [the *Informed Choice* leaflets] there's actually a lot more written than you'd normally tell them. So no, I don't think they have helped really.' (Community midwife, site 1.3)

Insufficient time in which to convey information to women about antenatal screening processes was reported as being problematic some years ago (Green, 1994). Since then, the amount and complexity of information on most pregnancy-related topics has greatly increased and there is now considerable pressure on health professionals to assist service users to participate more fully in decision-making and to offer (informed) choices in their care. There has been no concomitant increase, however, in the time available for antenatal consultations. Indeed, many areas of the UK, including some of the study sites, have adopted a reduced schedule of antenatal care (Sikorski *et al.*, 1996).

The pressures of time, and the imperative for women to be offered only local normative choices, were identified as key factors in midwives' overall failure to discuss the contents of the *Informed Choice* leaflets with their clients. Furthermore, during consultations midwives often (mis)took women's lack of questioning as evidence that they had no questions to ask, whilst women took the midwife's demeanour as evidence that they should not ask: a truly vicious circle which enabled the service to continue in circumstances which would otherwise have been intolerable.

Midwives and their clients were very aware of the pressures of time during antenatal consultations. This frequently produced a situation where women 'did not like to ask' questions; midwives responded by offering women limited and/or selective information. As illustrated by the following quotation, many midwives resorted to the security blanket of documenting their actions as protection against future chastisement:

'I only pass on the information that I have to now and I make dead sure it's all documented … To be honest, I only give them the stuff I'll get the rap for if I don't … I haven't the time for anything else.' (Midwife, site 1.2)

This behaviour also, however, led to inequality in the information midwives offered to women:

'Giving information to women takes so much more time. … I have to be selective with it … there isn't the time to do it well for all the women.' (Midwife, site 1.2)

Women with more formal education were more likely to ask more questions during consultations with health professionals who, in turn, felt obliged to answer. Hence, women who were already more knowledgeable were given more information. More knowledgeable women were also most likely to be given the *Informed Choice* leaflets. Time pressures on midwives thus served to favour their more articulate clients and to further disadvantage those who were less well educated and less articulate. The conduct of antenatal consultations, under the pressure of time, resulted in striking inequalities in care; the 'inverse care law' (Tudor Hart, 1971) was very evident (Kirkham *et al.*, 2002).

Recent work (Ball, Curtis and Kirkham, 2002) shows the shortage of midwives exacerbating the pressures upon the time of those who remain and thus decreasing further their job satisfaction. The shortage of midwives in the UK has worsened since this data was collected and hence the pressures on those remaining can only increase. However, recent events now stress the need for all health professionals to create working arrangements which permit 'the necessary time to communicate with patients' (Bristol Royal Infirmary Inquiry, 2001).

Rhetoric and resistance

The climate of fear and blame and the resulting emphasis on doing things 'right' led midwives and obstetricians to adopt the language of current Department of Health documents. 'Informed choice' and 'evidence-based practice' were, therefore, frequently mentioned by health professionals participating in this study. In clinical practice, however, this rhetoric tended to be interpreted very narrowly. Appropriate local practice was derived from the authoritative knowledge of the consultant. Sometimes, the climate of blame and fear led consultants to stick rigidly to their tried and tested experience rather than taking the risk of acquiring new skills or changing their practice in line with evidence. Thus 'right' practice became that which was tried and tested and with which obstetricians felt skilled and secure, such as with the previously mentioned tendency to perform an elective Caesarean section on any woman with a breech presentation. Informed choice meant making the locally defined 'right' choice.

Sometimes 'right' choices were described as being 'dictated by economics', such as when limited antenatal screening options were offered, or the provision of a home birth or Domino service was withdrawn or dramatically reduced.

The midwives observed were all fluent in the required rhetoric. Thus midwives of all grades equated the presence of the informed choice leaflets with the implementation of informed choice, though they did not discuss the leaflets with women nor differentiate them from leaflets, which were not evidence based, or which contained advertising. Midwives spoke of 'facilitating informed choice' whilst ensuring that women made the 'right' choices. Similarly midwives spoke of 'woman-centred care' whilst their clinical behaviour was routinised and rule governed.

Antenatal midwifery tasks have proliferated in recent years. Midwives speak the rhetoric of care whilst concentrating upon the routine tasks since the omission of these tasks would leave them culpable. In such circumstances midwives' best endeavours keep the conveyor belt of antenatal consultations operating and, for most women, individualised care does not appear as a real option.

Childbearing women's response to the maternity service

'You don't like to ask'

The vast majority of service users expected to conform with the care offered by doctors and midwives and were anxious to avoid 'troubling' or 'bothering' staff. Many saw the midwives caring for them as 'stressed out' or 'too frazzled' and this deterred them from accessing midwifery advice outside of their scheduled appointments. Even when they were extremely worried or upset about things, they rarely contacted a midwife because they 'didn't want to trouble her'.

Checking not listening

In the antenatal consultations observed, service users were largely silent. These 'silent' women voiced clear and perceptive views, however, when interviewed by the researchers. Their expectations of doctors and midwives were different. Most women expected doctors to undertake physical 'checks' in silence but the vast majority felt that discussion should be possible with midwives. Whilst many felt this was achieved, a number of women of all social classes spoke of midwives placing undue emphasis on tasks rather than the listening and facilitation required for support and informed choice.

> Researcher: 'You mentioned earlier that the midwives did a lot of "checking"…?'

> 'Yes that was it. Not how I was myself emotionally or any of my feelings I had from losing my second child. Again, that was very much always on my mind. But they never asked me about that. It was just have you remembered your urine sample, let's have a feel of the baby … things like that to do with my body, not about how I was feeling.' (Service user, intervention site)

> 'I don't think midwives know how to handle that [emotional] stuff. They can't handle when you get upset so you don't tend to show them. You tend to keep that for your friends and partner. The midwives are good for checking the baby and making sure all your tests get done.' (Service user, intervention site)

Thus the physical tasks of monitoring the pregnancy, as well as local imperatives on monitoring choices, acted as obstacles to establishing and meeting women's needs. Women were also aware that midwives were often very busy and pressed for time and this inhibited their ability to listen, to pick up cues and to give individualised information.

Sympathy in powerlessness

Many women praised their midwives and showed considerable insight into their situation.

> 'I was very impressed. I thought the midwives were excellent. I think they were incredibly hard-worked. Some people got annoyed that maybe they weren't getting their painkillers when they should have done – on the dot of when it was due. But I just thought they were so busy there. They never seemed to get off for a break and they often had to stay on because the next shift were short. They were really stressed out some of them. One of the junior ones sat on my bed and cried with me one day ... We cried together.' (Service user, intervention site)

> 'I think it's a shame that the midwives haven't got enough say and they're not listened to ... It is a shame that they're not listened to more.' (Service user, intervention unit)

Thus, whilst women sympathised with their midwives, they saw them as powerless, not as capable of changing the system within which they worked.

Contrasts in scale and culture

This final section introduces data from some of the smaller maternity units. The aim is to briefly describe some of the key factors which were identified as being pivotal in enabling these practitioners to 'do midwifery' differently. The observational work and interview data collected from these smaller units supports recent research (Churchill and Benbow, 2000) which suggests that there may other factors (besides size) within the local culture of these units which enhances women's sense of participation in the decision-making process. The remainder of this section describes a number of such factors which emerged from this data-set.

Background

The smaller midwifery units were mainly in rural locations and all had delivery rates of under 500 p.a. Staffing arrangements varied for both midwifery and medical staff. Some units were staffed by midwives on a 24-hour basis with 24-hour obstetric (GP) and/or anaesthetic cover on call a short distance away. Other units had neither in-house obstetric nor anaesthetic cover, and/or were situated some distance from a consultant unit and/or were staffed by midwives only when a woman was in labour. All the smaller units accepted women as postnatal transfers from the neighbouring consultant units. Many of the midwives working in the smaller units worked part-time. A substantial number worked in a dual-role capacity as midwife and/or district nurse and/or family planning nurse and/or school nurse and/or health visitor.

The participants working in these units usually described them as rural units, midwife-led units or as General Practitioner (GP) units; occasionally the establishment was described as a 'birth centre'. In order to maximise the anonymity for participants, these units will simply be referred to as 'small units'. For a more detailed description of terms, definitions and stories of small scale maternity units, see Kirkham (2003).

Unless otherwise indicated, all quotations are from participants working in the small maternity units. For reasons of confidentiality only generic terms such as midwife, service user, GP, etc. are used to indicate participants' professional role.

Differences in the research process

The majority of participants in these smaller units appeared to be less threatened by the researcher undertaking formal observation work or, indeed, in just 'hanging about' in the time-honoured way required of ethnography. Interviews with participants tended to be livelier, participants spoke with more spontaneity and for longer periods than elsewhere, and more humour was expressed. Childbearing women often spontaneously reflected on their previous experiences of the maternity service in consultant units, recalling busy, harassed staff and impersonal, fragmented care. These memories compared negatively with maternity care received in the context of a small unit. This is not to denigrate the efforts of midwives and other health professionals working in large, centralised maternity units who deliver care in traditional ways. Nor is it intended to romanticise the efforts of those providing maternity care in alternative settings. Neither is it implied that maternity care provided by staff working in the smaller units was always of a higher standard than that provided by their colleagues elsewhere. What became very apparent during the research process, however, was that the 'personalising' of relationships between women and their care providers seemed to reduce the need for fearful and defensive behaviours. The mutual sharing of trust and confidence generated a strong, and palpable, sense of positive belief in women's capacity to 'do' birth successfully; midwives seemed to enjoy, and value, being 'with' women!

Time

A small number of childbearing women, in all phases of this research, reported that their information and decision-making needs had been accommodated within their own time-frame, rather than having to fit in with that imposed by an individual health professional or organisation. Such women were more likely to be receiving care from midwives working in the smaller maternity units. Here, time pressures seemed to be less dominant in client–staff interactions and this may account for observed differences in emphasis on some aspects of the antenatal consultation. For example, at the booking visit midwives were less likely to give women 'the routine spiel' about food prohibitions in pregnancy but to take account of women's actual dietary intake. No midwife on any of the research sites, however, was observed to enquire about women's eating patterns in a systematic way.

Women attending the smaller maternity units seemed particularly appreciative of the greater degree of responsiveness and flexibility demonstrated by midwives:

> 'The midwives don't push you to make decisions. They let you change your mind and then change it back again. [laughs] … When the midwife came to my house to book me she asked me if I wanted to have the baby at home. I was shocked. I'd never thought about it before. I said no because I thought it was too dangerous. But I've thought about it a lot more … my partner is all for it. The midwives have given me a lot to read … Last week I saw the midwife [at 38 weeks gestation] and we talked about it again. I said I still didn't know what to do so she told me I could wait and see how I feel when I go into labour. I can make up my mind then to stay at home or go to the hospital.'

A number of women receiving care from midwives based in the small units commented on their 'all rounded' quality .The attitude these midwives adopted in their interactions with women seemed to convey to them a less harassed, more welcoming and accommodating, message:

> 'Y [rural unit] is a lovely situation because you've got half a dozen midwives who do everything. They're all real all-rounders so it doesn't matter who you see. The midwives at X [consultant unit] were far too busy. I hardly saw them apart from doing my basic blood pressure.'

The following quotation is somewhat unique, being a description of a midwife giving birth at home and being cared for by a colleague. The chameleon-like qualities of the attending midwife, who appears able to suspend time and to 'be' with the labouring woman rather than having to 'do' to her, are emphasised:

> 'She just blended into the atmosphere… She took her time… She just arrived without any of the hustle and bustle you come to just expect as part of the midwife package… I'd had a home birth before but this time there was none of that awful nattering of midwives in the corner and rustling paper and … There was none of that midwife looking at you and just praying there'll be a problem so she can whip you into hospital. I felt like she wasn't there a lot of the time and yet I felt like she was very there all the time… In the end I think the only equipment she used was a pair of gloves and the scissors to cut the cord.'

There may also be economic advantages to the maternity service if more midwives mimicked the minimalist approach described here with regards to the use of equipment.

Many of the midwives, including the participant 'speaking' in the following quotation, *'moonlighted'* at consultant maternity units. A number of them volunteered that such work afforded them an opportunity to reflect upon their own clinical practices and to compare them with what they observed in the consultant unit. The differences highlighted by the midwives indicated some important and distinguishing features of medicalised, and midwifery, models of care:

> 'We don't intervene unless there is a reason. I think our understanding of what an intervention is, though, is very different here. Taking the blood pressure [in labour] is an intervention we think carefully about. We don't do routine things. We don't do four hourly vaginal examinations. We don't have this idea that if they don't progress in a certain time then they get the drip up. We don't have a CTG machine in the unit so we can't do the 20-minute admission trace. We do everything on merit really, on how things are. We have a different idea of what's normal here. We don't have frightened doctors breathing down our necks and freaking us out so we don't go out there and freak the women out.'

An issue of concern, which emerged from this data set, was the reduction in the quality of midwifery care endured by women when they were required to transfer to consultant unit care. After a series of discussions with previous service users who had experienced this, the midwives in one unit instituted a new arrangement whereby they continued to provide the same pattern of antenatal consultation whilst also initiating regular phone contact with medical staff in the consultant unit. Maintaining this level of contact was, however, very time-consuming for the midwives concerned.

Working within a flattened hierarchy

Many of the participants who contributed their views to this data-set spoke about the importance, and relief, of working in an environment where 'there isn't that sense of hierarchy around '. Midwives who worked in units without on-site medical staff, and where local GPs no longer involved themselves in antenatal care, were the group who spoke most expressively about how this translated into practice. Improved communication, greater equality in status and a willingness to find mutually acceptable solutions rather than a need to 'have all the answers' were frequently mentioned aspects of working in a flattened hierarchy. The following quotations are illustrative:

> 'What I've noticed most is that we talk things through. We don't always agree, in fact we often don't agree [laughs] but we're not afraid to say we don't agree and go from there.

'… There isn't the same need to be the top dog any more … the one who's in the right. … You don't have to have all the answers … I don't feel so ashamed to say when I don't know here. I don't need to cover up as much.' (Midwife)

Better communication between professional groups, and with maternity-related agencies, was also mentioned by participants. Some described a more egalitarian process of decision-making whereby the more cautious members of staff were accommodated, rather than pressured:

'We do have regular meetings with the midwives and we do really discuss things. We also have regular meetings with our maternity liaison committee and they really give us a run for our money. [Laughs] … We tend to reach a consensus which is probably based on the more cautious end of the spectrum because we can't afford to take huge risks with anybody feeling that they're in a situation that's out of their depth. We do disagree about things but usually we agree to disagree and settle for a more cautious point of view. I don't think anybody wants to make any of the others feel uncomfortable with their skills. … We all know that there are differences of opinion within the group. We're quite open about the differences but over the years we've found a way of working with those differences rather than being confrontational and making people feel more guilty and inadequate.' (GP)

The previous quotation is notable for the absence of blame and stereotyping.

With the exception of this data-set, the authoritative voices of supervisors of midwives were noticeably absent from this study. Throughout the study, supervisors and the supervisory process were hardly mentioned as a potential framework for support. In the following quotation, a supervisor attributes the midwives' willingness to access supervision in one of the small units to the absence of a hierarchy within that unit:

'They're a little family of midwives there [in the rural unit] and they do support one another. They also have a positive view of supervision and use the supervision process to its full advantage and that doesn't happen everywhere. I think it's because there are no hierarchies, there's no specifically designated team leader. They all take the initiative. They all practice very differently as well – some are quite conservative and some are very radical so they certainly don't agree about everything all the time but what they do is to meet very regularly and thrash things out and then reach some sort of consensus of agreement.' (Supervisor of midwives)

It appeared that a flattening of the hierarchical structure was really only possible when midwives enjoyed a greater degree of autonomy and were not required to defer to medical staff. External features of this included midwives carrying their own caseloads, running their own clinics, and providing intrapartum care for their clients. In the following quotation, a midwife describes the 'difficult atmosphere' which pervades her small unit, where GP obstetricians exercised considerable power:

'It's very medically dominated here compared to Y [small unit described in the previous quotation] so there's a split in the camp here. There's those midwives who follow the medical model and there's the few in the minority who follow a more holistic model of care. It's a very difficult atmosphere.'

Relationships

Women booked at these smaller units appeared to enjoy close and supportive relationships with all of the midwives. Whilst each woman was usually assigned a 'named midwife' from whom she received the majority of her antenatal care, this arrangement was often nominal in that women were observed approaching the midwife on duty with a similar degree of confidence and familiarity to that which had been observed during one to one consultations. The fact that women who were observed and interviewed appeared to enjoy a similar quality of care from all the midwives in the unit echoes the findings of earlier researchers (Waldenstrom, 1998; Green *et al.*, 1998), who suggest that continuity of care was more important to women than continuity of carer.

Including male partners

Throughout the observation work, midwives often displayed patronising and/or dismissive attitudes towards male partners, regardless of whether the consultation took place in the woman's home or in the antenatal clinic. On occasions, the researchers observed midwives 'invisibilising' menfolk who were present during their consultations with childbearing women, by not asking them their names nor ascertaining their relationship status. This was not generally the case, however, in the small units, where midwives were often observed greeting male partners by name and actively including them in the consultation process. Women welcomed their inclusion and, as is implied in the following quotation, this may have increased men's degree of co-operation and level of contribution in the postnatal period:

'I think they're all lovely. These ones here [at small unit] are just lovely. They have been really, really helpful. My boyfriend thought so as well. They were lovely with him too. They included him in everything. He was very quiet at first but then he opened up to them after a while. He's been great with the baby too. He's changing him 'n all. I didn't think he'd do that.' [Laughs]

Standing up to doctors

Women expressed their gratitude when midwives interceded on their behalf with medical staff. This often required that the midwife accompany the woman to the consultant unit and speak on her behalf to the obstetrician. These occasions frequently called for the midwife to construct a case for the woman concerned to continue her pregnancy without recourse to intervention or, as illustrated by the second quotation, without being labelled 'high risk' simply on the basis of physical characteristics.

> 'I think you get really spoiled at here [at small unit]. You don't realise how much the midwives do behind the scene for you. You don't realise how strong those midwives are. They have to be I suppose to stand up to the doctors. One of them came over with me when I had to see the consultant. She stood up to the consultant too. He was one of those "doctor knows best types" so if I hadn't had the midwife with me, he'd have signed me up for an induction there and then.' (Service user (term+7days))

> 'You feel the midwives here would always stick up for you. One of them argued with the doctor for me. He said I shouldn't be having my baby here [in the rural unit] because I'm high risk ... I'm too short (4′9″) and I'm too young (aged 15) and it's my first one. The midwife came with me [to see the consultant]. She argued for me to come here. I had my baby here and everything was fine.'

A number of midwives spoke about the dilemmas of their advocacy work on behalf of women, especially when this involved confronting medical colleagues with whom they worked on a day-to-day basis. Not all midwives were able, or willing, to do this work and this sometimes created tensions and rivalries.

Taking worry home

Some health professionals described themselves as having a 'more intimate' relationships with childbearing women and, whilst most regarded this as a positive feature, a small number volunteered that having a greater degree of 'closeness' also had its less attractive aspects insofar as clinical autonomy was concerned. This was most evident when women exhibited signs and symptoms which the professional interpreted as indicative of the pregnancy becoming 'higher risk'. It was at this point that staff appeared to feel their professional isolation most keenly and, as the following quotation illustrates, worry was a common manifestation of their concern:

> 'You can't help worrying if they start showing signs that they're becoming higher risk. It's difficult not to [worry] because you don't have access to facilities if they suddenly do take a dive ... But you don't want to be worrying them with your worry either ... I do tend to take the worry home with me in those cases ... It's a different sort of relationship when you're a GP in a rural community and I think you worry about your patients more because you know them so much better.' (GP)

In the following extract from a recent paper on this subject, the author conflates the two issues so that 'care' and 'worry' become inextricably fused; an inevitable consequence perhaps of relationships in which continuity and 'knowing' are valued components.

'Caring responsibility increases in proportion to the measure that it is assumed. The more I care for this person, the more I worry, and the more I worry, the stronger my desire to care. Why? Because care *is* worry.' (Van Manen, 2002, p. 270)

Relationships between staff and women in the smaller units seemed to be more relaxed and informal and their interactions with one another were generally observed to be relaxed and spontaneous; touch and laughter were prominent features. Respect for 'boundaries' was, however, commented upon by both parties. As has been reported elsewhere (Reed, 2002), relationships which are based on 'knowing the women well' seem to simultaneously protect midwives against women (inadvertently) transgressing private/professional limits.

Trust

Women and staff used variations on the word 'trust' when referring to their relationships with one another. Sometimes women reflected on their previous experiences of maternity care when, in retrospect, they realised they had not trusted their care-provider:

'I was living in another part of the country when I had my first baby… It was a big hospital … I didn't realise it was so bad until now when I've had the chance to look back on it. Something to compare it with. I didn't feel the need this time to be so well informed. I think because of the support I've had from the midwives. I trust them. Looking back on it, I didn't trust them last time. I felt this time we were all coming from the same place so I didn't have to make any decisions as such because what I wanted to do was how they did it anyway. I felt they would tell me about anything I needed to know and protect me from the things I didn't need to know.'

Trust enabled women to ask questions, to become more actively involved in decision-making and to feel protected against unnecessary intrusions, including being given irrelevant information and being asked to make inappropriate decisons. Trust also enabled women to believe that they did indeed have the capacity to carry, birth, and mother their babies. Such affirming feedback was especially appreciated by women pregnant for the first time:

'That's why I think the midwives here are so good … They keep telling you to listen to your body before you listen to what anyone else says. It's good. It's helps you to not believe all the horror stories. I think it helps you to believe you really can do it.'

Midwives who believed in women's 'ability to be her own and her baby's expert' (Leap, 2000, p. 6), and who were able to reflect that trust back to individual women in their care, seemed more confident in their professional roles and less likely to defer unnecessarily to medical authority. Trust, faith and belief in the midwife's own 'self' were also seen as essential to personal autonomy and integrity:

Researcher: 'This idea of the woman having faith in her decisions. Is having faith of any importance for the midwife?'
'Yes I think it does really. I don't mean faith as in a religious meaning. I mean in a sense of you believing in yourself. Of trusting yourself… If you have a belief in yourself then you'll have faith in knowing and doing what's right by someone else. You'll trust their decisions and you'll trust your own decisions. … Knowing what to do for the women. Trusting them … Sometimes I think we have lost that faith in ourselves as midwives and that's why we let doctors tell us what to do and then we tell the women what to do.'

Listening to women's feedback was considered by some of the midwives working in the small units to be an essential link in the 'trust' cycle. The voices of the women, when midwives' were able to hear them, appeared to be something of a counterbalance to their own critical, and sometimes incorrect, versions of clinical events:

'I think sometimes we are overly critical of ourselves. I think self-criticism, being critical of your own self all the time, can have adverse effects on you. You start to lose your trust in yourself … I think midwives are very bad at that. We're always blaming ourselves and criticising the way we've done things. We're always questioning ourselves. If you think what you've done is a pig's ear but the woman doesn't think that then maybe you should listen to the woman's voice instead of your own voice.'

Some women related trust to 'knowing' their midwives and valuing their expert knowledge:

Researcher: 'So the "just in case something goes wrong" argument that the consultant used when you saw him didn't persuade you?' [to book at the consultant unit]
Service user: 'No, because I know all the midwives here. I trust them to know that if there was really anything wrong, they'd send you there [to the consultant unit] straight away. They wouldn't keep me here if they were really worried. But they don't make up things either. I know they'll not send me there just to get me out of their hair!' [Laughs]

Trust enabled women to respect their midwife's clinical judgment, although, as is implied in the previous quotation, this was conditional to the midwife remaining honest and open in her interactions with the women in her care.

Valuing the 'troublemakers'

The smaller units appeared to be much more tolerant of difference and diversity within the workforce than the larger centralised units where there was more pressure on staff to comply with the 'corporate image' projected by their employing organisation. Difference of opinion, whilst not always easy to integrate, nor necessarily welcomed at the time, was nonetheless seen as integral to the continued development of the smaller units:

'Thankfully I have a few troublemakers in my patch and thank goodness for them or we'd have lost some of those [small] units years ago. The problem is there aren't enough midwives overall who are prepared to stick their necks out so that the few who do are branded as troublemakers and have a hard time of it. Whereas if we were all prepared to do that, if we were all prepared to be branded as troublemakers, we could be a force to be reckoned with.' (Supervisor of midwives)

Staff working in the smaller units appeared to be more flexible in their attitudes and there appeared to be less resistance to change, perhaps because so many had endured substantial change over the years simply to avoid closure.

Conclusion

Informed choice must start with listening to women if midwives are to learn about women's knowledge, values and preferences. This was much more likely in the small, isolated units. In consultant units those few midwives who really listened to women found this put them in very vulnerable positions since listening to individuals made it very difficult to 'go with the flow' of local obstetric opinion. The majority of the midwives studied spoke of 'informed choice' yet their practice was centred upon 'checking'. There was relatively little attention paid to the views and needs of individual women in the consultations observed and routinised care was accepted as normal by all concerned. This was logical within the culture of the maternity services in which they worked. If, however, we seek to be 'with women', we cannot uncritically accept authoritative knowledge, for when women are listened to they voice many ways of seeing maternity care and many definitions of safety (Edwards, 2002).

Midwives, in the privacy of the research interview, were eloquent in their description of the culture within which they worked. Most described a professional setting within which their voices were muted or silenced. Experience of a culture of powerlessness left midwives ill equipped to empower their clients, as they lacked the confidence or sense of their own power that is needed before power can be shared.

There was little evidence that participants in this study had engaged with the wider philosophical dimensions underpinning the provision of informed choice at the clinical coalface. This was particularly so where decision-making was pressured by emotionality and perceptions of risk. Only a tiny minority of staff were heard questioning whether it was possible, or indeed appropriate, to engage in non-directive counselling with women (Williams *et al.*, 2002), the demarcations between choice and coercion (Michie *et al.*, 1997) and the social and psychological structures governing 'how we think, what we value and what we see as legitimate' (Davies, 2001).

It is widely accepted that being 'with woman' largely defines the role, and purpose, of the midwife. What the midwifery profession has yet to acknowledge, let alone resolve, are the conflicts midwives must resolve if they are to be 'with women' in providing them with evidence-based information where it is in conflict with obstetric policies. Clarke (1995) adds a further dimension to this conundrum in describing the additional, but opposing, demands on midwives to fulfil the requirements of their professional organisation. In declaring that 'Information is an evident political good. It has the power to help consumers protect their interests...[it] is contentious', Williamson (1992, p. 80) makes a case for midwives taking a political stance. Political activism is not, however, commonly associated with the midwifery profession and may be counter-productive because of the risk of professional alienation and social exclusion. The examples of horizontal violence described in this chapter illustrate the cultural reality of resistance to change in the maternity services. Describing, and accounting for, 'discrepant views' (Kleinman *et al.*, 1978) of health and illness, traditionally the preserve of anthropology, may thus be a useful prelude to implementing and managing change within the clinical environment.

With the exception of the small rural units, the culture observed in this study was not one of being 'with women' nor of informed choice. Most of the midwives observed nurtured the maternity service and their employing organisation. They acted as the shock absorbers which took the stress within that service and made its routinised system able to continue.

Notes

1 The word manipulation is used here with reluctance because of its negative connotations. We have been unable to find another word which primarily means 'to handle with some skill, to control or influence cleverly or skilfully' but will extend to 'to falsify for one's own advantage' (Collins Dictionary, 1987). The word 'engineer' does not seem to work grammatically and words with military origins such as strategy or manoeuvre imply a power which the women do not have. We are very aware that such actions were seen by the women as the only way to achieve their aims and wish to avoid the value judgement which is linguistically in-built.
2 The breech multi-centre trial (Hannah *et al.*, 2000) was in progress at the time of our research although the results were published after the intervention period. Obstetricians and midwives on the research sites, some of whom were enrolled in this trial, did not cite it as a possible influence on their clinical decisions and no woman with a breech presentation was observed being given information about the trial. On intervention sites, despite the fact that staff had access to an evidence-based information tool on this topic (the *Informed Choice* leaflet number 9), there did not appear to be any significant change in clinical practice nor in the information given to women.

References

Ball, L., Curtis, P. and Kirkham, M. (2002) *Why Do Midwives Leave?* London: Royal College of Midwives.
Bristol Royal Infirmary Inquiry (2001) *Learning from Bristol: The Report of the Public Inquiry into Children's Heart Surgery at the Bristol Royal Infirmary 1984–1995.* London: Stationery Office. www.bristol-inquiry.org.uk

Churchill, H. and Benbow, A. (2000) Informed choice in maternity services. *British Journal of Midwifery*, **8(1)**: 41–7.

Clarke, R.A. (1995) Midwives, their employers and the UKCC: an eternally unethical triangle. *Nursing Ethics*, **2(3)**: 247–53.

Davies, C. (1995) *Gender and the Professional Predicament in Nursing*. Buckingham: Open University Press.

Davies, H.T.O. (2002) Understanding organizational culture in reforming the National Health Service. *Journal of the Royal Society of Medicine*, **95**: 140–2.

De Ville, K. (1998) Medical malpractice in twentieth century United States; the interaction of technology, law and culture. *International Journal of Technology Assessment in Health Care*, **14(2)**:197–211.

Dobson, R. (2002) Doctor's bad behaviour makes nurses quit. *British Medical Journal*, **324**:1477.

Edwards, N. (2002) *Women's Experiences of Planning Home Births in Scotland: The Birth of Autonomy*. Unpublished PhD, University of Sheffield.

Finlayson, B. (2002) *Counting the Smiles: Morale and Motivation in the NHS*. London: Kings Fund.

Green, J. (1994) Serum screening for Down's syndrome: experiences of obstetricians in England and Wales. *British Medical Journal*, **309**: 769–72.

Green, J.M., Curtis, P., Price, H. and Renfrew, M. (1998) *Continuing to Care: The Organisation of Midwifery Services in the UK: A Structured Review of the Evidence*. Hale, Cheshire: Books for Midwives Press.

Hadikin, R. and O'Driscoll, M. (2000) *The Bullying Culture*. Books for Midwives, Oxford: Butterworth-Heinemann.

Hannah, M.E., Hannah, W.J., Hewson, S.A., Hodnett, E.D., Saigal, S. and Willan, A.R. (2000) Planned Caesarian section versus planned vaginal birth for breech presentation at term: a randomised controlled trial. *Lancet*, **356**:1375–83.

Hart, T.L. (1971) The inverse care law. *Lancet*, **1**: 405–12.

Jordan, B. (1997) Authoritative knowledge and its construction. In R. Davis-Floyd and C. Sargent. *Childbirth and Authoritative Knowledge: Cross-Cultural Perspectives*, pp. 55–79. Berkeley: University of California Press.

Kirkham, M. (1999) The culture of midwifery in the NHS in England. *Journal of Advanced Nursing*, **30(3)**, 732–9.

Kirkham, M. (ed.) (2003) *Birth Centres: A Social Model for Maternity Care*. Oxford: Butterworth-Heinemann.

Kirkham, M. and Stapleton, H. (2000) Midwives' support needs as childbirth changes. *Journal of Advanced Nursing*, **32(2)**, 465–72.

Kirkham, M. and Stapleton, H. (eds) (2001) *Informed Choice in Maternity Care: An Evaluation of Evidence-based Leaflets*. NHS Centre for Reviews and Dissemination, University of York.

Kirkham, M., Stapleton, H., Curtis, P. and Thomas, G. (2002) The inverse care law in antenatal midwifery care. *British Journal of Midwifery*, **10(8)**: 509–13.

Kitzinger, J., Green, J. and Coupland, V. (1990) Labour relations: midwives and doctors on the labour ward. In J. Garcia, R. Kilpatrick and M. Richards (eds), *The Politics of Maternity Care*. Oxford: Clarendon Press.

Kleinman, A., Eisenberg, L. and Good, B. (1978) Culture, illness and care: clinical lessons from anthropologic and cross-cultural research. *Annals of Internal Medicine*, **88**: 247–59.

Leap, N. (1997) Making sense of 'horizontal violence' in midwifery. *British Journal of Midwifery*, **5**:11.

Leap, N. (2000) The less we do, the more we give. In M. Kirkham (ed.) *The Midwife–Mother Relationship*. London: Macmillan Press.

Levy, V. (1999) Protective steering: a grounded theory study of the processes involved when midwives facilitate informed choice in pregnancy. *Journal of Advanced Nursing*, **29(1)**: 104–12.

Michie, S., Bron, F., Bobrow, M. and Marteau, T. (1997) Non-directiveness in genetic counselling: an empirical study. *American Journal of Human Genetics*, **60**: 40–7.

MIDIRS (1996) *Informed Choice leaflets*. MIDIRS and The NHS Centre for Reviews and Dissemination.

Quine, L. (1999) Workplace bullying in an NHS community trust: staff questionnaire survey. *British Medical Journal*, **318**: 228–32.

Rapp, R. (1992) *Commentary on 'Birth in Twelve Culture: Papers in Honour of Brigitte Jordan'*: a symposium at the annual meeting of the American Anthropological Association, San Francisco.

Reed, B. (2002) The Albany midwifery practice. *MIDIRS Midwifery Digest*, **12(2)**: 261–4.

Sikorski, J., Wilson, J., Clement, S., Das, S. and Smeeton, N. (1996) A randomised controlled trial comparing two schedules of antenatal care visits: the antenatal care project. *British Medical Journal*, **312**: 546–53.

Stapleton, H., Duerden, J. and Kirkham, M. (1998) *Evaluation of the Impact of the Supervision of Midwives on Professional Practice and the Quality of Midwifery Care*. London: English National Board for Nursing and Midwifery.

Stein, L. (1967) The doctor–nurse game. *Archives of General Psychiatry*, **16**: 698–703.

Stein, L., Watts, D. and Howell, T. (1990) The doctor–nurse game revisited. *New England Journal of Medicine*, **332(8)**: 546–9.

Tinsley, L. (2000) Industrial relations in Wales. *RCM Midwives Journal*, **3(1)**: 8.

Tudor Hart, J. (1971) The inverse care law. *Lancet*, **1**: 405–12.

Van Manen, M. (2002) Care-as-Worry, or 'Don't Worry, Be Happy', *Qualitative Health Research*, **12(2)**: 262–78.

Waldenstrom, U. (1998) Continuity of carer and satisfaction. *Midwifery*, **14**: 207–13.

Williams, C., Alderson, A. and Farsides, B. (2002) Is non-directiveness possible within the context of antenatal screening and testing? *Social Science and Medicine*, **54**: 339–47.

Williamson, C. (1992) *Whose Standards? Consumer and Professional Standards in Health Care*. Buckingham: Open University Press.

CHAPTER 7

Information Used by Pregnant Women, and their Understanding and Use of Evidence-based *Informed Choice* Leaflets

MEG WIGGINS AND MARY NEWBURN

Chapter Contents

- Study participants and methods

- Approaches to obtaining information

- Approaches to obtaining information: typology

- Women's understanding and attitudes towards evidence-based information

- Planned use of the *Informed Choice* leaflets

- Discussion

- Conclusion

The maternity services are different from many other healthcare services in that they provide care for women during a physiological process which for most is normal and without complication (Department of Health, 1993). In addition, pregnancy and the birth of a baby mark a life transition of major social and emotional significance for the mother, father and the child. Despite the normality of the process and the social significance of the transition to motherhood, the 1992 report of the UK's Health Select Committee concluded that maternity care had become highly medicalised and that women tended to see a succession of care providers in unfamiliar places, leaving them feeling powerless and undervalued (House of Commons Health Select Committee, 1992). The Government's Expert Maternity Group responded by saying that the first principle of the maternity services should be that 'the woman must be the focus of maternity care. She should be able to feel in control of what is happening to her and able to make decisions about her care (Department of Health, 1993). This vision, which has become known as 'woman-centred care', continues to be supported by Government a decade later (Department of Health, 2003). If women are to be fully involved in decisions about their care then they need to have a sense that alternative courses of action can be taken, that these are equally accessible, and to have reliable information about the advantages and disadvantages of alternatives so that they can make informed choices.

While the notion of informed choice has enjoyed the support of all political parties, as well as the whole spectrum of health professionals and user groups, when examined critically it is apparent that providing for informed choice in practice is a considerable challenge. By the mid-1990s there was increasing discussion about how adequately maternity services were providing reliable, evidence-based information. Studies since the 1970s had shown that women wanted 'more information' about maternity care (Fleissig, 1993; Cartwright, 1979; Jacoby, 1988; Green et al., 1988) but there still appeared to be barriers in the way: poor communication, conflicting advice, a scarcity of written information and inadequate time for discussion (Gready et al., 1995). Although evidence-based information leaflets had been published by MIDIRS and the NHS Centre for Reviews and Dissemination using systematic reviews of clinical research findings, drawing on the work of the UK Cochrane Collaboration, the leaflets were not widely available. The leaflets had to be bought by health authorities, maternity units or GP practices, and few prioritised expenditure in this way. There were also many gaps in the available information, because of a lack of evidence or because no leaflet had been produced. At that time, for instance, while information was available on place of birth, support in labour, and the evidence for keeping upright and mobile, there were no widely available booklets or leaflets on the combination of factors that would increase a woman's chances of having a straightforward vaginal birth (Newburn, 2002; Rosser, 2002). Furthermore, there was a lack of consensus about the conclusions that could be drawn about outcomes associated with different forms of treatment from the available studies and meta-analyses (Oliver et al., 1996). Similarly, there were some who doubted the appropriateness of providing this type and degree of information to pregnant women, for fear that it might cause anxiety or create unrealisable expectations (Oliver et al., 1996; Levy, 1999a). Tellingly, there was evidence in some areas of the country that only just over half of the women felt that they had been 'fully involved' in decision-making about their antenatal and intra-partum care (Gready et al., 1995).

In this chapter, we will be discussing a qualitative study that was designed to explore some of these apparent barriers, concentrating on women's approach to obtaining information during pregnancy and their expectations of maternity care. We will focus particularly on women's understanding of evidence-based information on three aspects of care and behaviour during labour, and the use they were able to make of the information while having their baby. The study posed the question: To what extent can access to evidence-based information enable women to negotiate care which is both clinically effective and responsive to their needs, care which is genuinely women-centred?

Study participants and methods

The study was based on a longitudinal series of three focused discussions with eleven groups of women. Two of the discussions were held during pregnancy (at 5–6 months and then at 7–8 months) and one held approximately eight weeks after the participants had given birth. A key purpose of the first discussion was to explore women's approaches to obtaining information during pregnancy. At the end of the focus group each woman was given three of the evidence-based *Informed Choice* (MIDIRS, 1996) leaflets to take away with her. The three leaflets were: *Positions in labour and delivery; Support in labour;* and *Listening to your baby's heartbeat during labour.* At the second discussion we explored the women's understanding of research and the degree of importance that they placed on having evidence-based information. There was discussion about whether the women had attempted, or intended, to use the information in the leaflets in discussions with health professionals or in planning for the birth. The purpose of the third discussion included finding out to what extent the leaflets, and other information, had influenced decision-making during labour.

Following ethics committee approval, women were recruited from two maternity units in Essex and two in London. Letters were sent to 511 pregnant women due to give birth in July or August 1996, inviting them to participate in three group discussions about information in pregnancy. No incentives were offered for participation, but travel costs and childcare expenses were reimbursed. Seventy-three women replied (14 per cent) and 54 women participated.

Two of the eleven groups were for 'Asian' women and nine were comprised of white British women. Thirty group discussions were carried out, plus 27 individual interviews when a woman's participation in a stage of the group discussions was not possible. An interview schedule was developed for each of the three stages, and was used both in the group and individual interviews.

At the end of the first discussion the women were asked to fill in a demographic questionnaire (see Table 7.1). The discussions were taped and transcribed, and then theme analysis was carried out across the groups. The participants were not told until the end of the third session that the National Childbirth Trust was involved in the research, to ensure that this did not bias responses.

Table 7.1 Sample of 54* women who attended focus group discussions

Parity		Age	
No children (currently pregnant)	48%	15–19 years	2%
1 child	35%	20–24 years	9%
2 children	15%	25–29 years	43%
4 or more children	2%	30–34 years	32%
		35 years or older	15%

Highest level of educational qualifications obtained		Ethnicity	
No formal qualifications	6%	White British	80%
GCSE or O Level	36%	Indian	9%
A level	31%	Pakistani	6%
Degree level	27%	White Irish	4%
		White – other	2%

Housing tenure		Employment	
Own home/mortgage	75%	Full-time employment	51%
Rent – private	11%	Part-time employment	24%
Rent – housing association	8%	No employment	26%
Rent – local authority	4%		
Other	2%		

Living arrangements		Is English your first language?	
With partner (and children)	93%	Yes	87%
Live with parents	4%	No	13%
Live with other people	7%		

Note:
*Includes three women who dropped out of the study after the first discussion.

The results of the study will be discussed in three sections: women's approaches to obtaining information; their understanding of and attitudes towards evidence-based information; and their use of the *Informed Choice* leaflets.

Approaches to obtaining information

Previous research has found evidence of a high demand for information during pregnancy and around birth. One of the interesting questions that is frequently taken as a given is 'what counts as information?' We found that many of the things women want to know about when they are pregnant do not coincide neatly with the questions clinical researchers ask and investigate. They have practical concerns about what equipment to buy, feeding their baby when away from home or when they go back to work, and how their partner feels about choices they might want to make. Much of the information that women value and feel they can rely upon is the embodied knowledge they have from personal experience or see family and friends acting on and reproducing around them daily (Hoddinott, 1999). Indeed, one woman commented that she had gained confidence from her mother's and mother-in-law's birth stories but had also seen a lot of animals give birth. She said, 'I think animals were as much help as the grandmothers!'

Formal information or theoretical knowledge (Hoddinott, 1999), from written sources and verbally from health professionals, represent just two among many sources of knowledge and beliefs. Some of the topics that theoretical knowledge can elucidate are not high on most women's list of priorities. It would not necessarily occur to many women expecting their first baby to question the method by which their baby's heart should be monitored during labour. Many other questions relating to their social world and emotional lives would be more pressing. It is often only when they have given birth or talked to other women who have had a baby that women become aware of the details of the process of labour and how it is managed in hospital. One woman explained how misleading she felt ideas picked up from television could be:

> 'I don't think you are given any indication that you are going to be left alone ...When you see somebody [on TV] giving birth with three midwives round her, you think to yourself – if you haven't had a baby – that the whole of the time you're in labour that you've got these people round you, and you haven't.'

Most importantly, there is great diversity amongst pregnant women in terms of their information interests and perceived needs and in their strategies for trying to obtain this information. In analysing the first two focused discussions, patterns emerged from these differences. We developed a typology to represent the key characteristics of five different groups from those who wanted most information and spent most time and energy obtaining it, to those who were inclined to feel anxious about information and did not want to know more than they felt they would need in the short-term. The typology, which forms a continuum, included: 'voracious gatherers', 'readers', 'listeners', 'old hands' and 'waiters'. While not every woman fitted neatly into one group or another, the typology was both developed from women's descriptions of obtaining information, and it helped us to question and understand the women's differing feelings, attitudes and behaviour.

It became clear that a woman's view of the maternity services was fundamental to her approach to obtaining information. Those women who felt that there were alternatives to choose from, that they could potentially access or negotiate, were more inclined to want to obtain information to assist then in discussions with health professionals and making decisions. Those women who were less committed to obtaining information tended to be those who felt they would be less actively involved in decision-making. They included women who felt they would probably just get on with what came their way using what they knew already; women who believed that they couldn't become 'experts' so it was better to take advice; and women who expressed a feeling of being powerless to influence what went on around them, and what was done to their body and their baby.

The study was qualitative and involved just 54 women, however the sample was broadly representative of the profile of childbearing women, in terms of parity, educational attainment and age, with a higher than average proportion of Asian women. Given its representativeness, it is therefore of interest to note that there were small numbers of women in the groups at the extreme ends of the typology, with most having characteristics belonging to one or other of the three middle groups.

Approaches to obtaining information: typology

Voracious gatherers

There were a few women whom we felt could best be described as 'voracious gatherers'. They were prepared to invest a great deal of time and effort in pursuit of the information they felt they needed. They visited libraries, found research papers, arranged interviews with specialists, attended more than one course of antenatal classes, and contacted voluntary support organisations. In this study, all the 'voracious gatherers' were women having their first baby. One said:

'I found it very difficult to get good books on nutrition. There are no books on the market with the top ten sources of calcium or Vitamin B12. I looked. I even looked in academic sections in bookshops. It became a challenge and I couldn't find anything.

I eventually managed to prise some information out of the health visitors which they got from the dietician at the hospital, and I wrote to the Vegetarian Society.'

Readers

A greater number of women, around a quarter of those involved in the study, we described as 'readers' because they wanted a considerable amount of information and expected to get a lot of it by reading. They tended to be familiar with different sources presenting information in contrasting and sometimes conflicting ways. They bought books and magazines, some used the public library, and, if they were given leaflets, they were likely to read them. They were enthusiastic attenders of antenatal classes and might phone a helpline if the number was readily accessible. The group included women having their first baby:

'I read a lot, what ever I could get my hands on to start with, books, library books, even before I got pregnant ... Most of my information comes from books. But it's nice to talk to other people because even if you know the medical facts and things behind things, it's nice to get other people's experiences ... I think you can't get too much information.'

There were also those having a second baby who had been voracious gatherers in a first pregnancy but had different needs now.

'With the first baby I read quite a lot of books about pregnancy and I felt political about it ... I think it was more necessary then, they were more interventionist, bossier, then. I felt I needed to clarify my own ideas ... It feels more self-indulgent reading this time. I read about the progress of the pregnancy ... it's just time I can spend thinking about the baby. Whereas last time I was reading for a purpose which was to clarify my ideas and provide myself with ammunition, if necessary.'

Listeners

We called the next group 'listeners' because they relied quite heavily on what their midwife or doctor told them. There was a higher proportion of the total sample in this group than in any of the others, around two fifths of the participants, including both primiparous and multiparous women. They had a fairly relaxed attitude to information; they would 'take it as it comes'. Most of them had read quite a few 'pregnancy and birth' magazines, they might have a pregnancy book or two that they dipped into and they might read the leaflets given to them. They also got information from experience, family and friends and picked things up from television, but they looked to health professionals to give them appropriate information and the reassurance they needed. Generally, they expected not to have to go out and look for information. They wanted to know about new developments, but they were fairly dependent upon the knowledge provided and time for discussion allowed by their midwives or obstetrician. Some of the comments from women in this group include:

'Rachel, the midwife, has been good in explaining the domino scheme … I saw her for my other two kids, so I know her quite well. That's nice, to have the continuity … [She's] really nice. She listens. You think, "They know what's going on". She gives me confidence.'

'You want somebody in authority, that's got the right qualifications, to turn round and go, "You're absolutely right, you're getting heartburn because the valve at the bottom of your stomach is opening", or whatever. It's like, 'Alright, I've read it right, I've understood it right, that's it.'

'My mum, the very first time I was pregnant, she actually bought me the Dr Miriam Stoppard book … and I found it very handy 'cos if anything cropped up, at any of my scans or anything like that I could go back and refer to the book. And if I didn't understand that, I must admit, I could discuss it with the midwife when I saw her and she would tell [me].'

Old hands

Some women – all of them having their second or a subsequent baby – seemed best understood by the phrase 'been there, done that', so we called them 'old hands'. This was about a fifth of the sample. They were not particularly interested in information during this pregnancy because they felt that they had heard most of it before, or that their own experience and knowledge was more relevant than things they might read or be told.

'Basically, I know it all, you know. I just don't want them to come up with any new procedures, I suppose. I'm quite happy to stick to pethidine, I had that the last two times.'

Waiters

Some women – about a tenth of the group – were reticent about finding out a lot about pregnancy and birth. In particular, they did not want to know about unpleasant things that might happen. Their way of coping tended to be to wait; to take things as and when they came, and not anticipate the future. They could hope to avoid some possible complications altogether and believed that they would face new challenges as they occurred. Some were less confident than other women that they could determine what happened to them or influence the outcome of their care, therefore they did not see much point in gathering a lot of information. Others did not want the hard responsibility of making difficult choices.

'I didn't realise that an epidural actually numbs your body and you don't feel anything. I wouldn't have known if I hadn't gone to parentcraft … I haven't read up on [pain relief]. I thought I'd reach each thing as I came to it. I didn't want to know too much in advance – or know too little. Do each stage as I come to it. I don't want to know too much too far in advance. I don't really want to become an authority on something I don't really know anything about, like some people.'

Women's understanding and attitudes towards evidence-based information

Fundamental to understanding the use women were able to make of evidence-based information was ascertaining the level of importance that they placed on information of this kind. This tended to be affected in turn by their degree of understanding about the quality of the research on which it is based. These issues were explored during our second group discussions when the women were 7–8 months pregnant. The women were also asked their views of the three *Informed Choice* leaflets and, following discussion of their content, to comment on the ways, if any, that they felt they might use the information during labour.

Levels of understanding

The women ranged from those who were familiar with research and had some knowledge of different methodologies, to those who had very limited under-standing. The most informed women predictably tended to be 'voracious gatherers' and 'readers'. Among 'listeners' and waiters' there was a good deal of confusion about methodological issues; some participants assumed that the *Informed Choice* leaflets were based simply on women's views. Perhaps this is not surprising, as much of the research in the public domain is based on surveys of attitudes rather than on an experimental design. Furthermore, even those who have participated in a randomised controlled trial tend to be confused about concepts such as 'trial' and 'randomisation' (Featherstone and Donovan, 1998).

Attitudes to evidence-based information

Many positive comments were made about evidence-based information. Most of the women felt that it had the potential to be more reliable than information from a health professional or the experiences of family and friends.

> 'It meant more to me that they had researched it, that it wasn't just what some doctor had decided on, and that they had actually looked into it. Especially with the positions and the pros and cons with being upright, it meant a lot more to me that it had been based on research and not just somebody spouting on.'

They were more likely to trust research that was carried out by a person, or institution, that they held in high regard. However, a lot of scepticism was also expressed. The women said research could be 'subjective', 'slanted' or 'biased' and that 'science' was far removed from real experiences. Some women were familiar with market research being used in advertising to sell a product and this made them question the motive behind healthcare research. Was it really to help them make informed choices or was it to serve someone else's agenda? These women and others doubted the legitimacy of some research and questioned whether it had been 'faked'. These views echoed findings in a review of public attitudes to science carried out in Britain in 2000, which found that more than two thirds of those surveyed felt concerned about what researchers did 'behind closed doors' and that scientists should listen more to 'real people' (Office of Science and Technology and Wellcome Trust, 2000).

> 'I'd like to think that it was done with real people, by real doctors in a real hospital or wherever, but it probably isn't. I'd like to think it was, but I think I'm probably kidding myself.'

Some women also said that they distrusted research on women's issues that had been carried out by men. There was a tendency among the women to feel that research is not based on women's experiences – or does not reflect them accurately.

> 'I'd rather believe what other women have been through.'

> 'Medical research is based on the experience from a medical person's point of view. I think at the end of the day what reassures is that someone can tell you that they've been through it as well. You're automatically going to be more responsive to what they tell you.'

The women also felt that it was difficult to apply the results of research to themselves as individuals when it had been carried out on another group of women.

> 'I think the thing is with childbirth, it's so individual and then it's very difficult to have any leaflet really. You know something can say "well this is what happens to 800 women out of a study of 850" and you could be one of the fifty that you know it all goes the other way for.'

Sometimes the women were resistant to research because they intuitively doubted the conclusions or found that the results clashed with their preferences.

> 'But you know at the end of the day I think you've always got your own opinion anyway …You always weigh something up anyway. If you read something that says research has proved whatever, then you think, no that can't be right, I'm not having that.'

Women wanted to know

In order to assess the credibility of information which claims to be evidence-based, the women wanted to know:

- the kinds of research methods used
- who carried out the research
- the number of women involved
- when it was carried out.

They also wanted an explanation of conflicting or confusing findings and an indication of the strength of the evidence where one approach to care was significantly more effective than another.

Planned use of the *Informed Choice* leaflets

The *Informed Choice* leaflets aim to provide women with the most reliable evidence-based information available to help them make informed choices. Most study women intended to have one or more supporters with them during labour prior to reading the *Support in labour* leaflet, and they did not anticipate any conflict between their wishes and hospital policy. In the main, therefore, the information was seen as uncontentious. However, one woman, who had said it was her preference to be unaccompanied during labour, said she felt the leaflet put women under pressure to have a supporter.

The *Positions in labour* leaflet suggested to women that they might consider moving around and adopting upright positions during labour. The information related primarily to an aspect of their own behaviour rather than care provided for them. Depending on their hospital and their midwife, some of those who said they might like to move around freely, felt they might need to challenge cultural expectations that most women would labour on a bed in a semi-recumbent position. This would demand that they assert themselves against the norm during labour, at a time when women need to be able to feel relaxed and secure as possible (Lundgren and Dahlberg, 1998; Anderson, 2002). The leaflet on *Listening to your baby's heartbeat during labour* related directly to clinical care. Not only do women have less control over clinical care than over their own behaviour, but also it was current practice in the study maternity units at the time, as in many other units, for most women to have at least a period of continuous electronic foetal monitoring (EFM). The information in this leaflet was therefore contentious. Those women who felt they would like to have intermittent monitoring of their baby's heartbeat rather than EFM would need to be involved in decisions about their care and challenge both cultural expectations and clinical protocols. If they were to 'choose' intermittent monitoring, they would have to refuse to go along with what was usual. Their decision might raise questions of safety in the minds of midwives or doctors and challenge the unit's risk management strategy (Oliver *et al.*, 1996).

The leaflets were generally well received by the women, however one criticism was that they were 'nice, but not reality'. The women felt they were put in a difficult position when faced with a discrepancy between the evidence in the leaflets and what they were told occurred or had previously experienced in practice. This highlighted a gap between the vision of woman-centred services, in which women would feel at ease to do what felt right for them, particularly when this was known to be clinically effective, and the continuing influence of a medical model of care. Individuals' intentions for using the information led us to devise a second typology which reflected women's reaction to the conflict that so many anticipated: 'crusaders', 'the cautiously optimistic', 'the resigned but regretful', and 'the unmoved'.

Intentions for using evidence-based information: typology

Crusaders

Approximately one in ten of the women were 'crusaders' who were determined to use the information to get the advantages described in the leaflets. They were willing to challenge standard practice and do battle with health professionals, if necessary.

> 'I would definitely go in and say that I don't want to be strapped down, I want to be able to walk around. I couldn't care less if they're going to be horrible to me afterwards, I want to be able to move around.'

Cautiously optimistic

Another group, about one fifth of the women, were 'cautiously optimistic'. They were interested in acting on the information in the leaflets, and were willing to question health professionals and the standard practice. But they were prepared to accept that it might not be possible to make their preferred choices in labour.

> 'All of these things are brilliant for what I'm thinking of, I'd be quite happy to go in there and say 'no I don't want an EFM ... yes I do want to be mobile this time, and I do want support in labour, etc. But my whole experience of what happened was completely different, so beforehand I think it is a really good idea all of these decisions, but I do think you have to keep an open mind.'

Resigned but regretful

'Resigned but regretful' women, a third of the total sample, would accept the care provided by health professionals, but having read the leaflets would sometimes wonder whether this treatment was the best option. Many of these women felt that they were powerless to change the course of events in labour, despite the knowledge that there might be advantages if things were done in a different way.

> 'If you're in hospital if a health professional says "this is going to happen" you're bound to say yes because they are supposed to know. It is very unlikely that I would start questioning anything they say to me, unless I really knew what I was talking about and I haven't got a clue, so if they said "we're going to give you a Caesarean" I'd obviously ask why, but they could say anything and if it sounds right to me, that's what I'll have to have.'

> 'I thought [the leaflets] made you think you had choices that in reality weren't there. The health professionals controlled the show. I'm not saying the information isn't true, it just made you believe you had a choice when in my [previous] experience you didn't.'

The unmoved

The remaining third of the women did not anticipate conflict or regret. For some, including those anticipating a planned Caesarean section or having an epidural, limited movement and continuous monitoring was not an issue. For them, the advantages of the pain relief outweighed the possible disadvantages. Some others were sceptical about the evidence provided on outcomes or were content for health professionals to guide them.

Reflecting on decision-making in labour

When we met the participants for the third time, in the postnatal period, we asked them to recount their experiences of labour and delivery, focusing specifically on the three areas covered by the *Informed Choice* leaflets we had discussed at the previous focus group. We asked them to reflect on whether the information covered in the leaflets had influenced their behaviour and decision-making in any way.

Supporters in labour

All of the women had at least one family member or their partner with them during labour. However, no one put this down to the evidence contained in the *Support in Labour* leaflet. They felt the information in the leaflet reassuringly reinforced their original intentions, but had no influence on their decision-making. One woman explained a positive effect reading the leaflet had had for her.

> 'One of the things actually I remember [from the leaflet] is how much difference having someone with you when you give birth makes to you afterwards.'

Positions in labour

Of the 47 women who went into labour, 14 specifically mentioned that they spent time during the first stage of their labour moving and adopting upright positions as ways to cope with the pain. The *Positions in labour* leaflet was credited by 10 women as having had some influence on the decisions they made. Other factors included previous experience, discussion with midwives, and other sources of written information.

> 'I think the positions one influenced me. I was determined this time to try and stay upright – as long as I didn't have an epidural … or pethidine. I did make an effort this time to stay upright. I did walk around for the first few hours and I'm sure that helped. So that did influence me.'

> 'Yeah, it made a difference – that picture that shows the positions. I got hold of the back of the bed and held on to it, I was kneeling. That made me feel more comfortable.'

A few women were able to go against the pressure to conform to norms in the unit having read the leaflet.

> 'I learned a lot about different positions. I hadn't got a clue until I read those. And they kept saying "Why don't you have a lie down?" and I was walking round.'

Other women did not feel comfortable using upright positions in labour, but they credited the positions leaflet with making them feel they had more options.

Monitoring your baby's heartbeat

All but three of the women who went into labour had EFM at some stage. Fourteen women said they had continuous EFM throughout labour, a further five said that they began with intermittent monitoring which then became continuous. Four women said that because of reading and discussing the leaflet they had asked for, and received, non-continuous monitoring with either the EFM or hand-held Doppler during labour.

> 'They put me on a monitor to begin with but I just said "no, I don't want a monitor, I just want you to check it every so often".'

> 'I must say that I found our session of monitoring the baby's heart whilst in labour very helpful as every time I was strapped up I asked how long it was for and then asked for it to be removed after the specified time. The midwives were more than happy to do this but I think they would have left me much longer if I hadn't asked.'

Intentions v. reality

Those who credited the leaflets with affecting what happened during labour were mostly the 'crusaders' and the 'cautiously optimistic' – those who had planned to make use of the evidence-based information they had received. In addition a couple of the 'resigned but regretful' women found that their labours were straightforward and they were able, to their surprise, to make choices.

But being a 'crusader' did not necessarily lead to the desired experience.

'The whole thing was completely opposite to how I wanted it. I was strapped to the monitor for the whole time and then he had a head monitor which I said I was going to totally refuse...They wanted to monitor him, I don't know why, because they don't really explain a great deal to you.'

Some women said the leaflets had been interesting to read, and that they had intended to discuss them with their midwives, but that the opportunity had not arisen. Others said that the experience had been 'out of my hands', that they had been unable to make decisions or influence the course of action.

Discussion

In this small-scale study, just over a quarter of the women credited the *Informed Choice* leaflets, or the group discussions about the leaflets, with having influenced in some way their decision-making or behaviour during labour. This is a more positive finding than others have been able to report (Kirkham and Stapleton, 2001).

However, our findings underline the fact that women's choices during labour and delivery remain limited. These results echo those of Kirkham, Stapleton and Oliver, and suggest that even when women's access to evidence-based information is not blocked, its usefulness can be undermined by the culture of the maternity unit (Oliver *et al.*, 1996; Kirkham and Stapleton, 2001; Stapleton *et al.*, 2002). Our participants were not offered an equal choice between options; and sadly by the time these women had reached the third trimester of pregnancy, they did not expect or imagine that they would be offered much choice during labour and delivery. Our typology on the intended use of evidence-based information was set in the language of conflict; pregnant women anticipated that if they wanted to use the evidence they had been given they would have to 'arm' themselves with it, rather than using it to help them make appropriate decisions as part of a collaboration with health professionals. Waterworth and Luker (1990) argued that avoidance of trouble and 'toeing the line' was of primary importance to patients in encounters with nurses; Levy found that on the whole, women are trying to 'maintain equilibrium' when making choices in pregnancy (Levy, 1999b).

Most women are not 'crusaders'; they do not want to do battle. It is not easy for women to argue or assert themselves when physically exposed, coping with pain and uncertainty, and dependent on the continuing support and care of the very people with whom they are in conflict. There are similarities here with the situation for women experiencing domestic violence (Stanko, 1985). In an attempt to minimise overt conflict, women deny the strength of their own feelings. The likelihood of evidence-informed decision-making is greatly reduced in a climate perceived to be either indifferent, or even hostile, to the principles of informed choice and consent.

The concept of informed choice depends not only on access to reliable information but also on the availability of genuine alternatives. If the rhetoric is to be realised, individualised care must be offered and this will involve ensuring that a range of diverse services are provided, with real opportunities for women to opt for what they feel is right for them. Where diversity is not even tolerated informed choice becomes a hollow phrase. One woman told us:

> 'He insisted, that doctor, that I have the injection to deliver the placenta. Now I've not had that before with the other two and I put in my birth plan that I didn't want it and they said "OK, no problem, you won't have to have it." Then they came with it to me when I was just giving birth and said, "The doctor said he insisted you have this". And I thought that was dreadful. "Why?" I said, "Oh, just do it!" I mean I know it wasn't going to harm anyone but I was really, I thought it was bad to come, you know, when you were so vulnerable ... I should have said no, but I didn't.'

For women having a baby, the maternity services are just one small part of their continuing lives. Yet, what the services provide or fail to deliver can have far reaching consequences. While many women are fairly independent, drawing on their own previous knowledge and on the experiences and beliefs of those around them in their families and communities, as a society we have come to expect expert knowledge from health professionals about pregnancy and birth (Stapleton *et al.*, 2002; Bluff and Holloway, 1994). When health professionals' information and clinical care falls short of what is expected, or their advice contradicts what women believe and value, women can feel let-down, angry with themselves, at worst suffering depression or post-traumatic stress disorder, with repercussions for many years (Church and Scanlon, 2002). Women's confidence in themselves and also in health professionals can be seriously undermined.

What is the value of evidence-based information for pregnant women?

This study has found that having become aware of evidence-based information a significant minority of pregnant women reported that it influenced subsequent events in some way. For most of these women the reported effects were positive, though there were times when the information added to the women's sense of conflict or uncertainty. The information on intermittent versus continuous fetal monitoring was expected to be most contentious, challenging both the informal culture in most maternity units at the time, and also the formal rules and protocols. As information on the effects of alternative forms of treatment is necessary in order for informed consent, many would argue that this alone justifies the need to disseminate evidence-based information more widely to pregnant women. Recent evidence shows that for healthy women with a normal pregnancy, exposure to EFM as a routine part of admission to hospital increases the chance of their labour ending in an emergency Caesarean section (Mires *et al.*, 2001).

Evidence-based *Informed Choice* leaflets are sometimes used by health professionals, but in many areas of the NHS these high-quality published leaflets are either not purchased and provided or, despite being available, are not seen as an integral tool for midwives and others in meeting women's needs (Kirkham and Stapleton, 2001). The relevant health departments in England and Wales, Scotland and Northern Ireland provide information for all first-time pregnant women (Health Education Board for Scotland, 2002; Health Promotion Agency, 1999; Health Promotion England, 2001; Khoner, 1999), but little of this is explicitly evidence-based, despite investment having been made through MIDIRS and the NHS Centre for Reviews and Dissemination in developing summaries of available evidence in a format and in language designed for parents.

In this study the *Informed Choice* leaflets were provided to women by the research team with a structured opportunity to discuss evidence-based information and the ideas and outcomes reported in the leaflets. Some of our participants were dubious about the information; the findings seemed counter-intuitive, or they were worried that the studies were biased. As the concept of using evidence-based information for decision-making in maternity care is still relatively new to pregnant women, it is hardly surprising that there were misunderstandings and some scepticism. An introduction to these leaflets by a supportive health professional, who could explain the methods used and clarify uncertainties, might allay some of these misgivings and help women to see how the leaflets might best help them. We are aware that this was the process originally intended when the *Informed Choice* leaflets were developed, but there is evidence that this does not always happen in practice (O'Cathain *et al.*, 2002). In addition, efforts need to be made to familiarise young people and adults with evidence-based health information, so that people of all ages can understand and use it.

Those women in the study who credited the leaflets with influencing their birth experiences said the group discussions about the leaflets were what made the difference to them. The groups varied in size from two to eight women with a facilitator. These interchanges had a lasting impression beyond just reading the information itself. It is quite possible that without this focus, a smaller number would have credited this information as having an influence. Potentially this is one reason for the discrepancies in the findings between this and the large scale RCT using these leaflets, where decision-making was unaffected (Kirkham and Stapleton, 2001). Also, in our study, all participating women were made aware of the information to some extent through the research. Further work is needed to replicate this method of using evidence-based leaflets, evaluating outcomes.

Women and their partners have access to more information on pregnancy and birth now than ever before, with more magazines and TV channels, helplines, such as NHS Direct, and the internet. Yet, as supply increases so does demand (Wiggins *et al.*, 2000; Singh *et al.*, 2002) and the quality of what is most easily available may be unreliable (Henderson *et al.*, 2000). The strategies women employ to acquire information vary considerably. Our typology of women's approaches to obtaining information in pregnancy serves as a reminder of this. Subsequent work by this research team involving a large, national representative sample has been able to show the proportion of women who identify with these types: most women expecting their first baby (70 per cent) and a third of those in a second or subsequent pregnancy (35 per cent) described themselves as 'wanting to know as much as possible – a great deal of information required' (Wiggins *et al.*, 2000). Also in the follow-up study, only 8 per cent of the first-time mothers wanted less than 'quite a lot' of information, including just one per cent who said they wanted 'very little – I'd rather not know too much'. Among women who had had a baby before, the demand for information was significantly lower with a third saying, 'I know what I need to know'. The follow-up study showed that women and men in lower socio-economic class groups, those under 20 years of age and those belonging to minority ethnic groups had greater unmet information needs than older, more advantaged and white expectant parents.

Providing written evidence-based leaflets may be an appropriate means for 'voracious gatherers' and 'readers' to gain this information, but many women and men are highly reliant upon opportunities to discuss information in relation to their own symptoms, experiences or anxieties with a professional or other parents. For 'listeners' and 'waiters' inter-personal contact is especially important. They depend upon health professionals for information in the right depth, at the right time, as well as affirmation and reassurance. It is clear from this study, and from other work (Curtis *et al.*, 2001) that some women 'regulate information' (Levy, 1999b), actively avoiding what they feel is inappropriate or comes at the wrong time for them. Midwives have a particularly important role to play in finding out about each woman's preferences, the extent and causes of any anxiety, offering appropriate information and opportunities for discussion. Sources of reading can often usefully reinforce face-to-face discussion. For those managing their own caseload there are more opportunities to get to know the needs of individual women and their partners.

As midwives' time is often short and the groups of parents who find it most difficult to access information are less likely than others to attend antenatal classes, midwives need to devise new ways of engaging with parents in a time-efficient way. Often significant opportunities can be opened up for discussion during limited consultation time, particularly if a clear signal is given that the midwife is ready to listen. The woman and her feelings and needs should be the absolute focus of the time that is available. It is all too easy for form-filling and a pre-occupation with screening and monitoring to intervene (Harris and Green, 2002). In addition, midwives could be more creative in inviting small groups of similar women or couples to meet with them for discussion at a relevant time in pregnancy, such as in early pregnancy to discuss screening and later pregnancy to discuss birth. There is no reason why there should be the rigid division between antenatal care and antenatal classes that still exists in some services. References to 'classes' may have negative associations, particularly for disadvantaged groups. Midwives should be prepared to ask women about information they have found interesting or useful and stop to think how it relates to the local service culture. Anything midwives can do to minimise the conflict women currently face when they enter hospital would be a positive step forward.

Conclusion

This qualitative study adds to the literature demonstrating that there is still some way to go before woman-centred care becomes a reality (Anderson, 2002). Surprisingly frequently, the women in the study, who came from a range of educational, social class, and ethnic backgrounds, used language that suggested that they felt that they had little control.

Communication could be improved in a number of ways. The chance to discuss the *Informed Choice* leaflets was generally welcomed by women, so they could be used more with groups during pregnancy, such as antenatal class groups. The women in the study felt the leaflets could be improved by explaining the kinds of research methods used and the number of people on which the conclusions have been based. Requests were also made for an indication of the strength of the evidence where outcomes differed with different treatment or behaviour.

While two of the *Informed Choice* leaflets enabled a minority of women to take care of themselves more actively in labour, we believe that they would have a positive influence on care for more women if the information in the leaflets was consistent with usual practice in the labour ward and supported by midwives and doctors.

It is arguably unethical to provide women with evidence-based information about choices if current practices and culture in the maternity service deny women that choice and create additional conflict for them at a time when they need care and rely on what the service is offering. On the other hand, it is surely unethical to deny women access to information without which they cannot make informed decisions or give informed consent to treatment. The only solution to this impasse is for maternity services to 'raise the game' through improved team working; better communication; support for clinical governance, including critical questioning and audit of practice; as well as a more rigorous approach to informed consent. Evidence-based information is certainly not sufficient to enable women to negotiate care that is both clinically effective and responsive to their needs. Maternity unit protocols and culture need to be evidence-based and woman-centred too.

References

Anderson, T. (2002) The misleading myth of choice: the continuing oppression of women in childbirth. *MIDIRS Midwifery Digest*, **12(3)**: 405–7.

Bluff, R. and Holloway, I. (1994) 'They know best': women's perceptions of midwifery care during labour and childbirth. *Midwifery*, **10**: 157–64.

Cartwright, A. (1979) *The Dignity of Labour? A Study of Childbearing and Induction.* London: Tavistock.

Church, S. and Scanlon, M. (2002) Post-traumatic stress disorder after childbirth. Do midwives have a preventative role? *Practising Midwife*, **5(6)**:10–13.

Curtis, P., Thomas, G., Stapleton, H. and Kirkham, M. (2001) In *Informed Choice in Maternity Care: An Evaluation of Evidence-based Leaflets*, edited by M. Kirkham and H. Stapleton. York: NHS Centre for Reviews and Dissemination, University of York.

Department of Health (1993) *Changing Childbirth*, Part 1: *Report of the Expert Maternity Group.* London: HMSO.

Featherstone, K. and Donovan, J.L. (1998) Random allocation or allocation at random? Patients' perspectives of participation in a randomised controlled trial. *British Medical Journal*, **317**: 1177–80.

Fleissig, A. (1993) Are women given enough information by staff during labour and delivery? *Midwifery*, **9**: 70–5.

Gready, M., Newburn, M., Dodds, R., and Gauge, S. (1995) *Birth Choices: Women's Expectations and Experiences.* London: National Childbirth Trust.

Green, J.M., Coupland, V.A., and Kitzinger, J.V. (1988) *Great Expectations: A Prospective Study of Women's Expectations and Experiences of Childbirth.* Cambridge: Child Care and Development Unit, University of Cambridge.

Harris, M. and Green, K. (2002) In *The Rising Caesarean Rate – From Audit to Action. Report of the joint conference organised by the Royal College of Obstetricians and Gynaecologists, the Royal College of Midwives and the National Childbirth Trust in London*, 31 January. London: National Childbirth Trust

Health Education Board for Scotland (2002) *Ready, Steady, Baby!: A Guide to Pregnancy, Birth and Early Parenthood, revised 2nd edn.* Edinburgh: Health Education Board for Scotland.

Health Promotion Agency (1999) *The Pregnancy Book: Your Complete Guide to Pregnancy, Childbirth and the First Few Weeks with a New Baby.* Belfast: Health Promotion Agency.

Health Promotion England (2001) *The Pregnancy Book: Your Complete Guide to Pregnancy, Childbirth and the First Few Weeks with a New Baby.* London: Health Promotion England.

Henderson, L., Kitzinger, J. and Green, J. (2000) Representing infant feeding: content analysis of British media portrayals of bottle feeding and breast feeding. *British Medical Journal*, **321**: 1196–8.

Hoddinott, P. (1999) Qualitative study of decisions about infant feeding among women in the east end of London. *British Medical Journal*, **318**: 30–4.

House of Commons Health Select Committee (1992) *Second Report on the Maternity Services.* London: HMSO.

Jacoby, A. (1988) Mothers' views about information and advice in pregnancy and childbirth: findings from a national study. *Midwifery*, **4**: 103–19.

Kirkham, M. and Stapleton, H. (eds) (2001) *Informed Choice in Maternity Care: An Evaluation of Evidence-based Leaflets*. York: NHS Centre for Reviews and Dissemination, University of York.

Khoner, N. (1999) *The Pregnancy Book: Your Complete Guide to Pregnancy, Childbirth and the First Few Weeks with a New Baby*. Cardiff: Health Promotion Division National Assembly for Wales.

Levy, V. (1999a) Protective steering: a grounded theory study of the processes by which midwives facilitate informed choices during pregnancy. *Journal of Advanced Nursing*, **29**: 104–12.

Levy, V. (1999b) Maintaining equilibrium: a grounded theory study of the processes involved when women make informed choices during pregnancy. *Midwifery*, **15**: 109–19.

Lundgren, I. and Dahlberg, K. (1998) Women's experience of pain during childbirth. *Midwifery*, **14(2)**: 105–10.

MIDIRS and NHS Centre for Reviews and Dissemination (1996).

Mires, G., Williams, F., and Howie, P. (2001) Randomised controlled trila of cardiotocography versus Doppler auscultation of fetal heart at admission in labour in low risk obstetric population. *British Medical Journal*, **322**: 1457–62.

Newburn, M. (2002) A birth policy for the National Childbirth Trust. *MIDIRS Midwifery Digest*, **12(1)**: 122–6.

O'Cathain, A., Walters, S.J., Nicholl, J.P., Thomas, K.J., and Kirkham, M. Use of evidence-based leaflets to promote informed choice in maternity care: randomised controlled trial in everyday practice. *British Medical Journal*, **324**: 643–6.

Office of Science and Technology and Wellcome Trust (2000) *Science and the Public: A Review of Science Communication and Public Attitudes to Science in Britain*. London: OST and The Wellcome Trust.

Oliver, S., Rajan, L., Turner, H., Oakley, A., Entwistle, V., Watt, I., Sheldon, T.A., and Rosser, J. (1996) Informed choice for users of health services: views on ultrasonography leaflets of women in early pregnancy, midwives and ultrasonographers. *British Medical Journal*, **313**: 1251–3.

Rosser, J. (2002) Help yourself to a straightforward birth. *New Generation*, February.

Singh, D., Newburn, M., Smith, N. and Wiggins, M. (2002) The information needs of first-time pregnant women. *British Journal of Midwives*, **10(1)**: 54–7.

Stanko, E.A. (1985) *Intimate Intrusions*. London: Unwin Hyman.

Stapleton, H., Kirkham, M. and Thomas, G. (2002) Qualitative study of evidence-based leaflets in maternity care. *British Medical Journal*, **324**: 639–43.

Waterworth, S. and Luker, K. A. (1990) Reluctant collaborators: do patients want to be involved in decisions concerning care? *Journal of Advanced Nursing*, **15**: 971–6.

Wiggins, M., Singh, D., Newburn, M. and Burbidge, R. (2000) Chapter in *Access to Maternity Information and Support*, edited by D. Singh and M. Newburn, pp. 7–55. London: National Childbirth Trust, London, 2000).

CHAPTER 8

Integrating MIDIRS *Informed Choice* Leaflets into a Maternity Service

JILL DEMILEW

Chapter Contents

■ Introduction

■ Context

■ Processes

■ Learning from this experience

■ Conclusion

Introduction

In 1995, I rejoined the National Health Service in a new role as quality assurance manager in the midwifery management team at Tower Hamlets Healthcare Trust. This followed several years practising as an independent midwife in south-east London, which culminated in forming a caseload model of midwifery practice with my colleagues in the South-East London Midwifery Group Practice. This experience honed our philosophy and skills of working in partnership with women and families. The aim of enabling women to work towards continually making their own informed decisions underpinned this model of professional practice. Our particular organisation of work had features which made this possible which are shown in Box 8.1. We played an active part in work supporting the government policy report, *Changing Childbirth* (Department of Health, 1993). We fully supported developing maternity services to provide continuity of care(er), supporting women having the opportunity to make informed choices and have increasing control

---

Box 8.1 Organisational factors supporting 'informed choice'

- Midwives have personal caseload

- Midwives have control of the size of their caseload

- Midwives share same philosophy of professional practice and the Group Practice chooses who joins the practice

- Same two midwives share providing antenatal, labour and postnatal care for a named woman

- Provision of weekly antenatal and postnatal 'drop-in' groups, mixed and women only

- Provision of library with books, videos for loan

- Booking consultation as long as needed often 1–3 hours

- Midwife antenatal consultations 30 minutes

---

over their pregnancy, birth and early parenting experiences. We believed that this would improve the outcomes for women and their children as well as improving midwifery practice. Indeed the outcomes for women and babies booked with the midwifery practice were improved in comparison with other local maternity services Obstetric interventions, assisted and operative deliveries were lower, normal vaginal births and home births were increased with a lower perinatal mortality rate (Demilew, 1994).

I started working in Tower Hamlets with enthusiasm for an opportunity to work with midwifery management colleagues who had a similar philosophy of professional practice. Lynn Thomas was newly appointed as head of midwifery, having previously worked in Tower Hamlets as a community midwife and subsequently as a hospital manager. She was deeply committed to developing the principles of 'Changing Childbirth' in Tower Hamlets. The challenge was to explore the possibility of applying these principles to a whole health district rather than to one midwifery group practice. The two major aims were:

- To improve the options, experience and outcomes for all local women using the maternity service
- To improve professional knowledge and practice of maternity service professionals

Reflecting on the rich and varied experiences in Tower Hamlets, I recognise that I had embryonic skills in managing change and effective implementation. This was complemented with a great deal of naivety about organisational behaviour. It was a powerful and enduring time of learning. In this chapter I want to share the context, the processes and discuss the learning from this experience of trying to integrate the MIDIRS *Informed Choice* Leaflets into the maternity service.

Context

Commissioning

In April 1995 Tower Hamlets Healthcare NHS Community Trust was established in East London. The East London and City Health Authority made a decision to change the usual pathway of commissioning maternity services from an Acute Hospital Trust to the Community Trust. All maternity service monies were directed through the new Community Trust which I believe was a unique arrangement in the UK. This included financing primary health, acute secondary and tertiary maternity services. The Acute Hospital Trust received monies from the Community Trust to provide obstetric, anaesthetic, and neonatal and theatre and intensive care facilities. All midwives transferred employment to the community trust. There were three separate maternity services commissioned by this Health Authority and differences in the populations served, the services offered and importantly in the outcomes for local women and families. Relative poverty was a unifying factor for a majority of all three maternity populations. The variance in the Caesarean section rates in East London at the time were between 13 and 25 per cent.

Maternity services

The main inpatient maternity unit was in The Royal London Hospital Whitechapel, with some antenatal midwifery services provided at Mile End Hospital. The locality served mainly socioeconomically deprived areas including the two poorest wards in the UK as well as newly emerging wealthy areas near the River Thames. About 80 per cent of housing was local authority owned and the population ethnically mixed. The ethnic majority using the maternity services were Bangladeshi women (55 per cent) principally from a region in Bangladesh called Sylhet, which has its own language.

The annual delivery rate was 3600 births having a midwifery establishment of approximately 105 WTE (whole time equivalents) and five Consultant Obstetricians two of whom, worked part time. A team of eight Bangladeshi women Health Advocates were an integral part of maternity and gynaecology services. This team had developed in response to the difficulties of providing effective and acceptable services to people who were not literate in English and often not literate in their own Sylheti language. A Health Advocate assisted a maternity service professional at every antenatal consultation with a Bangladeshi woman who needed an interpreter whether in hospital, primary care or in a woman's home. They had a roster, which included working on the maternity wards, but the team worked Monday to Friday office hours and Saturday mornings. They only worked in the labour ward with individual women who were in a crisis situation and were not present during 'normal' labours.

The maternity management structure was completely new (see Figure 8.1).

Maternity strategy and the programme of work

Integrating the MIDIRS *Informed Choice* Leaflets was *part of* an overall strategy to improve the maternity services. The strategy led to a programme of work for the maternity services. It included several related but independent pieces of work (see Box 8.2).

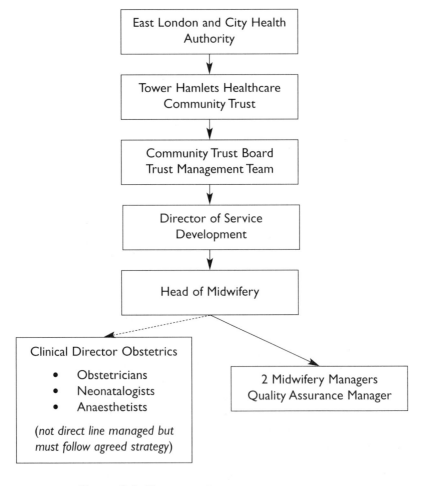

Figure 8.1 The maternity management structure

Box 8.2 Programme of work

- Develop philosophy of maternity care

- Reorganise midwives into group practices and hospital team

- Develop new woman held maternity record

- Develop clinical risk management system

- Develop maternity service clinical guidelines

- Change midwifery pay structure to minimum F grade

- Increase number of clinical Supervisors of Midwives

- Improve the fabric and décor of in patient facility

- Develop equipment review, replacement and financing system

Processes

It was clear from the beginning that integrating the MIDIRS *Informed Choice* leaflets would need several tasks to be completed for successful implementation. There was no *formal* project management. The leaflets were viewed by the midwifery management team as a potentially useful, good quality tool to support increasing the opportunities for women to make informed decisions when using the maternity service. The main aim was that the implementation process assured the sustained and appropriate use of the leaflets. We believed that:

- It supported professionals in the development of clinical skills which enable women to make informed decision.
- The leaflets are an exemplar of presenting information to support women making informed decisions.
- It supported service development which is actively informed by women's choices.

The processes of implementation are summarised in Box 8.3.

Stakeholders agreeing objectives

The Health Authority was committed to supporting the use of evidence-based knowledge in service provision. They had commissioned a review of maternity services in East London which was ongoing during the time of introducing the leaflets. They had purchased a set and carrying pack of MIDIRS *Informed Choice* leaflets for every GP practice in East London and distributed them.

Box 8.3 Processes of implementation

1. **Objectives agreed by all stakeholders**

   - Commissioners

   - Trust Management Team

   - Maternity Care Professionals (Community & Hospital)

2. **Agree the resources (£)**

   - Supplies of leaflets and wallets (initial and ongoing)

   - Training costs (initial & ongoing)

   - Time needed for staff training and cost of replacement of staff to maintain service provision in their absence

3. **Agree implementation programme**

   - Identify separate pieces of work (tasks)

   - Identify who needs to be involved

   - Identify quality indicators

   - Identify risks and contingency planning

   - Identify evaluation

   - Identify timetable including start date of using leaflets

---

The Community Trust Board and Management Team was committed to the development of user involvement in service development as well as enabling service users to make informed choices and decisions about their healthcare.

The agreed maternity service philosophy included the commitment to supporting woman-centred, individualised provision of care and supporting women making informed choices and decisions about their care.

Meetings were held individually with professional 'leaders' to discuss the project and to gain commitment. The intention to introduce them was also an agenda item in all unit administrative and professional meetings in the three months prior to their introduction. For example, Clinical Director for Obstetrics leads for anaesthetics, neonatology and the ultrasonographer supervisor. We also attended and presented at GP locality meetings.

Agreeing the resources

It was agreed to fund all initial and ongoing training in the use of the leaflets as well as the cost of a wallet and complete set of professional and women's leaflets for every individual midwife, obstetrician, neonatologist, ultrasonographer and health advocate. The ongoing supply of leaflets was costed and this with initial costs was placed in the service annual business plan which was an integral part of the Trust Annual Business Plan. This assured the financial commitment. The provision of time for staff to be trained and replacement staff for service provision proved problematic. It proved difficult to replace staff with bank or agency staff. There was also a lot of staff training being undertaken during this time which included introducing a new maternity record.

Agreeing the implementation programme

The midwifery management team and supervisors of midwives identified the main tasks (see Box 8.4).

Some of the tasks relating to other projects in the overall programme of work (Box 8.2) were allocated to the individual leading the project. Midwifery manager colleagues were heading project teams responsible for completing new guidelines, the education contract and staff induction. I also had responsibility for heading the team working with the new maternity record which included reviewing information currently being given to women.

The easiest task was completion of ordering and distribution of MIDIRS *Informed Choice* leaflets packs for each individual professional. A comprehensive

---

Box 8.4 Tasks identified for implementation programme

- Review all information currently being given to women for consistency and coherence with MIDIRS leaflets

- Review in house and contracted education programmes for consistency and awareness of information in MIDIRS leaflets

- Review the maternity service guidelines to include use of MIDIRS leaflets and consistency of information content

- Arrange initial training for all relevant staff groups in use of MIDIRS leaflets and how to access supplies * to include Health Advocates

- Arrange training in use of and being given a set of MIDIRS leaflets as part of formal induction of new staff in maternity service

- Arrange distribution of complete sets/wallets of MIDIRS leaflets to individual professionals

- Ensure that new maternity record prompts professionals in the appropriate use of the leaflets and that their use may be audited

information pack handout titled, *The informed choice initiative, what does it mean?* was included in the initial package. The leaflets had been discussed individually with the clinical lead in obstetrics, neonatology, anaesthetics and with the ultrasonographer supervisor. They had agreed to support the project and release colleagues for training.

An open half day training facilitated by MIDIRS was arranged and widely advertised. In the event only nine midwives, the midwifery managers, clinical director, head of midwifery and one ultrasonographer attended. This was a very disappointing response. It may have been influenced by the location not being in the main acute hospital although good quality refreshments were provided. The training was excellent, using videos demonstrating good and inappropriate practice in the use of the leaflets. The facilitator led a discussion regarding customising the use of the leaflets into our maternity service. For example, we discussed at what gestation certain leaflets should be used and how to access supplies.

Training was a major issue. Everyone had a copy of the Information Pack Guide which explored definitions of informed choice, the rationale for using the leaflets and examples of clinical scenarios. This did not guarantee time was taken to read or discuss any issues arising. A minority of group practices or ward staff met regularly for clinical discussion. Most met on an ad hoc basis for administrative reasons or as a response to a critical problem. There was little evidence of a culture of valuing regular time to review care, clinical practice or to reflect, discuss and plan. There was a mistaken assumption that most midwives and doctors understood what informed choice is, had the professional skills to support it and agreed with the philosophy. This is also in an environment with pressurised conditions of work which at times were relentless. We arranged designated times with each Group Practice of midwives and antenatal clinic staff. This reached a limited number, dependent on who was on duty at the time. One session of junior doctor training was used on a Friday afternoon to introduce the medical staff to the leaflets. The ultrasonographer supervisor was grappling with severe staff shortages and was unhappy with some of the contents of the Antenatal Screening and Ultrasound screening leaflets. During the training sessions, common themes of concerns raised emerged:

- We don't have the time, especially with the Bangladeshi women when working with the health advocates.
- Are they culturally appropriate for 'our' population? Many of the women turn up too late for the scans anyway.
- How am I going to carry all these leaflets when I am walking in the community?
- 'I don't agree with ....'
- Some of this is going to cause unnecessary worry to women.

These discussions were welcome, healthy and appropriate. However, once more it increased the awareness of how much bigger this project of introducing an information tool was. This was particularly around familiarity with evidence-based knowledge, dealing with uncertainty, being open about what is not known as well as what is known. The huge limiting factor of time available became a real but greatly magnified barrier. Reality for the majority of committed but overworked professionals in this busy maternity service was that most had not experienced the improved outcomes possible through sharing information freely with women and enabling them to make informed choices. Some professionals had experienced this usually with individual women in specific situations.

I had most training time with the health advocate team. They had a weekly team meeting for administration, professional training and case discussion. Individual members could leave at any point for urgent advocacy work but they all recognised that this meeting was a vital part of sustaining their over stretched team. During this time the focus of their daily work changed from being mainly hospital-based to community-based. They were struggling with allowing time to travel between greatly increased numbers of community clinics. We discussed at length the contents and use of the leaflets. They had the advantage of familiarity with informed choice as a norm in their professional practice. During the previous year it was acknowledged that they were not just 'mechanical' interpreters but actually advocates for Bangladeshi women. A lot of team meetings had been used for case discussion around how to advocate in situations where women did not fully understand all the issues or options or perhaps were choosing not to do something that a professional advised. We explored themes such as who were they accountable too?

Documentation in the new maternity record included places which indicated using the MIDIRS *Informed Choice* leaflets. There was a page in the antenatal section called 'Planning for labour/birth and first days'. The intention was that all women would have the opportunity antenatally to discuss this. The pages have sections addressing support in labour, monitoring your baby in labour, labouring well (maintaining energy, eating, drinking, positions, mobility), living with the pain of labour and specific issues in normal labour (third stage, perineum) the first feed and finally a section for labours and births which may have special needs. There are prompts in the documentation for using the leaflets and signing if given. The intention was that they be used with Bangladeshi women if the health advocate was present at the consultation. This documentation would also serve as a way of auditing the use of some of the leaflets at a later date.

Finally a start date for using the leaflets was given and we had checked that every relevant staff member had signed that they had received their MIDIRS pack and information guide. We ensured that half of the midwives had attended a training session before the launch. A lot of project work continued following the launch, including checking that there was coherent information in the maternity guidelines, with any other information given to women and in professional education. We secured a successful bid with the Trust Clinical

Audit department for an audit of the use of the *Informed Choice* leaflets in the following year. It should be noted that we started using the *Informed Choice* leaflets *before* the new maternity record was being used.

Learning from this experience

We had the belief, we had the commitment, we had the money, we had an initial awareness that implementation would involve multiple strands of work. Yet introducing the MIDIRS *Informed Choice* Leaflets into this maternity service at this time had limited or unknown effect, due to changes in maternity service contracting processes and service provision. I do not have all the answers but we can examine some insights in the context of current knowledge.

Informed choice

There are several definitions available and often this term is used inter-changeably with informed decisions. They have two core characteristics. The decision should be based on relevant, good-quality information and the choice made should reflect the decision-maker's values. It becomes clear from this that maternity care professionals should ensure that women have access to all the appropriate information and the opportunity to clarify discuss further and to make a continuing choice. The MIDIRS *Informed Choice* leaflets present knowledge in an accessible way to professionals and women. They are explicit and open regarding the extent and robustness of the evidence as well as inviting women to actively consider what is important to them.

Philosophy of professional practice

The authority of the clinical expert still appeared to be paramount in most professionals working lives. The concept of evidence-based practice and knowledge being used to inform and assist women to make decisions about their care was in its infancy in everyday clinical practice. Few professionals appeared to be absolutely comfortable with sharing uncertainty about various interventions and being able to easily articulate relative risks and benefits of these interventions. Despite the maternity service having a published philos-ophy and a professional press which eschewed these concepts as a 'good thing', there was a huge gap with working reality. We underestimated the size of this gap and the time needed to support professionals to be competent and confident in understanding and working with these concepts in clinical prac-tice. This was the reality even though many midwives and doctors readily subscribed verbally to the philosophy of informed choice.

MIDIRS leaflets as a 'decision aid'

There are two particular systematic reviews about methods of assisting people to make informed decisions about their healthcare, which provide helpful information for reflection. Bekker *et al.* (1999) completed an annotated bibliography of 547 articles which included 336 RCTs, 114 non-randomised concurrent studies, 34 historical and 63 before and after same sample studies. Only 51 of the RCTs had a low risk of bias and few studies provided adequate descriptions of the intervention materials used to support informed decisions. They concluded that information and education are relatively ineffective ways of facilitating decision-making compared with context and social influences. They noted that studies reporting manipulation of information and provision of feedback were the most likely to report an effect. Women may or may not read widely, they will have their own sources of information, which may be well informed or poorly informed. The opportunity for women to make informed decisions with midwives and doctors during standard maternity care at the time of the project was:

- A booking interview which was crammed with information and task completion usually with very limited time, maximum of an hour. More than half of consultations were assisted by a health advocate.
- Time-limited antenatal consultations during busy antenatal clinics. Extra time was usually given if a problem was perceived. Usual allotted time was a maximum of 15 minutes, which included checking the history and a physical examination. The context did not encourage a woman to ask questions or support a midwife to answer them.

Other factors that need to be considered besides the limitations on time:

- The service information booklet which centred on contacts, geography, processes and some limited information about pregnancy and birth and breastfeeding.
- There was a plethora of poor quality local information sheets, Bounty booklets and Emma's Diary given to women.
- Antenatal classes/groups were variable in content, access and appropriateness. A very small percentage of women attended these.
- There was a barrier due to language, culture and access issues: 55 five per cent of women were Bangladeshi, the majority of whom were not literate in English or Sylheti.

O'Connor *et al.* (2001) systematically reviewed the use of 'decision aids'. These are interventions designed to help people to make specific and deliberate choices among options by providing information on the options and outcomes relevant to that individual's health status. Eighty-seven decision aids were reviewed, twenty-four of which had been evaluated in twenty-three

RCTs. They concluded that the use of decision aids are superior to usual care interventions in improving knowledge and sharing realistic expectations of the benefits and harms of options. They are also superior in reducing passivity in decision-making and lowering decisional conflict resulting from feeling uninformed. They were no better in affecting satisfaction with the decision-making process or in decreasing anxiety. Perhaps a degree of anxiety is a normal adaptive and helpful response to uncertainty. MIDIRS *Informed Choice* leaflets could be categorised as a decision aid. They present information that is relevant to professionals and to women as well as giving the option for women to access both leaflet versions. There is an expectation of feedback and of a decision being made. The evidence suggests that decision aids are superior to usual care interventions, which are not individualised, and there are demonstrable benefits from using them.

Implementation process

We assumed as a midwifery management team that we had the resources to undertake this project. Overarching this was the assumption that we had the resources to complete a wholescale re-engineering of the maternity services. The Health Authority and the Community Trust were completely committed to this. We were actually learning 'on the job'. There are skills which are beyond common sense to initiating, supporting and completing larger-scale projects. Integrating the *Informed Choice* leaflets into the maternity service turned out to be a much larger project than just arranging the continuing distribution of a variety of information leaflets. This required the recognition that they are decision aids, more than 'just another leaflet' and successful integration is dependent on new knowledge and new competencies in professional practice. We gained this knowledge as we went through the process of implementation.

The project scale demanded a competency in project management methodology. The Community Trust Management Team recognised the need for this training. Everyone with responsibility for leading different projects in the Trust was funded to complete four-day training in a formal accredited project management course. They also provided the IT technology needed to support the efficient running of the projects, which occurred after the launch of the leaflets.

Organisation of maternity care

During the implementation process, barriers to successful implementation emerged and maternity service professionals clearly articulated specific issues. These included organisational barriers of time, opportunity, too heavy a workload and professional practice barriers of differing philosophies, lack of knowledge, lack of skills. It is pertinent to revisit the organisational factors which support women being encouraged and able to make continuing informed choices about their maternity care (Figure 8.1). These group practice midwives agreed and had commitment to a philosophy of professional practice of partnership with a woman. They had the requisite knowledge and skills to enable a woman to make informed decisions. They had the structures in their working lives which provided several and repeated opportunities to support women making these decisions. For example, the use of written and visual resources in a practice library with a loan system and the provision of facilitating groups every week for discussion and learning. The learning was equally from other women sharing their experiences, which contributed to informing the local social culture of birth. They provided a lengthy antenatal consultation equivalent to the booking visit around 36 weeks gestation. This was known as the birth talk and was the time to review the pregnancy, share knowledge and help a woman to make informed decisions about labour, birth and infant feeding based on her unique situation. They had control systems in place to maintain the quality of their practice. Crucially these centred on assuring that there was time to listen to women and for discussion at every consultation. They controlled the number of women they cared for so that they were not required to continually overstretch their resources. Organising care through midwifery provision by the same two midwives throughout antenatal, labour and postnatal period maximises the opportunity for a relationship of trust in which a woman is more likely to ask questions, voice uncertainty and expects a helpful response. Systematic reviews of some of the interventions that the midwives used have been linked with a significant reduction in various obstetric interventions including operative and assisted delivery (see Box 8.5).

Box 8.5 Interventions that decrease maternal morbidity

- Partnership model of caseload practice midwifery (Page *et al.*, 2001)

- Continuity of midwifery care (Waldenstrom *et al.*, 1997)

o Sharing information and actively supporting informed choice regarding interventions which support an increased chance of spontaneous vaginal birth and a reduction in obstetric interventions

1. Offering planned home birth (Olsen, 1997)

2. Delayed admission to labour ward through home assessment in labour (Hodnett, 2001)

3. Mobility in labour and upright positions in second stage (Gupta and Nikodem, 1995; Albers *et al.*, 1997)

4. Use of waterpool for labour/birth (Burns, 2001)

I think that a key factor in this particular organisation of maternity care was that the women using their service had the opportunity to be cared for by professionals whose clinical practice was aligned with the evidence that was being shared with the women. There was coherence between, information, policy and practice as well as several guaranteed opportunities for each individual woman to receive information, discuss and clarify prior to making informed choices.

The evidence on the process of implementation of any change to secure an improvement is that it usually needs to be a package of interventions rather than a single intervention. Grimshaw and Russell (1993) commented that the effectiveness of implementing clinical guidelines in improvements in outcomes was dependent on several variables which included use of a local strategy for use, specific education package and a reminder for use with individual patients at the time of consultation. Burr *et al.* (2001) undertook an RCT using an 'intervention package' to promote the increased use of ECV at term in women with babies presenting by the breech. The package consisted of literature, practice guidelines and a workshop for consultant obstetricians on ECV. The intervention resulted in a significant increase in the percentage of women being offered an ECV with an increase from 19 per cent to 36 per cent. This was still the minority of women. The authors commented that the intervention was less effective because only one consultant obstetrician was targeted in each maternity unit and that to increase the effect more professionals needed to be targeted.

Conclusion

The decision to integrate the MIDIRS *Informed Choice* leaflets into Tower Hamlets maternity service was supported by government policy, the local health authority, the trust board and by the maternity management team. Funding was secured for set-up as well as ongoing costs of leaflet supply. We identified and experienced many of the published barriers to successful implementation. We made too many assumptions about professional culture and practice, grossly underestimating the cultural shift required as well as the scope and size of professional skills and competencies that needed to be learnt. Introducing a decision aid such as the MIDIRS *Informed Choice* leaflets exposed the gap between rhetoric and reality which needs to be bridged before successfully integrating this or perhaps any decision aid.

References

Albers, L.L. *et al.* (1997) The relationship of ambulation in labour to operative delivery. *J.Nurse Midwif.*, **42(1)**: 4–8.

Bekker, H., Thornton, J.G., Airey, C.M., Connelly, J.B. *et al.* (1999) Informed decision-making: an annotated bibliography and systematic review. In *Health Technology Assessment*, **3(1)** (executive summary).

Burns, E. (2001) Waterbirth. *MIDIRS Midwifery Digest,* **11** supplement 2: 10– 13.

Burr, R., Johansen, R., Wyatt, J. *et al.* (2001) A randomised trial of an intervention package designed to promote ECV at term. *European Journal of Obstetrics and Gynaecology and Reproductive* Biology, **100(1)**: 36–40.

Demilew, J. (1994) South East London Midwifery Group Practice. *MIDIRS Midwifery Digest,* **4**: 3.

Department of Health (1993) *Changing Childbirth* Part 1: *Expert Maternity Group.* London: HMSO.

Grimshaw, J.M. and Russell, I.T. (1993) Effect of clinical guidelines on medical practice. A systematic review of rigorous evaluations. *Lancet,* **342**: 1317–22.

Gupta, J.K. and Nikodem, V.C. (1995) Position for women during the second stage of labour. (Cochrane Review) *The Cochrane Library,* **2**. Oxford: Update Software.

Hodnett, E.D. (2002) Continuity of caregivers during pregnancy and childbirth. (Cochrane Review) *The Cochrane Library,* **2**. Oxford:Update Software.

O'Connor, A.M., Stacey, D., Rovner, D., Holmes-Rovner, M. *et al.* (2001) Decision aids for people facing health treatment or screening decisions (Cochrane Review). *The Cochrane Library,* **4**. Oxford: Update Software.

Olsen, O. (1997) Meta-analysis of the safety of homebirth. *Birth,* **24(1)**: 4–13.

Page, L., Beake, S., Vail, A., McCourt, *et al.* (2001) Clinical outcomes of one-to-one midwifery practice. *British Journal of Midwifery,* **9(11)**.

Waldenstrom, U., Nilsson, C.A., Windblach, B. (1997) The Stockholm Birth Centre Trial: maternal and infant outcomes. *British Journal of Obstetrics and Gynaecology,* **104(4)**: 210–18.

CHAPTER 9

Should Doctors Perform Caesarean for 'Informed Choice' Alone?

SUSAN BEWLEY AND JAYNE COCKBURN

Chapter Contents

- Introduction

- Ethics

- Risk/benefit?

- Mother

- Baby

- Basic medical concepts

- Professional vested interests

- Women's changing status

- How should we respond to 'requests'?

- Unanswered research questions

- Conclusion

Introduction

A powerful debate is taking place in the medical (Paterson-Brown, 1998; Amu *et al.*, 1998; Belizan *et al.*, 1999) and lay press (Corrigan, 1997; Fisk and Savage, 1997; Hope, 2000) regarding elective Caesarean section (CS) for 'maternal request' even in normal uncomplicated pregnancy. As two obstetricians who are motivated by a desire to help and empower women through ensuring their best possible health, we have struggled intellectually and professionally to understand and deal with this new phenomenon.

It is normal (indeed rational) for women to fear childbirth. Childbirth is inherently unpredictable and painful, and accompanied by a small risk of serious morbidity or even death for both the mother and child. Most women cope with, and overcome, their fears. A small minority have extreme fear or anxiety, or request a Caesarean section (CS) in the absence of a medical problem. Conversely, some women are unable to consent to wanted intervention in the face of a compelling indication (e.g. a refusal of CS due to needle phobia) (*Re MB*, 1997). Whilst obstetricians have taken women to court for interventions in the fetal interest (Kolder *et al.*, 1987), they have not been so critical of elective CS on 'request', despite concerns that it is unethical and harmful to both mothers and babies (FIGO, 1999; Wagner, 2000). What should an obstetrician do if a woman presents to the antenatal clinic asking for CS, claiming to have made a well-balanced rational decision with plenty of information, maybe even having discussed it with her midwife (e.g. because she has a family history, 'big baby' or previous CS). If she denies that the request is fuelled by anxiety, should an obstetrician acquiesce, or is it 'paternalistic' to suggest that nature should generally be left alone?

Traditionally, interventions (instrumental or CS) with known and accepted complications are offered when the benefits outweigh risk. CS rates are rising worldwide. 'Request' CS has been proposed as a prophylactic means to avoid the small risks and uncertainties of labour (Paterson-Brown, 1998) and as a fulfilment of women's informed choices. Others argue that elective CS is not safer than labour (if it were, it should be offered to all), and that the duty of care does not encompass surgery on request. Presently, obstetricians are caught in a dilemma. If they believe surgery requires a medical indication, they must reassure, talk anxious women into facing their fear (without proper training) or get into conflict with their patient (a person who attends a doctor for care). If they accede to requests, they may have listened to the presented problem but be performing unnecessary surgery, wasting resources and failing to deal with underlying trait fear and anxiety. The implicit message of CS on 'request' (as surely doctors would not knowingly harm patients) is that it must be better, thus reinforcing cultural apprehensions.

Women want a healthy baby, to emerge from childbirth physically and psychologically intact and to avoid perceived problems. It is moot whether obstetricians wish to avoid interventions per se (as the need for medical skills vindicates their profession). On the other hand midwives too have vested interests; in non-interventionist childbirth as they cannot offer otherwise. The undisputed existence of complications in a minority of labours does not justify medical intervention or 'prophylaxis' (Paterson-Brown, 1998) as non-indicated CS might cause more harm than good. Definitive evidence from randomised trials or complex decision analysis (using Bayesianism, neural networks and/or systematic reviews) does not yet exist.

What we want to do in this chapter is firstly to look in detail at ethical arguments about 'informed choice' (which we do not find exists for obstetric interventions), and then the medical arguments. There are two distinct arguments any party proposing elective CS for 'request' might use; either (1) elective CS is *safer* than labour or (2) safety is not the issue but women's *informed choices* should be paramount, even if choosing a harmful operation without a medical indication. Proponents tend to use both arguments though only one is necessary and sufficient. The real debate thus gets confused for both professionals and women.

Ethics

Interventions with inevitable harms have to be justified by doctors, and patients have to give valid and informed consent to them. Doing nothing in the face of normality does not have to be justified. Thus the onus of both ethical and clinical proof is on the interventionist side.

Traditional versions of obstetricians' ethical duties

Professionally, doctors have an ethical and legal duty of care. That means making judgements about individuals in the light of real information (which is often incomplete). The General Medical Council states that patients have a right to decide whether or not 'to undergo medical intervention even where a refusal may result in harm or death' (General Medical Council, 1998). That negative right is quite different from a positive right to insist upon an intervention that the doctor is obliged to give. It is unclear whether any such positive ethical or legal right exists. Because society has great respect for bodily integrity and the right not to be interfered with, obstetricians cannot perform a CS to save the life of a baby of a competent mother (or her own life) without consent (Dyer, 1997). Obstetricians have become confused about negative rights to refuse intervention (the CS without consent) and non-existent but postulated positive rights to have non-indicated intervention (the CS on request). The International Federation of Obstetrics and Gynaecology (FIGO) Committee for the Ethical Aspects of Human Reproduction has submitted that it is unethical to perform a CS without a medical indication because of inadequate evidence to support a net benefit (FIGO, 1999). It has been even been suggested that 'a physician who merely spreads an array of vendibles in front of the patient and then says, "go ahead and choose, its your life" is guilty of shirking his duty, if not of malpractice' (Ingelfinger, 1980).

Putting traditional arguments and governing bodies aside, the ethical arguments are:

(1) If elective CS is genuinely safer than labour it is both medically indicated and ethically vindicated on a risk-benefit assessment (as with traditional indications). Doctors should do good and avoid harm (beneficence and non-maleficence). Indeed, it would actually become unethical for obstetricians not to offer CS to all women (within resource allocation and justice

constraints). The maternal request is almost immaterial (though a woman could still refuse the offer and choose the riskier path of natural childbirth);

(2) Alternatively, a doctor's duty is to respect women's requests (respecting her autonomy) even when harmful. If safety is no longer the issue, doctors must have a duty to fulfil an 'informed choice' (paid for privately or by the NHS), even if the operation is not medically indicated and more dangerous.

(3) A third claim is sometimes made: that information is inadequate to be clear about which sets of risks are preferable and therefore choice can reasonably be included in the equation. Doctors should acquiesce to requests rather than dictate to patients and risk being paternalistic. Illustrations from history are an embarrassing reminder to any doctor who feels they know best. However, (3) is not a distinct argument. It is a claim that CS appears as safe as not (1) and that women's choices should be respected (2). Paucity of information does not introduce a new issue. Individual circumstances will be included in doctors' assessment of risk-benefit, and the risk of harm will factor in women's decision-making. But either 'first of all, do no harm' or 'respect autonomy' must prevail. If medical risks are evenly weighed or unknown then there is enough uncertainty for (and ethics demands) further research and trials. When tested, one option may prove to have more, less or equivalent benefit and harm. The language of 'choice' is used as rhetoric to persuade. Lessons from history do not solely concern paternalism, but also fads and unanticipated damage.

We will look at safety issues later but analyse 'informed choice' first.

Is 'informed choice' paramount?

If obstetricians really believed informed choice was the paramount duty then it would be appropriate, indeed obligatory, to deliver by CS for maternal choice, after full discussion, whether at 34 weeks with painful anterior fibroids or in normal multiparas in progressive labour. Obstetricians presently do not agree to every request for early induction or CS precisely because of the known harms to both mother and baby. When put in stark terms, most doctors consider that not causing harm outweighs fulfilling informed choices. Taking women's views seriously is ordinary good clinical practice but it is not the overriding consideration in decision-making. When doctors offer choices, or a range of treatment options, but confine them to within a certain set of risks, then the basic ethical principle is still non-maleficence, not autonomy.

'Autonomy' is used as some kind of trump card as if it was a simple, linear and undisputed concept. Frankfurt (1971) has written eloquently about different and competing levels of desire and characterises true human freedom of the will as the ability to formulate second-order desires (to want to want something). Uncomplicated childbirth is not an unreasonable desire, but keeping this a second-order desire allows other factors (modes of delivery) to be considered and the reality of complications can be entertained and coped with without them being seen as a major threat to personal identity. Babies are only born via two routes and women (should rightly) have fears about both.

It is important to understand that numerous things may interfere with autonomy (ranging from illness, delirium and impaired mental capacity to misinformation, phobias, prior abuse and fears). It is unprofessional not to take these into account, especially if there are medical remedies, and unethical to exaggerate the dangers. It would be wrong, manipulative and potentially dangerous for midwives or obstetricians to claim to be pro-women and yet reinforce fears (whether the fears are about childbirth or interventions) rather than acknowledge the problems and manage them appropriately. One woman may want a CS to save her baby but be overcome by her phobia of needles. Another woman may want to deliver a baby vaginally but be overwhelmed by guilt and fear from a past history of herpes. It is more complex than the simplistic words of 'choice' or 'request' imply.

In addition, there is a difficult interplay between safety and choice, particularly if a woman anticipates labour or experiences a refusal of CS as a harm in itself. The woman who is frightened and unwilling to labour might well become psychologically or psychiatrically damaged if she does (e.g. post-traumatic stress disorder or tokophobia) (Hofberg and Brockington, 2000), but this may then revert to a medical (or psychological) indication and doctors should obtain appropriate assessments and treatments.

Even if doctors genuinely believe in fulfilling informed choices regardless of other ethical considerations, there is presently inadequate unbiased literature to help women. There are no standard evidence-based (or even uncertainty-based) leaflets (such as the MIDIRS *Informed Choice* leaflets) to help women make any postulated choice. Work from other areas suggests very poor quality counselling about choices (Abramsky *et al.*, 2001). Who knows what properly informed and assessed women prefer? CS rates, especially for 'request', are very variable, suggesting that women presently are not given full unbiased information and so remain susceptible to cultural, media and medical fashion.

Ethical consistency (personal and professional)

Another complexity that has been brought into the debate is that of consistency of professional and personal practice. One lone small study on London obstetricians has captured the popular imagination, and is repeatedly misquoted to back the 'choice' side of the debate (Al-Mufti *et al.*, 1997), despite its finding that the vast majority of obstetricians would choose labour as do other studies (McGurgan *et al.*, 2001), and as would midwives (Dickson and Willett, 1999). The argument runs that if a few obstetricians want, and obtain, elective CS then it should also be offered to patients, presumably because otherwise we are behaving hypocritically. But why? If a minority request CS, so what? Obstetricians may not be personally objective: they may be self-selected by their mothers or families' obstetric disasters; they are vulnerable human beings who may be biased by their exposure to the complications of childbirth. There is no need to have consistency between professional and personal lives. An insistence on an ethic of consistency actually leads to the conclusion that doctors who cannot objectively balance risks for themselves or their families should not be allowed to practise. That surely cannot be the conclusion intended by constantly quoting the survey?

Comparing harms to mothers and babies

Further complexity arises when comparing harms to babies and mothers, only one of whom can make a 'choice' that might harm the other. It would be easy if medical risks and benefits lined up with one another, but is more difficult as they do not. Let us imagine that it was universally agreed that elective CS was better for babies than labour yet harmful to women. Generally people cannot be compelled to harm themselves on behalf of another. However, if a woman made an 'informed choice' to harm herself on behalf of her child this could not be seen as selfish, but commendable and altruistic. On the other hand, if elective CS was proven to be better for mothers but dangerous for babies, with short and long term mortality and morbidity, most obstetricians would be reluctant to participate in deliberate harm, and 'informed choice' would not make it right to do so.

As mothers generally want to do their best for babies and doctors would not knowingly harm them, the mere discussion of 'informed choice' in a public arena sounds as though the medical risk-benefit argument is concluded. It can give the impression that elective CS is conclusively better for the baby (which we discuss later) and that obstetricians are convinced labour is dangerous.

Even taking CS for fetal indications (e.g. severe premature growth restriction or the term breech) there are further technical and ethical questions; (1) How many CSs are necessary to save one life? (2) How much maternal mortality, morbidity and future risk justifies saving the life of one baby? The only situations in which the ethical balancing is easy is where a foetus is considered of no worth (so mothers' views about harm come into play) or infinite worth (thus every attempt must be made to save). If a mother is of lesser moral worth than her baby then the more harmful route (whether that is CS or labour) will be easily justified on fetal grounds. An automatic presumption for the baby, dismissing maternal harm, can be interpreted as misogynist (a negative image the obstetric profession does not need).

It is not even mother *v.* baby in an isolated pregnancy. There are issues for other children and future pregnancies (with their increased risk). If a CS caused postnatal harm or discomfort, distracting women from mothering (e.g. less ability to care for small children, or lower breastfeeding rates) then this brings child harm issues onto both sides of the ethical weighing scales.

Risk/benefit?

Within the safety assessment there remain ethical issues. The relevant outcomes are mortality and morbidity (physical and psychological, short- and long-term) for both the mother and the baby. Trading outcomes against one another presents a complex matrix. Does our professional view matter? Would individual women have a different ranking, and how easy is it for them to be objective before the event? This comes back to good quality information, such as it exists, and how it is interpreted and imparted. There is plenty of research about the harms of childbirth and its interventions and yet it is being distorted on both sides of the debate. To maintain objective decision-making in the face of a barrage of medico-legal, media and emotional concerns is difficult and it would be easy for women and doctors to slip into a short-term approach of doing CS as the easy way out. Clement (1995) suggests that 'the belief that a Caesarean delivery is the easy way does not appear to come from facts about Caesarean birth itself but rather from deeply rooted fears about vaginal childbirth'. Is it fear, or simply that obstetricians are rightly more relaxed about the dangers of CS and focusing more on the recently and incompletely researched complications of vaginal delivery (Bump and Norton, 1998)?

Mother

Maternal mortality

Unusually, the 1994–6 Confidential Enquiry did not attempt a case fatality rate for CS (Department of Health 1994, 1997; NICE 2001) restricting the safety debate. Lilford *et al.* (1990), trying to isolate mortality due to elective CS in previously healthy women found a 3.8 relative risk (elective *v.* vaginal delivery: 23:6 deaths/100,000). This would equate to a 1 in 4262 maternal death rate for mothers having elective CS which seems high, particularly compared to unproven claims of avoidable intrapartum fetal death. A more recent study from the Netherlands (Schuitemaker *et al.*, 1997) found a similar relative risk of 3.25 (and death rate of 13/100,000). Extrapolated estimates (Table 9.1), show that elective CS death rates can be up to as much as eight times higher and in the last Confidential Enquiry period would be at least three times higher (Hall and Bewley, 1999) than vaginal delivery. Numerous studies have recorded the higher risk of CS delivery, not all of which can be accounted for by the complications which necessitated the operation (Frigoletto *et al.*, 1980; Pettiti *et al.*, 1992; Moldin *et al.*, 1984; Rouse *et al.*, 1996). Proponents of CS point out that the relative risk of elective CS might fall further with increasing safety procedures, e.g. use of epidural anaesthesia, antibiotics, thromboprophy-

Table 9.1 Case fatality rate by mode of delivery for last three Confidential Enquiries

	1988–90			1994–96			1997–99		
Mode of delivery	Number (000s)	Direct deaths	Rate per million cases	Number (000s)	Direct deaths	Rate per million cases	Number (000s)	Direct deaths	Rate per million cases
Vaginal	2,082	37	17.8	1,846	38	20.6	1,710	29	16.9
Elective CS	128	19	148.3	154	9	58.5			
							413 *	34	82.3
Emergency CS	150	38	252.7	198	36	182.0			

Note:
* New classification system used. Maternal death rate per million cases for elective CS = 38.5, scheduled CS = 12.8, urgent CS = 102.2, emergency CS = 202.9.

laxis, etc. However we must use what figures we have, as vaginal delivery too becomes less mortal with increasing use of the same procedures in an increasingly healthy population. There are rare risks in multiple medical interventions, such as allergic anaphylaxis, which may become more significant in the future and maternal mortality must be watched particularly in countries with the highest and rising CS rates.

Even if vaginal delivery is safer than elective CS, the real risk-benefit calculation is between labour (which might end in an emergency CS) and elective CS, and thus becomes critically dependent on the emergency CS rate. The only hard data on this comes from a meta-analysis of all the randomised breech trials which found an increased risk of maternal death or severe early morbidity (RR 1.29, 95 per cent confidence interval 1.03 to 1.61), and this despite a high emergency CS rate of 45 per cent in the labour arm (Hofmeyer and Hannah, 2001). This nearly 30 per cent increase is likely to be an underestimate for cephalic presentation with its higher vaginal delivery rate. A laissez-faire attitude to elective CS sends a mistaken signal to the public and professionals alike that all CSs are safe and the 'request' debate can be misinterpreted as such. A reduction in the threshold for emergency CS increases the dangers for labouring women (Waterstone *et al.*, 2001) in this and future pregnancies (as 67 per cent of women will have further CSs) (Thomas and Paranjothy, 2001). A vicious cycle can be set up whereby high emergency CS rates fuel further loss of confidence and raise CS rates, making elective CS relatively more attractive. Working towards optimum safety in childbirth must mean increasing the rate of uncomplicated vaginal delivery. As emergency CS in labour is the worst mode of delivery in terms of maternal morbidity, concentrating on the quality of intrapartum care should be our priority. Surely, the real obstetric debate today, with the highest intervention rates on record, is how to achieve this.

Morbidity

New, unexpected long-term risks of CS continue to be reported such as ectopic pregnancy (Hemminki and Merilainen, 1996), haemorrhage and hysterectomy following uterine evacuation (Lo *et al.*, 2000), latex allergy (Chen *et al.*, 1999), cutaneous endometriosis (Scholefield *et al.*, 2000), adenomyosis (Whitted *et al.*, 2000), increased hospital readmission and even an increase in gallbladder disease and appendicitis (Lydon-Rochelle *et al.*, 2000). Straightforward tables of complications could be formulated with inclusions depending on the severity and degree of risk. However these do not rank risks e.g. risk of UTI *v.* potentially life threatening haemorrhage. Nor are there tools to help us agree how much low risk should be accepted in order to avoid a rarer but potentially serious or lethal complication. Whilst some work has begun to look at decision analysis (Rouse and Owen, 1999) we do not have an ethical framework. Without this preparatory analysis, all counselling is personal and biased, affected by clinical experience. Using a more research based approach to reviewing complications reveals a voluminous amount of information on the complications of different modes of delivery but it is variable in quality and coverage and can be biased by enthusiasm or omission of negative trials. Whilst the medical profession debates the risks and benefits for different modes of management, the press and the public hear that the debate is about 'rights and wrongs' and so popular beliefs, myths and dogma are generated.

Morbidity of mythological proportions

Problems arising after birth are often attributed to labour and delivery. This scares and undermines women's ability to successfully undergo a normal process. Often this blaming occurs without good supporting evidence or, worse still, when opposing evidence suggests it is the pregnancy or life event changes that are contributory. Doctors must be sympathetic to women injured during vaginal delivery, but should distinguish between morbidity occurring after birth and that caused by it. A good example is the belief that childbirth inevitably damages the pelvic floor, often makes women incontinent of urine, and that CS is protective. Evidence suggests that much pelvic floor weakening is due to pregnancy, most incontinence settles or is treatable and CS is not completely protective. Nevertheless the dogma sticks.

The two common reasons for urinary incontinence in women are genuine stress incontinence (GSI) and detrusor instability (DI). Whilst pregnancy is likely to be a factor for GSI there is no known cause for DI in healthy women. Researchers have found that women in whom stress incontinence develops late in life are probably destined to do so from an early age. Heredity and pregnancy, rather than parturition, reveal the defect (Iosif, 1981; Beck and Hsu, 1965). The damage that is inflicted appears to be in those predisposed (King and Freeman, 1998) by development of antenatal stress incontinence

(Dimpfl *et al.*, 1992; Marshall *et al.*, 1998) or collagen disorders (Keane *et al.*, 1997). 62 per cent of primigravidae with incontinence say it started in pregnancy (Wilson *et al.*, 1996; Viktrup *et al.*, 1992; Beck and Hsu, 1965) and other workers find incontinence rarely if ever starts after childbirth (Francis, 1960; Stanton *et al.*, 1980). Where women are continent, CS is only 20 per cent protective and only for the first CS. Where repeat CSs are performed the protection is lost. By the third there is no benefit with 35 per cent of women suffering the symptom (Wilson *et al.*, 1996). The mechanism is thought to be due to vesical denervation (Parys *et al.*, 1989) which also increases the risk of detrusor instability, actually more important when looking at incontinence in old age. In older women DI (probably due to age changes in both the central nervous system and in the lower urinary tract) is the main cause for incontinence, made worse by immobility and sub-optimal nursing. 10 per cent of old people have GSI and DI (Royal College of Physicians, 1995).

So, whilst there might be an argument about diminution of incontinence (still as yet unproven) it would only apply to a minority of women. Future work should address these women and information should be given about possible treatments whichever route delivery takes. Antenatal pelvic floor exercises are helpful in prevention but not widely promulgated (Wilson *et al.*, 1996). Other risk factors for incontinence are having more than 4 children (Wilson *et al.*, 1996) and obesity consistent with non-pregnant weights of >120 per cent average weight (Wilson *et al.*, 1996; Dwyer *et al.*, 1988). If CS were to be proven protective, evidence-based incontinence prevention might be to offer it to the more obese planning large families whilst obstetricians could reassure slim women planning one child they are low risk.

Another recent concern is that women will become incontinent of faeces. Sultan *et al.*'s work (1994) has shown a 0.6 per cent frequency of documented anal sphincter tears and demonstrated a disappointing inadequacy of primary repair. However, there is confusion about symptoms and ultrasound findings. An ultrasound finding in normal controls of 33 per cent anal sphincter disruption (Sultan *et al.*, 1993) does not mean a third of women will have faecal incontinence (just as 100 per cent rectus sheath disruption at CS does not mean all suffer abdominal wall morbidity). It has been suggested that a moratorium on episiotomies would have greater impact on women's faecal continence and quality of life than further increases in CS rates (Girard, 1999). Whilst recent researchers blame anal sphincter tears, others blame long second stages with consequent nerve damage (Smith *et al.*, 1985) though the role of pudendal nerve damage and its recovery is now debated (Snooks *et al.*, 1985; Allen *et al.*, 1990; Sultan *et al.*, 1997). The role of constipation has currently been left out. It worsens with increased parity, and straining may have an effect on the pudendal nerve (Marshall *et al.*, 1997). The 'protective effect' of CS even after sphincter repair is debated by researchers in this field (Tetzschner and Lose, 1997; Nygaard *et al.*, 1997). Long-term, the incidence of faecal incontinence in older men is as high as in women, suggesting other mechanisms apart from childbirth are important (Johansen *et al.*, 1997; Read *et al.*, 1995; Johansen and Lafferty, 1996). Awareness of risks and targeting high-risk women for anoendoscopy and neuro-physiology should help ensure women do not live with chronic incapacitating symptoms, with most women benefiting from normal delivery (Sultan and Stanton, 1996). Undoubtedly, we are nowadays more aware of pelvic floor problems but are not yet doing enough to prevent and obviate them. Despite randomised trial evidence of antenatal perineal massage preventing trauma, few units practise this routinely (Labreque *et al.*, 1999). If concerns about childbirth damage are overplayed, anxiety in both obstetricians and women will be increased.

A related fear about damage to the perineum is that of dyspareunia and wrecking of sex life and relationship. The myth has grown that CS keeps the vagina 'honeymoon fresh' and presumably therefore relationships intact. Apart from the contradiction of 'honeymoon fresh' in a pregnant woman, what does this belief reveal? How much of a woman's identity and self-esteem reside in her vagina? What factors in men's and women's sexuality make them adapt or fail to adapt to the change childbirth brings? Whatever the culturally based attitude, what approach should doctors take? Recent work on postnatal symptomatology shows that dyspareunia and failed resumption of sexual intercourse at six months post childbirth are the same whether delivery is spontaneous vaginal, instrumental or CS (Barrett *et al.*, 2000). Something more complex is going on. If a doctor does a CS purportedly to keep the vagina the same, not only may it fail to preserve a fragile relationship (threatened by the new family member, sleeplessness and prior commitment), it may inadvertently reinforce problems of adaptation post birth. Offering surgery as the primary treatment of normal anxiety around childbirth does not acknowledge the genuine concerns around changing relationships and the loss of control of daily life that children bring. If concerns are not addressed, men are left out, couples are not aided through this life transition and parents may be less well prepared for childrearing.

New work on anxiety offers an insight to the importance of deep listening, and some common ground rather than polarisation. Anxiety has been associated with pregnancy complications (Wadha *et al.*, 1993; Kurki *et al.*, 2000), emergency CS in labour (Ryding *et al.*, 1998), postnatal depression and impaired bonding (Denyttenacre *et al.*, 1995; Neilson Forman *et al.*, 2000). Attention has focused on early identification of anxiety, intervention and effective treatment. In a recent Finnish study (Saisto *et al.*, 2001), 178 anxious low-risk women with no contraindication to vaginal delivery were identified, either by CS request or a specific screening questionnaire. Women were studied at recruitment, 36 weeks and 3 months postpartum, received information about the pros and cons of vaginal and CS delivery, and had routine appointments with the study (psychotherapeutically trained) obstetrician. The study was powered for a primary endpoint of 50 per cent reduction in CS rate from intensive *v.* conventional therapy; the intervention included three additional 45-minute appointments for cognitive therapy with the obstetrician, a 90-minute appointment with the midwife and visits to the ward for practical information. Of the 117 women who initially requested CS, 62 per cent chose to deliver vaginally (a non-significant decrease in elective CS for psychosocial reasons in the intensive and conventional groups, 24 per cent *v.* 29 per cent). Intention-to-treat analysis of other outcome measures showed lower birth concerns, lower pregnancy anxiety scales and shorter labours (6.8 *v.* 8.5hrs, p = .039) in the intensive therapy group, but no difference in use of epidural or postnatal depression. Although intensive therapy did not significantly reduce CS rate, treatment effects may have been contaminated by the relationship with the same obstetrician in both groups. The group of women avoiding the intervention had the highest CS rate. Although this is a small RCT, the findings are consistent with previous work, and powerful through the demonstration of anxiety reduction and shorter labour (thus making it safer, less painful and more likely to end with a normal vaginal delivery and satisfied mother).

At its extreme, for example after sexual abuse, a bad experience of health care or previous labour, a woman may be petrified of labour. In these situations, the primary appropriate management would be psychological support and only then consideration of a CS for preventative mental health indication. It has been documented that in some instances refusal of CS results in severe psychiatric problems (Hofberg and Brockington, 2000). Referral to an interested psychologist or psychiatrist should be performed in the same way as referral to medical colleagues for medical problems affecting pregnancy. If women with extreme fear of delivery are referred to a psychosomatic clinic for individualised counselling as many as 56 per cent opt for trial of vaginal delivery and 44 per cent for elective CS (Sjogren and Thomassen, 1997). Within the group of women requesting elective CS are some with bizarre attitudes who may bring forward the date of delivery by request, emotional pressure or deceit (Anwar and O'Mahoney, 2000). To perform CS for 'request' or anxiety without first offering professional midwifery and psychological support is unethical as there is evidence they work. On the other hand, to refuse a CS for a woman who has unresolvable severe anxiety, previous traumatic experience or genuine tokophobia is also unethical and cruel – but these women too may benefit from the same professionals even if having elective CS. The need for pain relief, length of labour and assisted delivery are decreased with continuity of carer (Hodnett, 2000). This leads to a practical and realistic way to handle women, by the setting up of multi-disciplinary services, for individualised assessment and planning. Psychologists could lead initiatives to train others to screen, offer simple therapy or make referrals. With a little time and inclination, we can use cheap and effective tools to intervene with long-term effect. If vulnerable pregnant women do not have the option of psychological treatments they will not be empowered to take control of their lives and bodies during this most defining of life changes.

It is hard enough for women to give birth and become mothers, let alone cope with the loss of control of emotions, sleep, daily life, relationships, finances and career progress. CS may give an illusion of control (to mother and surgeon), but miss what is really going on and make postnatal adaptation worse. We need continuing research, and in the meantime devise appropriate care for women and guidelines for midwives and obstetricians. Services should be designed around early screening or detection and prompt referral. It takes time and skill to elicit complex fears or histories of sexual abuse or to devise plans for women with previous stillbirth or traumatic labour. Intrauterine death, premature labour and precipitate delivery may supervene, so all women still have to contemplate and plan for vaginal delivery. Obstetricians have to take requests seriously, but not necessarily accept them at presented face value. The danger in not recognising fears and phobias but renaming them 'requests' or even 'rights' is that they remain unaddressed and reinforced. If obstetricians consider labour destructive and dangerous they will not be able to pass on any confidence in women to labour.

The evidence to date for normal delivery with minimal complications is that women do better with continuity of care and supportive companions. Good obstetricians who recognise our respective contributions should be working with and fighting for midwives, doulas, psychologists and other support staff. There is a national shortage of midwives, compounded in London by inexperience and high turnover. Insufficient midwives is a dismal indication for CS but may be part of the explanation of why this debate has come from the capital.

Baby

Mortality

There has been a consistent reduction in the perinatal mortality rate (PNMR) over the last 100 years, though this is as likely to be due to improved social conditions, healthier mothers and neonatal intensive care as obstetric practice (Savage, 1979). The relationship between rising CS rates and the PNMR is not consistent, questioning whether CS benefits the neonate (Thiery and Derom, 1986). In the United States, where CS rates have increased year on year since 1965, there is no evidence that maternal and child health has improved as a result (Department of Health and Human Services, 1991). The World Health Organisation pointed out in 1985 that the countries with some of the lowest perinatal mortality rates in the world had CS rates under 10 per cent and that thus there was no justification in any specific geographical region to have more than 10–15 per cent CS births (WHO, 1985).

The current UK PNMR is 7.9 per thousand births (CESDI, 2001), largely still related to prematurity and congenital abnormality and with a propensity to occur in lower social classes. It is odd that the current vogue for elective CS has come from the more affluent south-east and social classes not traditionally associated with high PNMR.

The antenatal stillbirth rate has remained static compared to the overall reduction in PNMR. Proponents of 'request' CS have speculated that elective CS at 38 weeks could be offered to prevent one intrauterine death (IUD) between 38 weeks and delivery per 600 pregnancies (Hilder *et al.*, 1998) (or 1 in 730 unexplained stillbirths)(Cotzias *et al.*, 1999). It is even postulated that 1 death per 1500 births of babies of >1.5kg in labour (CESDI, 1997), 1 term intrapartum stillbirth per 5000 births, 1 case of hypoxic-ischaemic encephalopathy per 1750 births and 10 per cent of cases of cerebral palsy would be avoided by a policy of elective CS (Paterson-Brown, 1998). Seductive though this sounds, the logic is that considerably more stillbirths and late pregnancy complications would be avoided by offering CS at 32 weeks. This is not suggested because it is more obvious that iatrogenic damage has been left out of the calculations. The assumption that CS is protective for babies is neither robust nor proven. Perinatal deaths occur even in normal babies after elective CS at term (as high as 1.6 per cent in the term breech trial (Hannah *et al.*, 2000) and 0.5 per cent in an observational study of repeat CS (McMahon *et al.*, 1996)). The analytical difficulty is that elective CS numbers are smaller than emergency, statistics are not available and CESDI does not analyse by mode of delivery. With less than 10 per cent of deliveries occurring by elective CS, and even less in low-risk pregnancies, rare adverse outcomes and death would not be immediately apparent.

In addition, there might be an excess infant morbidity or mortality in the first year and beyond, which we presently will miss. Imagine two babies conceived on the same day, with the same due date. If the first is delivered electively by CS at 38 weeks and the second by spontaneous labour at 40 weeks, the first has to live to a year and 2 weeks to reach the same time point as the second for a true comparison of stillbirth and infant mortality risks. Assessing the first at one year post-birth artificially decreases the time period of risk by 4 per cent. Infant mortality statistics cannot pick up the effect of iatrogenic early delivery if the reduction in born life is not accounted for. Conventional measures of infant mortality or cot death (known to be associated with prematurity) (Malloy and Hoffman, 1995) will underestimate any adverse effects as the extra born life after pre-labour delivery is not being taken into account in current audit or research calculations.

Morbidity

Whether CS prevents death, fails to prevent death, or even causes death, this is separate from immediate and long-term effects of premature abdominal delivery on children's health. Cerebral palsy has not been shown to have fallen as a result of an increasing CS rate (Stanley and Watson, 1992). Regression analysis of 17,000 vertex births stratified by 500gm birthweight found no impact of CS on outcome (Rosen and Chil, 1984). 'Brain damage' occurs without difficult labour or perinatal hypoxia and CS is no guarantee against it. We have been warned before that 'it is irrational to ascribe a child's so-called brain damage to labour or delivery without considering other factors. There is an interaction of numerous factors, prenatal, perinatal and postnatal and it is simplistic to ascribe "brain damage" to single factors without considering the antecedent causes of these factors' (Illingworth, 1985; International Cerebral Palsy Task Force, 1999). The corollary is also true. Birth depression and severe hypoxia/acidosis at birth are not in the great majority followed by evidence of 'brain damage' (Andres *et al.*, 1999; Ingermarsson *et al.*, 1997).

Performing an elective CS before the onset of labour inevitably leads to the baby being born earlier and of lower weight. Does harm flow from this? There is a doubling of respiratory morbidity with each week earlier that elective CS is performed between 37 and 40 weeks (Morrison *et al.*, 1995), more transient tachypnoea and respiratory distress (Annibale *et al.*, 1995). Even though a doubling of morbidity with each week earlier is highly significant as elective CS rates rise, reports also exist of fourfold increases in intermediate or intensive nursery care, mechanical ventilation and oxygen therapy (Annibale *et al.*, 1995) and up to 120-fold increase in mechanical ventilation after CS at 37–38 weeks (Madar *et al.*, 1999). Maybe as many as 1 in 18 (5.5 per cent) babies born by elective CS as opposed to 1 in 63 (1.6 per cent) after vaginal delivery cannot support themselves in room air (Annibale *et al.*, 1995), a fact that might worry mothers-to-be, were they informed. Gestational age calculation is not accurate, and up to 9 per cent of babies born by elective repeat CS are thought to be <38 weeks (Hook *et al.*, 1997). As there is no possibility of iatrogenic prematurity and the undisputed immediate respiratory sequelae are less if CS is performed in labour (Madar *et al.*, 1999) those who want to protect babies should consider the rational policy of planned CS at labour onset. Convenience comes into conflict with optimising the safety for babies.

Along with respiratory compromise and SCBU admission, elective CS brings associated risks such as maternal separation and anxiety, poor feeding, jaundice, cannulation and cross-infection, sometimes with multi-resistant hospital-acquired organisms. Scalpel lacerations have been reported as 1 per cent with cephalic presentation, up to 8 per cent with abnormal lie (Smith *et al.*, 1997). We have no idea of the longer-term consequences. Increasing work on programming in early life brings understanding of how small changes can cascade or be amplified with time. Seemingly small differences in respiratory health, birthweight or breastfeeding might well make significant differences to long-term health or development. For example, long-term follow-up of term infants treated for severe persistent pulmonary hypertension (a condition associated with elective CS (Heritage and Cunningham, 1985)) shows ongoing problems with neurodevelopmental disability, reactive airways disease and slow growth (Rosenberg *et al.*, 1997). Other work shows Caesarean section exacerbates maternal–neonatal discordance in gut flora (Gronlund *et al.*, 1999), which may be related to rising incidence of atopic disease (asthma and eczema), potentially relievable by perinatal probiotics (Murch, 2001).

Basic medical concepts

Good medicine starts with an understanding of physiology. Normal pregnancy and childbirth are physiological processes, though disorders exist.
Much, though not all, death and damage due to disease can be avoided or
treated. Doctors, with their powerful diagnostic tools and treatments for
pathology, can also cause harm. Risk-benefit changes with the prevalence of
disease, and interventions become relatively more harmful in the well rather
than the ill. In general, pregnant women are strong enough to bear children
and their babies are capable of surviving. It is true that the outcome of labour
is unknown and that nature is not perfect, but it is almost as if some think that
female physiology flawed and childbirth always pathological. There is plenty
of justifiable work, so is it well-intentioned, misguided or arrogant to think
obstetricians can improve on healthy physiology? Respected gynaecological
thinkers have written about the evolutionary mistakes of womankind, for
example with labour (Steer, 1998) or the menopause (Purdie, 1999; Lilford
and Bryce, 1991). Gynaecologists who wished to cure women of being female
would find much resonance in the 'CS for prophylaxis' argument. By seeing
the normal as pathology, the need for everyone to have a doctor is created.
Not only does this disregard the evidence about the better outcomes of
midwifery-led care (Hodnett, 2000) and diminish our sister profession, it
undermines those obstetricians trying to develop evidence-based practice in
complicated pregnancies. Focusing on elective CS for choice distracts from
the highest-risk women on whom the burden of complications of high CS
rates and repeated CSs will inequitably fall (e.g. older, high parity, high BMI,
socially disadvantaged, ethnic minority or medically complicated women).

Professional vested interests

Many reports have identified an individual obstetrician effect on CS rates
(Poma, 1999; DeMott and Sandmire 1990, 1992). The trend of 'request' intervention is more established in the private sector. It has been shown repeatedly
that CS rates are higher in the private sector (Gregory *et al.*, 1999; Roberts *et
al.*, 2000; Hopkins 2000; Belizan *et al.*, 1999; Potter *et al.*, 2001) with lesser
strength of indication (Peipert *et al.*, 1999). One explanation is that physicians
in private practice use different criteria for decision-making which would
support the changing rates being 'doctor-led'. There is a financial disincentive
for doctors to challenge their clients' requests, and incentives both to make the
well worried and perform procedures during office hours. Third-party payers
(State or insurance companies) also have an interest in the threshold for interventions, and, as in the USA, it is possible they may wish to step into standard
setting to control medical behaviour, as has happened in gynaecology.

It is interesting that trends that come from within, and suit, the profession
can be projected as coming from outside (the phenomenon of blaming the

patient or the lawyer), whereas detailed qualitative work actually demonstrates mechanisms whereby doctors induce the so-called demand for CS by choice (Hopkins, 2000; Potter *et al.*, 2000).

From the outside, and to historians of medicine, the elective CS debate might appear to be a simple professional boundary dispute about who should control normal pregnancy and childbirth. 'Turf wars' in Britain and North America have carried on through the centuries (Oakley, 1980; Williams, 1997) with little evidence to support obstetric claims of safety (Tew, 1990). The subject has changed, from the registration of midwives, introduction of forceps, or home *v.* hospital delivery debate to CS. After the limited midwifery success of *Changing Childbirth* (Cumberlege, 1993) it is fascinating to see how the powerful rhetoric of 'choice' and 'control' has moved from the naturalist to the interventionist camps.

The evidence base supports midwifery-led care for low-risk women which obstetricians should accept. There is a professional contradiction if an individual obstetrician supports elective CS on request and yet is not active on the delivery suite, helping women who 'choose' labour to get a good outcome from it. To their credit, some of the proponents of elective CS are also active practising obstetricians, but some are not.

Women's changing status

Women have made tremendous gains towards personal and financial independence in western societies in the last century. However, this new self-esteem, which has been hard to win and maintain in the male-orientated culture of work is fragile and brings new fears of loss of self-control. There is a paradox of the strong, controlled career woman who has succeeded by her brain and wits and yet who has lost confidence in her female body. If a generation of women are losing confidence in their innate abilities, this is a tragedy. If deep and genuine fears are driving the requests for CS, then doctors must address them sensitively, but it is difficult to envisage mass surgery as an appropriate solution.

Competing notions of good and bad motherhood are also at stake. It is intriguing that concepts of 'suffering on behalf of the child' and 'putting her own needs first' resonate on both sides of the debate. Women who want home births without interventions might be considered to suffer without drugs or pain relief for their babies or to satisfy personal needs. Elective CS with postoperative pain and restrictions might be perceived to be avoiding fetal risk in the last weeks of pregnancy and labour but is also requested to suit parental convenience and putatively protect the perineum for sex. As health professionals we should be wary about fashions that ignore physiology (e.g. remembering the harmful, and even fatal, historical fashions for wet-nursing and formula feeding). There are powerful psychological pressures on women and it is hardly surprising if they continue to feel anxious, guilty or dependent on one or other health professional with their individual ideology.

How should we respond to 'requests'?

1. The first response must be to listen. Why is this woman requesting a CS? What is her prior knowledge of childbirth and CS and what are the sources of that information? It may be that the obstetric history of her mother, sisters or friends is particularly relevant (and the relationships she has with them). What are her beliefs about her body and its capabilities? What happened in a previous labour?

2. Only then should unbiased information be given and management options explored.

3. Having a negotiated plan (that is open to renegotiation in late pregnancy or labour) helps women to have control, without being left with all the responsibility, and may help her believe that her professionals understand.

4. A proper discussion about labour, the realistic available local midwifery services and continuity of care by a known midwife should be undertaken by a senior midwife.

5. For women with a past bad labour experience, reassurance and a written negotiated plan to avoid a replay may be all that is required (for example: to avoid induction, set a maximum length of labour, different pain relief, avoidance of instrumental delivery, have a known midwife, consider a home delivery, etc.).

6. For women with non-recurrent stillbirth/neonatal loss, fears may be controlled with monitoring, plans for delivery at term or even admission.

7. For women with intractable anxiety or overwhelming fears referral to a psychologist or psychiatrist should be contemplated (whatever the decision re mode of delivery) since anxiety and fear can be disabling and continue after the baby is born.

8. There is evidence to support CS for psychological or psychiatric indications as a phobia realised can be very damaging. However, this is something that should be assessed with expert advice as there are other potential modalities for dealing with anxiety and phobia. Fear is not a rational emotion and the range of its manifestation means the obstetrician should be able to provide a range of managements rather than merely reach for the scalpel.

9. Doctors who in good conscience feel they cannot recommend a CS (or any other procedure) on demand should refer on. Examples of non-indicated elective CSs might be those in normal women, burnt out herpes, or explained non-recurrent perinatal death. A second opinion after a refusal would be good practice so that women are given kindly care even if not acquiescence. It is important to avoid conflict in the doctor–patient relationship and offering a referral to a colleague can be a way of continuing the dialogue with the patient, taking her seriously and avoiding any sense of bias or bullying (Harley–Avon Productions, 1999).

10. We are not suggesting obstetricians get in cahoots to refuse all 'request' CSs, as we consider a 'request' as merely the start of a continuing dialogue and process. However, a second opinion would appear a wise routine for any

doctor considering an operation with no medical indication. A mandatory second opinion would also be a means for doctors or society to demonstrate the seriousness of executing women's choice (generally good and thoughtful and concordant with the doctor) if that is what is to be done, in the face of a compelling countervailing consideration (e.g. safety, and especially that of her baby). A system with checks and hurdles can be the pragmatic compromise between 'first of all, do no harm' and 'fulfilling women's choice'. One private hospital currently charges self-payers £600 more for a CS with no medical indication. This is a crude way to say 'have second thoughts before treading this path' but may have a similar intention. On the other hand, the extra payment may make women think celebrities and those who can afford it are buying something better than is otherwise rationed on the NHS!

On a national level, it is imperative that we perform more and better research, especially about longer-term maternal and child outcomes of labour and delivery. The implication for longer-term funding needs to be taken seriously by grant awarding bodies. Obstetricians and midwives might improve their counselling and inform women better if good referenced information leaflets were available. To deliver good care to mothers and babies, obstetricians have to play a more active part in labour ward and take responsibility for emergency outcomes. Intervention rates can fall with simple audit and peer pressure methods (Sandmire and DeMott, 1994; Robson *et al.*, 1996; Lagrew and Morgan, 1996). The enthusiasm (and support) for this may be driven by the needs of clinical governance (Richman, 1999).

Unanswered research questions

The radical interventionist view has valuably drawn important research questions to our attention. What outcomes matter to women, and do their values change with age, parity, ethnicity and experience? What are the risks to mother and baby of each successive elective CS and how can both the natural and iatrogenic complications of labour be minimised? How can we predict problems and protect and repair the perineum? Can randomised trials be performed to get the information about the real differences in outcomes? Who 'requests' elective CS and why? What are women's fears and fantasies about labour and how are they altered by unbiased information? How do women perceive risk and assess information? How do professionals provide information properly? What is the midwife or obstetrician effect?

Conclusion

The Lancet noted recently that the UK governments National Institute of Clinical Excellence (NICE) is producing guidelines about CS and will have to bite the bullet about 'requests' (Feinmann, 2002). Some think that in a 'post-modern world' (Smith, 2002) doctors have to accept (even irrational) patient choices as medical expertise and authority hold less sway. But there remains a difference between rejection of medical advice and doctors being obliged to give unindicated treatments. There is a danger in accepting a new surgical ethic that doctors should perform CS on demand because of some purported (and controversial) 'right to choose'. Although this rhetoric was used to win women basic reproductive freedoms (to contraception and abortion and from marital rape), feminists might be suspicious about a debate about controlling women's bodies and self-confidence (again) where women are being treated en masse rather than a mass of individuals. We hope that NICE recommends that women get good one-to-one professional care in labour, that appropriate services are available for anxiety or prior trauma and that operations have medical indications. Senior midwifery and psychology referral should be made prior to decisions about non-indicated elective Caesarean. Obstetricians (or midwives or general practitioners) can say, 'I respect you and your request and views, but childbirth is normal and physiological. Operations (with complications) need justification. The facts do not support "prophylactic" CS. If you want to reduce your fears and dangers see a psychologist, have a midwife you know and an experienced companion in labour. There is good evidence these work. It is unprofessional not to refer you. However, if they don't work, come back after proper assessment and we can consider Caesarean for psychological indications.' Why isn't this happening? Is it too scary to label fear and phobia for what they are? Maybe, in the UK, with a shortage of midwives in an under-valued and demoralised profession more structural change is required to provide the basic care. Non-interventionist services are not in medical vested interests, and it is perhaps unsurprising that high CS rates are a recurrent feature in private systems worldwide. Obstetricians too can be traumatised by their experience of handling complications and their own unresolved fears may resonate with and exaggerate women's fears. If CS really was safer than labour (made more morbid by high emergency operative delivery rates) then it would be unethical for doctors not to offer them to all patients. Obstetricians do not offer CS to all women at term, nor in any circumstances or at any gestation, because they do not believe in unconstrained 'informed choice' – they want to give as much choice as possible but within the established frame-work of doing good and avoiding harm. Obstetricians who do not want to harm their two patients must be fact- rather than fear-based. There is presently no evidence that elective CS is safer than labour. If there were, all women would, and should, be offered elective CS. The infant risks and bene-fits have not been calculated and rapidly rising CS rates may harm women and the next generation. There is a paucity of evidence to counteract the known and inevitable increased risk of maternal death and morbidity following CS. The ethic of 'informed choice' for non-indicated surgery is not overwhelming and we have postulated other explanations for the recent fashion for elective CS without medical indication.

Acknowledgement

This chapter first appeared as commentaries in the *British Journal of Obstetrics and Gynaecology* 2002 (Bewley and Cockburn, 2002a and b) and the *Lancet* (Bewley and Cockburn, 2002) and appears with permission of the publishers/editor.

References

Abramsky, L., Hall, S., Levitan, J. and Marteau, T.M. (2001) What parents are told after prenatal diagnosis of a sex chromosome abnormality: interview and questionnaire study. *British Medical Journal*, **322(7284)**: 463–466.

Allen, R.E., Hosker, G.L., Smith, A.R. and Warrell, D.W. (1990) Pelvic floor damage and childbirth: a neurophysiological study. *American Journal of Obstet Gynecol*, **97**: 770–9.

Al-Mufti, R., McCarthy, A. and Fisk, N.M. (1997) Survey of obstetricians' personal preference and discretionary practice. *Eur J Obstet Gynaecol Reprod Biol*, **73**: 1–4.

Amu, O., Rajendran, S. and Bolaji, I.I. (1998) Should doctors perform an elective Caesarean section on request? Maternal choice alone should not determine method of delivery. *British Medical Journal*, **317**: 463–64.

Andres, R.L., Saade, G., Gilstrap, L.C., Wilkins, I., Witlin, A., Zlatnik, F. and Hank, G.V. (1999) Association between umbilical blood gas parameters and neonatal morbidity and death in neonates with pathologic fetal acidemia. *American Journal of Obstet Gynecol*, **181**: 867–71.

Annibale, D.J., Hulsey, T.C., Wagner, C.L. and Southgate, W.M. (1995) Comparative neonatal morbidity of abdominal and vaginal deliveries after uncomplicated pregnancies. *Arch Pediatrics and Adolescent Med*, **149**: 862–7.

Anwar, K. and O'Mahoney, F. (2000) Patient access to their records: rights or risks? *BJOG*, **107**: 141–2

Barrett, G., Pendry, E., Peacock, J., Victor, C., Thakar, R. and Manyonda, I. (2000) Women's sexual health after childbirth. *BJOG*, **107**: 186–95.

Beck, R.P. and Hsu, N. (1965) Pregnancy, childbirth and the menopause related to the development of stress incontinence. *American Journal of Obstet Gynecol*, **91**: 820–3.

Belizan, J.M., Althabe, R., Barros, F.C. and Alexander, S. (1999) Rates and implications of Caesarean sections in Latin America: ecological study. *British Medical Journal*, **319**: 1397–400.

Bewley, S. and Cockburn, J. (2002) Responding to fear of childbirth. *Lancet*, **359**: 2128–9.

Bewley, S. and Cockburn, J. (2002a) I. The unethics of 'request' Caesarean section. *Br J Obstet Gynaecol*, **109**: 593–6.

Bewley, S. and Cockburn, J. (2002b) II. The unfacts of 'request' Caesarean section. *Br J Obstet Gynaecol*, **109**: 597–605.

Bump, H. and Norton, P. (1998) Epidemiology and natural history of pelvic floor dysfunction. *Clinics of North America Obs and Gynecol*, **2**: 723–46.

CESDI (Confidential Enquiry into Stillbirths and Deaths in Infancy) (1997) *Fourth Annual Report*. London: Maternal and Child Health Research Consortium.

CESDI (Confidential Enquiry into Stillbirths and Deaths in Infancy) (2001) *Eighth Annual Report*. London: Maternal and Child Health Research Consortium. p. 25.

Chen, F. C.-K., von Dehn, D., Buscher, U., Dudenhausen, J.W. and Miggemann, B. (1999) Atopy, the use of condoms, and a history of Caesarean delivery: Potential predisposing factors for latex sensitisation in pregnant women. *American Journal of Obstet Gynaecol*, **181**:1461–4.

Clement, S. (1995) *The Caesarean Experience*. London: Pandora, p. 26.

Corrigan, S. (997) The benefits of a having nice clean cut (interview with Nicholas Fisk). *The Times* 15 July: 16.

Cotzias, C.S., Paterson-Brown, S. and Fisk, N.M. (1999) Prospective risk of unexplained stillbirth in singleton pregnancies at term: population based analysis. *British Medical Journal*, **319**: 287–8.

Cumberlege, J. (1993) *Changing Childbirth: Report of the Expert Maternity Group.* London: HMSO.

DeMott, R.K. and Sandmire, H.F. (1990) The Green Bay Cesarean section study. I: The physician factor as a determinant of Cesarean birth rates. *American Journal of Obstet Gynecol*, **162**: 1593–602.

DeMott, R.K. and Sandmire, H.F. The Green Bay Cesarean section study. II: The physician factor as a determinant of Cesarean birth rates for failed labor. *American Journal of Obstet Gynecol*, **166**: 1799–810.

Denyttenacre, K., Lenaerts, H., Nijs, P. and van Assche, F.A. (1993) Individual coping style and psychological attitudes during pregnancy predict depression levels during pregnancy and during postpartum. *Acta Psychiatr Scand*, **91**: 95–102.

Department of Health and Human Services. (1991) *Healthy People 2000.* (PHS) 91-500212. Washington DC: DHSS.

Department of Health, Welsh Office, Scottish Office Home and Health Department, Department of Health and Social Services, Northern Ireland. (1994) *Report on Confidential Enquiries into Maternal Deaths in the United Kingdom 1988–90.* London: HMSO.

Department of Health, Welsh Office, Scottish Office Home and Health Department, Department of Health and Social Services, Northern Ireland. (1997) *Why Mothers Die. Report on Confidential Enquiries into Maternal Deaths in the United Kingdom 1991–3.* London: HMSO.

Dickson, M.J. and Willet, M. (1999) Midwives would prefer a vaginal delivery. *British Medical Journal*, **319**: 1008.

Dimpfl, T., Hesse, U. and Schussler, B. (1992) Incidence and cause of postpartum urinary stress incontinence. *Eur J Obstet Gynaecol Reprod Biol*, **43**: 29–33.

Dwyer, P.L., Lee, E.T.C. and Hay, D.M. Obesity and urinary incontinence in women. *Br J Obstet Gynaecol*, **95**: 91–6.

Dyer, C. (1997) Appeal court rules against compulsory Caesarean sections. *British Medical Journal*, **314**: 993.

Feinmann, J. (2002) How to limit Caesareans on demand – too NICE to push? *Lancet*, **359**: 774.

FIGO Committee for the Ethical Aspects of Human Reproduction and Womens Health (1999) Ethical aspects regarding Cesarean delivery for non-medical reasons. *Int J Obstet Gynecol*, **64**: 317–22

Fisk, N. and Savage, W. (1997) Head to head: childbirth techniques. *NHS Magazine*, Summer: 8–9.

Francis, W.J.A. (1960) The onset of stress incontinence. *J Obstet Gynaecol Br Emp*, **67**: 899–903.

Frankfurt, H.G. (1971) Freedom of the will and the concept of a person. *J Philosophy*, **68**: 5–20.

Frigoletto, F.D., Ryan, F.J. and Phillipe, M. (1980) Maternal mortality associated with Cesarean section: an appraisal. *American Journal of Obstet Gynecol*, **136**: 969–70.

General Medical Council (1998) Seeking the patient's consent: the ethical considerations.

Girard, M. (1999) Episiotomy and faecal incontinence. *Lancet*, **354**: 2169.

Gregory, K.D., Ramicone, E., Chan, L. and Kahn, K.L. (1999) Cesarean deliveries for Medicaid patients: comparison in public and private hospitals in Los Angeles county. *American Journal of Obstet Gynecol*, **180**:1177–84

Gronlund, M.M., Lehtonen, O.P., Eerola, E. and Dero, P. (1999) Fecal microflora in healthy infants born by different methods of delivery: permanent changes in intestinal flora after Caesarean section. *J Pediatr Gastroenterol Nutr*, **28**: 19–25.

Hall, M.F. and Bewley S. (1999) Maternal mortality and mode of delivery. *Lancet*, **354**: 776.

Hannah, M.E., Hannah, W.J., Hewson, S.A. and Hodnett, E.D. (2000) A randomised controlled trial of planned Caesarean or vaginal delivery for the term breech. *Lancet*.

Harley–Avon Productions Ltd. (1999) *Caroline's Story*. A video made in Bristol about handling a request for CS after stillbirth.

Hemminki, E. and Merilainen, J. (1996) Long-term effects of Cesarean section: ectopic pregnancies and placental problems. *Am J Obstet Gynecol*, **174**: 1569–74.

Heritage, C.K. and Cunningham, M.D. (1985) Association of elective repeat Cesarean delivery and persistent pulmonary hypertension of the newborn. *Am J Obstet Gynecol*, **152**: 627–9.

Hilder, L., Cotesloe, K. and Thilaganathan, B. (1998) Prolonged pregnancy: evaluating gestation specific risks of fetal and infant mortality. *Br J Obstet Gynaecol*, **105**: 169–73.

Hodnett, E.D. (2000) Continuity of caregivers for care during pregnancy and childbirth (Cochrane Review). *The Cochrane Library*, **2**. Oxford: Update Software

Hofberg, K. and Brockington, I. (2000) Tokophobia: an unreasoning dread of childbirth. *Br J Psych*, **176**: 83–5.

Hofmeyr, G.J. and Hannah, M.E. (2001) Planned Caesarean section for term breech delivery (Cochrane Review). *The Cochrane Library*, **4**. Oxford: Update Software.

Hook, B., Kiwi, R., Amini, S.B., Fanoroff, A. and Hack, M. (1997) Neonatal morbidity after elective repeat Caesarean section and trial of labour. *Pediatrics*, **100**: 348–53

Hope, J. (2000) Caesareans 'are best'. *Daily Mail*, 11 May: 25.

Hopkins, K. (2000) Are Brazilian women really choosing to deliver by Cesarean? *Soc Sci Med*, **51**: 725–40.

Illingworth, R.S. (1985) A paediatrician asks – why is it called birth injury? *Br J Obstet Gynaecol*, **92**: 122–30.

Ingelfinger, F. (1980) Arrogance. *New Eng J Med*, **303**: 1507–11.

Ingermarsson, I., Herbst, A. and Thorngran-Jerneck, K. (1997) Long term outcome after umbilical artery acidaemia at term birth: Influence of gender and duration of fetal heart rate abnormalities. *Br J Obstet Gynaecol*, **104**: 1123–7.

International Cerebral Palsy Task Force (1999) A template for defining a causal relation between acute intrapartum events and cerebral palsy: International consensus statement. *British Medical Journal*, **319**: 1054–9.

Iosif, S. (1981) Stress incontinence during pregnancy and the puerperium. *Int J Gynaecol Obstet*, **19**: 13–20.

Johanson, J.F., Irizzarry, B.S. and Doughty, A.D. (1997) Risk factors for faecal incontinence in a nursing home population. *J Clin Gastroenterol*, **24**: 156–60.

Johanson, J. and Lafferty, J. (1996) Epidemiology of faecal incontinence : The silent affliction. *Am J Gastroenerol*, **91**: 33–6.

Keane, D.P., Sims, T.J., Abrams, P. and Bailey, A.J. (1997) Analysis of collagen status in premenopausal nulliparous women with genuine stress incontinence. *Br J Obstet Gynaecol*, **104**: 994–8.

King, J. and Freeman, R. (1998) Is antenatal bladder neck mobility a risk factor for post partum stress incontinence? *Br J Obstet Gynaecol*, **105**: 1300–7.

Kolder, V.E., Gallagher, J. and Parsons, M.T. (1987) Court-ordered obstetrical interventions. *New Engl J Med*, **316**: 1192–6.

Kurki, T., Hiilesmaa, V., Raitasalo, R., Mattile, H. and Ylikorkala, O. (2000) Depression and anxiety in early pregnancy and risk for preeclampsia. *Obstet Gynecol*, **95**: 487–90.

Labrecque, M., Eason, E., Marcoux, S., Lemieux, F., Pinault, J.J., Feldman, P. and Laperriere, L. (1999) Randomized controlled trial of prevention of perineal trauma by perineal massage during pregnancy. *Am J Obstet Gynaecol*, **180**: 593–600.

Lagrew, D.C. and Morgan, M.A. (1996) Decreasing the Cesarean section rate in a private hospital: Success without mandated clinical changes. *Am J Obstet Gynecol*, **174**: 184–91.

Lilford, R.J., Van Coeverden de Groot, H.A., Moore, P. and Bingham, P. (1990) The relative risks of Caesarean section (intrapartum and elective) and vaginal delivery: a detailed analysis to exclude the effects of medical disorders and other acute pre-existing physiological disturbances. *Br J Obstet Gynaecol*, **97**: 883–92.

Lilford, R. and Bryce, F.C. (1991) Teleology of the menopause. *Eur J Obstet Gynecol Reprod Biol*, **38**: 89–90.

Lo, J.Y., Hartley, C.C. and Wendal, G.D. (2000) Uterine evacuation complicated by hysterectomy: an association with prior Cesarean delivery. *Am J Obstet Gynecol*, **182**: S151.

Lydon-Rochelle, M., Holt, V.L., Martin, D.P. and Esaterling, T.R. Association between method of delivery and maternal rehospitalization. *JAMA*, **283**: 2411–6.

Madar, J., Richmond, S. and Hey, E. (1999) Surfactant deficient respiratory distress after elective delivery at 'term'. *Acta Pediatr*, **88**: 1244–84.

Malloy, M.H. and Hoffman, H.J. (1995) Prematurity, sudden death syndrome and age of death. *Pediatrics*, **96**: 464–71.

Marshall, K., Walsh, D.M. and Baxter, D. (1997) Faecal incontinence after childbirth. *Br J Obstet Gynaecol*, **104**: 870.

Marshall, K., Thompson, K.A., Walsh, D.M. and Baxter, G.D. (1998) Incidence of urinary incontinence and constipation during pregnancy and post partum: survey of current findings at the Rotunda Lying-in Hospital. *Br J Obstet Gynaecol*, **105**: 400–2.

McGurgan, P., Coulter-Smith, S. and O' Donovan, P.J. (2001) A national confidential survey of obstetrician's personal preferences regarding mode of delivery. *Eur J Obstet Gynecol Reprod Biol*, **97**: 17–19.

McMahon, M.J., Luther, E.R., Bowes, W.A. Jr and Olshan, A.F. (1996) Comparison of a trial of labor with an elective second Cesarean section. *N Engl J Med*, **335**: 689–95.

Moldin, P., Hokegard, K. and Nielson, T.F. (1984) Cesarean section and maternal mortality in Sweden 1973–1979. *Acta Obstet Gynaecol Scand*, **63**: 7–11.

Morrison, J.J., Rennie, J.M. and Milton, P.J. (1995) Neonatal respiratory morbidity and mode of delivery at term: influence of timing of elective Caesarean section. *Br J Obstet Gynaecol*, **102**: 101–6.

Murch, S.H. (2001) Toll of allergy reduced by probiotics. *Lancet*, **357**: 1057–8.

National Institute for Clinical Excellence, The Scottish Executive Health Department, The Department of Health, Social Services and Public Safety: Northern Ireland (2001) *Why Mothers Die 1997–1999. The Confidential Enquiries into Maternal Deaths in the United Kingdom.* London: RCOG Press.

Nielsen Forman, D., Videbech, P., Hedegaard, M., Dalby Salvig, J. and Secher, N.J. Postpartum depression: identification of women at risk. *Br J Obstet Gynaecol*, **107**: 1210–17.

Nygaard, I.E., Satish, S.C. and Dawson, J.D. (1997) Anal incontinence after anal sphincter disruption: A 30-year retrospective cohort study. *Obstet Gynaecol*, **89**: 896–901.

Oakley, A. (1980) *Women Confined: Towards a Sociology of Childbirth*, pp. 10–14. Oxford: Martin Robertson.

Parys, B.T., Haylen, B.T., Woolfenden, K.A. and Parsons, K.F. (1989) Vesico-urethral dysfunction after simple hysterectomy. *Neurol Urodynam*, **8**: 315–16.

Paterson-Brown, S. (1998) Should doctors perform an elective Caesarean section on request? Yes as long as the woman is fully informed. *Br Med J*, **317**: 462–3.

Peipert, J.F., Hogan, J.W., Gifford, D., Chase, E. and Randall, R. (1999) Strength of indication for Cesarean delivery: Comparison of private physician versus resident service labor management. *Am J Obstet Gynecol*, **181**: 435–9.

Pettitti, D.B., Cefalo, R.C., Shapiro, S. and Whally, P. (1992) In hospital maternal mortality in the United States: Time trends and relation to method of delivery. *Obstet Gynaecol*, **59**: 6–12.

Poma, P.A. (1999) Effects of obstetrician characteristics on Cesarean delivery rates: a community hospital experience. *Am J Obstet Gynecol*, **180**: 1364–72.

Potter, J.E., Berquo, E., Perpetuo, I.H., Leal, O.F., Hopkins, K., Souza, M.R. and Formiga, M.C. (2001) Unwanted Caesarean sections among public and private patients in Brazil: prospective study. *British Medical Journal*, **323**: 1155–8.

Purdie, D. (1999) The genesis line. *Lancet*, **353**: 404–5.

Read, V., Celik, A.F. and Katsinelos, P. (1995) Constipation and incontinence in the elderly. *J Clin Gastroenterol*, **20**: 61–70.

Re MB Adult: medical treatment [1997] 2 FCR 541.C.A.

Richman, V.V. (1999) Setting goals for reductions in Canadian Cesarean delivery rates: Benchmarking medical practice patterns. *Am J Obstet Gynecol*, **181**: 635–7.

Roberts, C.L., Tracy, S. and Peat, B. (2000) Rates for obstetric intervention among private and public patients in Australia: population based descriptive study. *British Medical Journal*, **321**: 137–41.

Robson, M.S., Scudamore, I.W. and Walsh, S.M. (1996) Using the medical audit cycle rate to reduce Cesarean section rates. *Am J Obstet Gynecol*, **174**: 199–205.

Rosen, M.G. and Chil, L. (1984) The association between Cesarean birth and outcome in vertex presentation: Relative importance of birthweight, Dubowitz scores and delivery route. *Am J Obstet Gynaecol*, **150**: 775.

Rosenberg, A.A., Kennaugh, J.M., Moreland, S.G., Fashaw, L.M., Hale, K.A., Torielli, F.M., Abman, S.H. and Kinsella, J.P. (1997) Longitudinal follow up of a cohort of newborn infants treated with inhaled nitric oxide for pulmonary hypertension. *J Pediatr*, **131**: 70–5.

Rouse, D.J., Owen, J., Goldberg, R.L. and Cliver, S.P. (1996) The effectiveness and costs of elective Cesarean delivery for fetal macrosomia diagnosed by ultrasound. *JAMA*, **276**: 1480–6.

Rouse, D.J. and Owen, J. (1999) Prophylactic Cesarean delivery for fetal macrosomia diagnosed by means of ultrasonography: a Faustian bargain? *Am J Obstet Gynecol*, **181**: 332–8.

Royal College of Physicians (1995) Incontinence: Causes, management and provision of services. Summary of a report of a working party of the Royal College of Physicians. *J Roy Coll Physicians Lond*, **29(4)**: 272–4.

Ryding, E.L., Wijma, B., Wijma, K. and Rydhström, H. (1998) Fear of childbirth during pregnancy may increase the risk of emergency Caesarean section. *Acta Obstet Gynecol Scand*, 77: 542–7.

Saisto, T., Salmela-Aro, K., Nurmi, J,-E., Kononen, T. and Halmesmaki, E. (2001) A randomized controlled trial of intervention in fear of childbirth. *Obstet Gynecol*, **98**: 820–6.

Sandmire, H.F. and DeMott, R.K. (1994) The Green Bay Cesarean section study. III. Falling Cesarean birth rates without a formal curtailment program. *Am J Obstet Gynecol*, **170**: 1790–802.

Savage, W. (1979) Perinatal mortality trends. *Medicine in Society*, **5**: 20–6.

Scholefield, H.J., Sajjad, Y. and Morgan, P.R. (2000) Cutaneous endometriosis and Caesarean section. *J Obstet Gynaecol*, **20**: S45–6.

Schuitemaker, N., van Roosmalen, J., van Dongen, P., van Geijn, H. and Gravenhorst, J.B. (1997) Maternal mortality after Caesarean section in the Netherlands. *Acta Obstet Gynaecol Scand*, 76: 332–4.

Sjogren, B. and Thomassen, P. (1997) Obstetric outcome in 100 women with severe anxiety over childbirth. *Acta Obstet Gynecol Scand*, 76: 948–52.

Smith, A.R., Hosker, G.L. and Warrell, D.W. (1985) The role of partial denervation of the pelvic floor in the aetiology of genito-urinary prolapse and stress incontinence of urine: a neurophysiological study. *Br J Obstet Gynaecol*, **92**: 824–8.

Smith, J.F., Hernandez, C. and Wax, J.R. (1997) Fetal laceration injury at Cesarean delivery. *Obstet Gynaecol*, **90**: 344–6.

Smith, R. (2002) The discomfort of patient power. *British Medical Journal*, **324**: 497–8.

Snooks, S.J., Henry, M.M. and Swash, M. (1985) Faecal incontinence due to external sphincter division in childbirth is associated with damage to the innervation of the pelvic floor: a double pathology. *Br J Obstet Gynaecol*, **92**: 824–8.

Stanley, F. and Watson, L. (1992) Trends in mortality and cerebral palsy in Western Australia 1967–1985. *British Medical Journal*, **304**: 1658–62.

Stanton, S.L., Kerr-Wilson, R. and Harris, G.V. (1980) The incidence of urological symptoms in normal pregnancy. *Br J Obstet Gynaecol*, **87**: 897–900.

Steer, P. (1998) Caesarean section: an evolving procedure? *Br J Obstet Gynaecol*, **105**: 1052–5.

Sultan, A.H., Kamm, M.A., Hudson, C.N. and Bartram, C.I. (1994) Third degree obstetric anal sphincter tears: risk factors and outcome of primary repair. *British Medical Journal*, **308**: 887–91.

Sultan, A.H., Kamm, M.A., Hudson, C.N., Thomas, J.M. and Bartrum, C.I. (1993) Anal sphincter disruption during delivery. *N Engl J Med*, **329**: 1905–11.

Sultan, A.H. and Monga, A.K. (1997) Anal and urinary incontinence in women with obstetric anal sphincter rupture. *Br J Obstet Gynaecol*, **104**: 754.

Sultan, A.H. and Stanton, S.L. (1996) Preserving the pelvic floor and perineum during childbirth. *Br J Obstet Gynaecol*, **103**: 731–4.

Tetzschner, T. and Lose, G. (1997) Anal and urinary incontinence in women with obstetric anal sphincter rupture. *Br J Obstet Gynaecol*, **104**: 753 & 754–5.

Tew, M. (1990) *Safer Childbirth? A Critical History of Maternity Care*. London: Chapman and Hall.

Thiery, M. and Derom, R. (1986) Review on evaluative studies on Caesarean section. Part 1: Trends in Caesarean section and perinatal mortality. In M. Kaminski (ed.), *Perinatal Care Delivery Systems: Description and Evaluation in European Community Countries*, pp. 93–113. Oxford: Oxford University Press.

Thomas, J. and Paranjothy, S. Royal College of Obstetricians and Gynaecologists Clinical Effectiveness Support Unit. (2001) *The National Sentinel Caesarean Section Audit Report*, p. 29. London: Royal College of Obstetricians and Gynaecologists, RCOG Press

Viktrup, I., Lose, G., Rolf, M. and Barfoed, K. (1992) The symptom of stress incontinence caused by pregnancy or delivery in primiparas. *Obstet Gynaecol*, **79**: 945–9.

Wadha, P.D., Sandman, C.A., Porto, M, Dunkel-Schetter, C. and Garite, T.H. (1993) The association between prenatal stress and infant birth weight and gestation age at birth: a prospective investigation. *Am J Obstet Gynecol*, **169**: 858–65.

Wagner, M. (2000) Choosing Caesarean section. *Lancet*, **356**: 1677–80.

Waterstone, M., Bewley, S. and Wolfe, C. (2001) A case-control study to identify the incidence and predictors of severe obstetric morbidity. *British Medical Journal*, **322**: 1089–93.

Whitted, R., Verma, U., Boigl, B. and Mendez, L. (2000) Does Cesarean delivery increase the prevalence of adenomyosis? *Obstet Gynecol*, **95**: S83.

Williams, A.S. (1997) *Women and Childbirth in the Twentieth Century*, pp. 198–9. Stroud, Gloucestershire: Sutton Publishing.

Wilson, P.D., Herbison, R.M. and Herbison, G.P. (1996) Obstetric practice and the prevalence of urinary incontinence three months after delivery. *Br J Obstet Gynaecol*, **103(2)**: 154–61.

World Health Organisation (1985) Appropriate technology for birth. *Lancet*, **24(2)(8452)**: 436–7.

CHAPTER 10

Negotiating Elective Caesarean Section: An Obstetric Team Perspective[1]

JULIA SIMPSON

The research

This chapter is based upon data gathered whilst conducting an ethnography within a large regional obstetric unit. One of the aims of the study was to identify the professional perspectives relating to elective Caesarean section. I intend to examine the way talk is used by obstetricians in their everyday interactions with their team colleagues. This analysis is developed from a recording of a naturally occurring discourse between a team of obstetric practitioners in the consultant's office within the antenatal clinic. Team members present include a consultant obstetrician, registrar, senior house officer (SHO) and two medical students. It is significant that both the SHO and the medical students were new to the team. I had been a participant observer in the unit for several months when the conversation occurred and the participants were familiar with the research and had consented to conversations between team members being recorded. I transcribed the tape, in full, myself.

This analysis will explore the team narrative as a medical story; guided by Wolcott's (1994) three major levels of analysing qualitative data: description, analysis and interpretation. The first level will explore the team narrative to illuminate the thematic content, identifying themes that closely reflect the participants' own categories of expression. The second level proceeds 'in some careful and systematic way to identify key factors and the relationships between them' (Wolcott, 1994, p. 10). The systematic procedures of both discourse and conversation analysis will be used to explore the way talk is actually used by obstetricians in their interactions and negotiations with team colleagues in the clinical environment. The third level of analysis will be concerned with elucidating the broader professional and organisational meanings and functions of the medical story and the language that the participants use to create it. There will be an attempt to show how professionals draw upon wider systems of meaning to construct and defend their own positions or perspectives. Medical storytelling will also be examined in terms of its political function relating to power, conflict and resistance.

Thematic analysis

Uncertainty of vaginal delivery

In Fragment 1, the registrar indicates to his team colleagues that uncertain aspects of their clinical work and decision-making are coming under increasing scrutiny from 'people' outside the medical profession.

Fragment I

R: In the next 4 or 5 years on, there will be people looking at a whole number   I
    of different aspects ... If you add that to the uncertainty of vaginal delivery   2
    that there is in the antenatal period compared to elective CS.   3

This suggests heightened awareness within the obstetric team of continuing external interest. Roth (1963) has argued that within the hospital as an organisation, medical timetables structure the physical processes and events, creating sanctions and medical controls. Timetabling is a significant key feature of everyday obstetric work. For example 'time limits' are usually set concerning the progress of the labouring woman. However, over time these limits can be revised (Boylan, 1989). Obstetric intervention can be modified in direct relation to temporal deadlines and timetables.

In Fragment 2 the registrar assumes that the timescale of labour must be controlled. He acknowledges ambiguity and real 'uncertainty' concerning the appropriate apportioning of time for length of labour where obstetricians cannot 'guarantee' and predict the precise timing of birth for their patients.

Fragment 2

R:	I mean you can't guarantee that a	217
	labour's not going to last four hours it might last longer. You're having to	218
	deal with that risk, it's not like a retrospective view, do you know what I	219
	mean? It's a matter of making a decision on risks and balancing it out and on	220
	the balance patient's would rather have an elective CS than a 12-hour labour	221
	and we can't guarantee that a patient is going to have a 12-hour labour. A	222
	great majority of our clients are going to have a 12-hour labour. And in that	223
	situation a certain proportion of patients are going to say, 'well if that on	224
	balance are my two options, you know a high risk of a 12-hour labour or an	225
	elective CS, I'd rather have the elective CS please'	226

In this fragment it follows logically that pregnant women may also be visualising their progress toward delivery and birth in terms of their personal expectations of the amount of time involved. Roth (1963) has suggested that both patients and physicians develop norms about how long given aspects of treatment should take – the patients to help them anticipate their future, the physician to help them make 'reasonable decisions' in a highly uncertain situation. The registrar appears to equate the view of 'a certain proportion of patients' with his need for control of time if not of decision-making.

In Fragment 3 the registrar defines his key outcomes. In these terms there are similar levels of risk attached to the two treatment categories plus the uncertainties of time in labour. It would seem that professionals perceive they are more at risk as labour lengthens. For the team members' time returns as an important factor effecting and dominating their clinical work.

Fragment 3

R:	...all I know in terms of simple language it's not	319
	affecting maternal mortality it's not affecting perinatal mortality so the	320
	patient can have want she wants, do you see what I mean? Unless you are	321
	going to start regarding other objectives then it becomes quite difficult and	322
	then you really have to look into it and think into it and reassess it every	323
	time you read something that might be partly related to it. And there might	324
	be so many things that might be partly related to it that every time you think	325
	about it, what you find is that there is very little in it between the two.	326

Roth (1963) suggests that professionals who control the careers of others must decide upon appropriate times for making changes in those careers.

These obstetricians are under pressure to regularise this process of definition. Therefore, indirectly, the obstetrician's inability to control and accurately predict the time agenda of delivery and birth poses a serious challenge to their professional authority and autonomy.

Ongoing persuasion

The dominant theme of the medical story re-emerges at regular intervals throughout the narrative: there is no overall professional consensus to distinguish between the two treatment categories. Conditions both external and internal to the profession have changed. A major consequence of these changes is that as obstetricians they cannot now simply inform a pregnant woman that she will have a vaginal delivery.

Fragment 4

SHO:	But the arguments for CS …	4
R:	I don't think there is an argument against an elective CS. I don't believe	5
	there is a very, very good argument against an elective Caesarean section	6
	compared to a difficult vaginal delivery. Now we don't have a very good	7
	argument against that.	8
SHO:	But nobody knows the arguments a year down the line about Caesarean	9
	sections.	10
R:	But what's happening over the last couple of years which never used to	11
	happen before? Now doctors are identifying more and more problems	12
	associated with vaginal deliveries, there are now in actual fact, more	13
	doctors arguing for the benefits, arguing for an elective Caesarean section	14
	because of the disadvantages of a vaginal delivery. There are more of those	15
	doctors around now than there used to be. In the past it was just a blanket	16
	statement from all obstetricians, 'you will have a vaginal delivery'. That's	17
	not the case any more.	18

In Fragment 5 it is possible to gain some appreciation of the intensity of the professional debate which the registrar presents as emotionally draining. The broad, general discussion occurring within the profession about 'correct' Caesarean section rates, he has decided do not concern him.

Fragment 5

R:	[I'm] not interested in trying to convince women. I don't want to spend the rest of	137
	my life arguing with colleagues, arguing with the college, arguing with	138
	patients trying to find out what the correct Caesarean section rate is. I don't	139
	want to spend the rest of my life finding the answer to a question which at	140
	the end of the day doesn't even need answering, who cares? At the end of	141
	the day all that matters is that that patient has got what she wants that's all	142

that matters whether by section or not is irrelevant. She's happy there's no   143
problem. But to spend the rest of my professional life getting involved in   144
discussions and heated debates about this is really just banging my head   145
against a wall. It's a stupid question.   146

As a profession medicine asserts its autonomy in defining what is an 'appropriate', 'effective', or 'good' service. Freidson (1988) suggests that the practitioner has to believe in what he is doing in order to practise. In Fragment 6, it would appear that there is a major dilemma for the registrar, given his commitment to action and practical solution, he is not convinced of the appropriate professional action therefore how can he advise his clients. The woman is described as in control of the practitioner/client encounter, for that reason the registrar defensively states, 'We are in trouble, it's not skewed our way, it's skewed their way.'

Fragment 6

Q: Some would say the situation is skewed in your favour.   198
R: It is when you're right; it is when you have got a good argument. The point   199
    I'm trying to make is that if we have an argument that the patient would find   200
    convincing then we haven't got a problem. But we don't have an argument   201
    that is going to convince the patient and for that reason we are in trouble.   202
    It's not skewed our way; it's skewed their way. Because now our argument   203
    does not convince the patient. It could be so simple …   204
    If I'm convinced I know that I'll be able to convince the patient, because I'll 205
    have thought through the benefits and disadvantages of the treatment for   206
    them. But when it comes to elective CS and difficult or possibly problematic   207
    vaginal deliveries and I'm trying to be honest about possible outcomes and   208
    possible risks, I'm not convinced, so how can I convince them if I am trying   209
    to be honest.   210

In Fragment 7 the theme of an ongoing argument has began to coalesce around the practitioner/client relationship. The consultation between practitioner and client forms a meeting between groups who differ in their knowledge, power and resources. There does appear to be the possibility of a relationship developing between the registrar and his clients, in which the client is an active participant, or where the pregnant woman is requesting an elective Caesarean section and the registrar is co-operating with her choice. In reality though, how far are they practitioners willing to bend to accommodate the preferences of the pregnant woman? Are the team members willing to face up to the possible loss of status and professional autonomy that this may involve? Part of the answer to this question lies behind the term 'eventually'. There are various forms of strategic interaction available that the experienced practitioner may yet utilise to maximise their own interests within the practitioner/client negotiation process.

Fragment 7

R: .... Now we don't have a	226
very good argument against that to try to dissuade them away from it	227
because it's not like we are magistrates in a court and we can lay down	228
sentences and things, we can't ... we obviously can't. I mean how far do we	229
draw the line, if a patient just says, 'I want a CS', and the obstetrician says,	230
'I don't want you to have a CS', and she goes, 'I really want a CS', the	231
obstetrician is going to have to give way at the end of the day, eventually.	232
They'd have to. If a patient is not prepared to budge at all the doctor has to	233
because he doesn't really have that strong an argument against it.	234

It is argued that obstetricians do not have a convincing argument or persuasive, discursive strategy that they can utilise when negotiating mode of delivery and treatment options with pregnant women. This dilemma places them as professionals in a particularly weak bargaining position. In this scenario, senior team members perceive pregnant women to have equal, if not greater, bargaining power in the negotiation context than they have as professionals. There appears to be a need to set up or construct a convincing professional argument which provides an illusion of client choice but one that also ensures that the choice being discussed is the choice or outcome that is supported by the obstetricians (see Fragment 4). The discursive strategy that the team are proposing is to convey labour as 'difficult and possibly problematic' and CS as controlled and problem-free. The team members now need to redefine and reshape their interactional opposition, if any, to a woman's requests regarding mode of delivery, if that request is for CS.

McClosky (1998, p. 96) has suggested that, 'talk establishes the relationships for doing business. That it establishes a repeated game, or at least some atmosphere of a repeated game, for reassuring people that they have implicitly promised to act as though they were friends with each other'. However, in interactions between lay people and professionals, the professionals usually retain the initiative. (Frankel, 1990; Linell *et al.*, 1988; Mishler, 1984). There is a fundamental distinction between the symmetry of ordinary conversation and the asymmetries of institutional interaction (Heritage, 1997). Billig (1991) has suggested that it is possible to inspect discourse for the way it is rhetorically organised to make argumentative, persuasive cases and for the way it is used to undermine alternative cases. This process involves exploring the participant's use of rhetorical strategies where recourse to arguments and persuasion may have been used. Examining the team members' use of rhetorical strategies therefore offers an opportunity to explore how they as professionals may attempt to persuade pregnant women of their preferred mode of delivery options.

Higher client expectations

In Fragment 8 the registrar explains the 'two-tier medical health care system operating generally, till now'.

Fragment 8

R: There generally has been a two-tier medical health care system, generally
    up till now. Those who could afford private health care were getting a   20
    different health care system to those in the NHS in a number of different   21
    ways. The CS rate under private health care has always been high, much   22
    higher than what it has been on the NHS, well over 25 per cent. The thing is what 23
    you're seeing is just what's happening in the north-east, very little private   24
    obstetric care going on in this region. If you go to Manchester, if you go to   25
    Leeds, oh I don't know about Leeds. A very high percentage of women in   26
    actual fact book privately for their obstetric care. I don't just mean antenatal 27
    care I mean for the actual labour as well. The CS rate for those patients is   28
    well in excess of 25 per cent, some people would say 50 per cent.
        What's happened over   29
    the last few years is the NHS has tried to improve the general standard of   30
    care to the general public approaching that to what women are generally   31
    getting, or were getting under private health care. There is very little   32
    difference nowadays between private health care and what you would get on   33
    the NHS in all specialities. The gaps closing. Now look at what that is going   34
    to do in obstetrics, it's going to: 1) reduce the high CS rate for those   35
    patients that were booking privately and 2) it's going to raise the CS rate for   36
    the NHS patients who are now going to expect care that other women were   37
    getting previously under private health care. I can truly imagine it hitting   38
    30 per cent I don't know about 50 per cent I can imagine it hitting
        25–30 per cent that's my   39
    upper limit of what could potentially occur. It could, but it certainly is in   40
    private health care. Would you not agree that generally the NHS is now   41
    providing better quality care to what it did 10 years ago? We are having to   42
    do now to a 100 per cent of the population what we were only doing to
        10 per cent of the   43
    population ten years ago. We were offering a two-tier system that's what's   44
    twisted all the figures.   45

It would appear that recently something has changed to alter the nature of the team members' relationships with their NHS obstetric clients. The cause of this change is attributed to rising standards of care in the NHS that are now at the level private clients were experiencing and receiving in the past. One of the challenges occurring both inside and outside the medical profession has been identified as the emergence of the patient as an active consumer of health care, rather then merely a passive recipient (Stevens, 1986). This trend is seen to mirror a general move toward a more consumerist society. The notion of consumerism in health care is problematic however; argue Wiles and Higgins (1996), because of the uniquely vulnerable position of consumers. In theory an 'active' patient-consumer would make choices about the hospital, the doctor, the timing of treatment and the treatment itself. Within the NHS however, such choices are limited due to the scale of demands made on the services and the lack of resources. What real choices are NHS obstetric clients now exercising that they possibly were not exercising in the past?

It would seem that lack of resources in the NHS, coupled with an increase in demand for better quality of obstetric care by NHS clients, are considered by the registrar to be factors that are having a critical effect upon the obstetricians' current workload. The registrar predicts paradoxically, that given similar standards in the future, the result will be higher Caesarean rates in the NHS and lower rates in private obstetric care. One possible explanation for this is that the relationships that doctors and clients have are dependent on structural constraints such as time. Research has shown that doctors experience fewer time constraints in the private sector and one would expect doctors to find this a more satisfying atmosphere in which to work (Higgins, 1988). In contrast the 'conveyer belt' system of the NHS, with greater time constraints demands a different sort of doctor–patient relationship to maximise throughput (Meredith, 1993).

Time and information

Freidson (1970) suggested that a profession can be distinguished from other occupations in that it has been given the right to control its own work. According to this perspective, doctors have power because of their professional status and autonomy over work, which is maintained by their control over medical knowledge (Freidson, 1970; Starr, 1982; Willis, 1989). Medicine is described as a form of collegiate control because of its ability to impose on the consumer its own definitions of need and how it should be catered for. Johnson (1972) argues that this ability of the provider to define needs is due in part to the problems consumers face in terms of knowledge on such matters, which help create consumer uncertainty and dependency, heightening the social distance between parties. It has been argued by Waitzkin and Stoeckle (1972) that this 'competence gap' (i.e. discrepancy in knowledge and information) leads to potential for exploitation and that the doctor's ability to control and manipulate information creates a basis of asymmetry in the doctor–patient relationship.

In Fragment 9, there is a continued contrast and focus upon two main categories of obstetric patients; private and NHS. Specifically the NHS patients are now asserting their needs and requesting 'long, discussions and explanations' before agreeing to the registrar's recommendations for treatment. There is no indication as to the content of the negotiations; therefore there is no way of telling if the NHS patients were dissatisfied or not with the professionals' knowledge and expertise on offer. However, the time available for the professionals to engage in discussions is limited. The medical staff are perceiving NHS patients requests for information as excessive demands on their clinical time. Rather than being viewed as 'active patients', NHS patients are becoming viewed as 'demanding patients'.

Fragment 9

R: ....There are more discussions going on now   102
    between doctors and patients within the NHS than there used to be10 years 103
    ago. There used to be discussions between consultant and patient,   104
    explanations, whatever else in private health care ten years ago, but not in 105
    the NHS. We are now having long discussions and explanations in the   106
    NHS, not just in obstetrics in all specialities. With that will come a higher 107
    Caesarean section rate. I have certainly had more discussions than that, I do 108
    know of two women that I was having repeated discussions with, the last   109
    time was actually on the day unit because she really wanted a full discussion 110
    about it, she was post dates and she did end up a CS at the end of the day, 111
    but eventually she did take my advice. Of the five or six I can remember, two 112
    ended up having an elective section out of maternal choice, two ended up   113
    having a labour and then ended up having an emergency CS due to failure to 114
    progress and one ended up having a vaginal delivery of the five I can remember 115
    having long discussions with and getting frustrated at by the end of the day. 116
    With each of them I ended up having long, long discussions with them   117
    about it and it's frustrating. Looking at it at the end of the day, of the three 118
    that still went for a vaginal delivery two did end up as a Caesarean section. 119
    At the end of the day it is their choice. Like I said in the past two years, I 120
    don't have an answer for it; there are more women, oddly enough in terms   121
    of long discussions, complications, going into all the aspects of routine and 122
    every detail it's just getting more complex, it really is. These are the   123
    discussions you would expect to get when a women books for antenatal care 124
    privately. Yes fine, you are quite happy to go through all that for a couple of 125
    thousand quid for it but when you're doing a NHS clinic, it's a busy clinic 126
    and you're having to get involved in that kind of discussion with virtually 127
    every single patient which will happen, then it's really getting difficult.   128
C: I say this with certain confidence it's just going to get worse and worse. ... 129

Time is a very different resource available to both patients and professionals in the different organisational settings. Spending a long time with patients and encouraging questions is not valued by professionals in the hospital or public clinic setting (Atkinson, 1981; Lazarus, 1988; Stein, 1990). Particularly in a busy NHS clinic, where the management of time is of the utmost importance for the medical staff who are in the position of having to deal with many patients in a short space of time. However, management of time can also be used by medical staff as a strategy for maintaining authority (Lupton, 1994). For the pregnant woman, lack of time for discussion with a professional can directly affect her access to information. Within the NHS, the appointment system and the period of waiting particularly serve to emphasise that the doctor's time is more important than the patients. Lack of information for the client, is however, closely linked to powerlessness. Decisions can only be made on the basis of information and if the woman is not properly informed about her diagnosis or treatment, her chances of making meaningful decisions are diminished.

The registrar and the consultant express frustration with NHS patients' requests for more information. The NHS patient asking for more discussions is perceived defensively by the registrar as trying to control their professional work. However, the power to frame the information still lies with the professional.

The obstetricians anticipate that private patients will expect long discussions. It has been argued that the theoretical ability to 'shop around' for health care puts private patients in a position of greater power than other groups, as these patients have the greatest potential for adopting a consumerist relationship with doctors (Wiles and Higgins, 1996). Superficially, this would seem to be confirmed by the registrar's comment, 'You are quite happy to go through all that for a couple of thousand quid'. Whilst there is ample evidence that financial incentives to perform Caesarean sections influence obstetricians' decisions about whether or not to perform the operation (Lomas and Enkin, 1989), what the private obstetric patients may be doing is buying professional time. The private patients are not challenging the professionals' clinical authority and autonomy. The control of the practitioner–client relationship in private care remains unchanged, unlike the loss of control that obstetricians are now experiencing in their relationships with their NHS patients.

'A healthy baby'

A particular theme of this story is that from the senior obstetricians' perspective, 'everyone now expects to have a healthy baby'. The interests of pregnant women and obstetricians' coincide with this common goal. So it would appear that the patients' position on choice is not necessarily in conflict with the professionals' aim. If clinical autonomy is the practitioners' freedom to offer advice about diagnosis and treatment based on knowledge and experience, it would seem theoretically at least, that an agreed decision rests as much on the patients' autonomy as on the practitioners'.

Fragment 10

R: Everyone now expects to have a healthy baby. An obstetric disaster is a   130
     nightmare, totally unacceptable. It has to be avoided at all costs, so it is still   131
     driven by them, it's coming from them. For that reason we are now doing   132
     sections for normal deliveries. I'll go along with the college; I mean I'm not   133
     going to stand on my own about it, I don't care one way or the other. If the   134
     general rate is 12 per cent I'd try to keep mine around 12 per cent. If the
          national rate was   135
     around 20 per cent then I'd keep mine around 20 per cent. I don't want
          to be alone.   136

Significantly however, the registrar speaks of increasing pressure to avoid an obstetric disaster and possible litigation. Such pressure, together with patient requests, increases CS rates. In this situation, the obstetricians seek to identify with their professional norm, rather than to negotiate with patients. Their patients are also applying external pressure as pregnant women are increasingly requesting elective Caesarean sections (Fragment 4). These pressures are perceived as threatening in that they diminish professional control. It could be argued that the obstetricians have 'relinquished' their clinical authority and autonomy to their patients and are now functioning as service providers.

The aim of a healthy baby specifically serves to provide the team members with a professional target or benchmark. The benchmark also provides a rationale for *routinised* treatment or clinical care that the team members agree to as a package, without the need to for individual discussion with each patient. The registrar supplies evidence for this when he states, 'I'll go along with the College, I mean I'm not going to stand on my own about it' (line 133). In an attempt to gain some measure of control and predictability in the management of multiple cases, the registrar's judgement is focused on the routinisation of treatment and care.

Routines constitute, in Konner's terms, the safety of the norm: you feel safe because you do what everybody else is doing (1988, p. 366). Berg (1992) suggests that the concept of routines supplies a structure in medical action together with 'economy of effort' (p. 170). Interestingly, Berg comments that stepping out of a routine implies that the action needs to be explicitly renegotiated. Such adoption of routines by the senior team members does raise questions about the extent to which the 'rule basis' of their clinical knowledge is able to structure the localised, individual negotiations and decision-making between themselves and pregnant women.

Fragment 11

C: If you actually were to look at outcomes, if the outcome you chose to   156
    measure is fetal well-being, then 100 per cent is the correct CS rate. Well maybe 157
    not, it will depend when you do it of course, there are suggestions that CS   158
    might increase the chances of respiratory distress syndrome. Leaving all that   159
    aside, the success outcome that you really should be measuring in pregnancy   160
    is a healthy baby. Caesareans are associated with a healthy baby more   161
    frequently than vaginal deliveries. It's up to the mother to decide what she   162
    wants. The mother can look after herself; the baby is not able to look after   163
    itself.   164

In Fragment 11 the consultant obstetrician provides his colleagues with some indication of the beliefs that guide his professional practice: 'Caesareans are associated with a healthy baby more frequently than vaginal deliveries'. This would suggest that as professionals the team members should aspire to orientate their obstetric practice to the success outcome of a healthy baby delivered by an elective Caesarean section. This benchmark provides clarity for the obstetric team members in terms of their goal for obstetric practice, but what are the possible implications and consequences of this collective, practical reasoning and medical decision-making for the individual pregnant woman?

How much choice does the pregnant woman really have to 'decide what she wants'? The birth of a 'healthy baby' from the senior obstetrician's point of view does not involve any reference to the individual woman's preferences and choices. The consultant appears to be of the opinion that he, as the professional, is best able to advocate and judge the interests and rights of the foetus. However, before the obstetric team's benchmark of a healthy baby delivered by elective Caesarean can be actioned, the team members will have to negotiate mode of delivery options with each individual pregnant woman and gain her informed consent.

Categorisation of pregnant women

In Fragment 12 the consultant obstetrician and the registrar explain to their junior colleagues that women in all class categories are increasingly taking an active interest in negotiating their obstetric treatment and care. These negotiations are occurring within an organisational context in which the registrar has already stated time is a limited resource and where they, as professionals, are beginning to feel pressured and threatened by their clients' demands.

Fragment 12

Q:	Would a woman have to wait for a consultant to suggest it? [elective	86
	Caesarean section]	87
C:	It depends on how articulate she is. A lot of women know that they can ask	88
	for an elective Caesarean section. It actually tends to be social class 1 and 2,	89
	with access to the Internet and all this sort of stuff. Sooner or later it affects	90
	the others.	91
R:	Yes, that's right, I mean everyone else will expect the same.	92
C:	I don't think it's class. I think it's education, they are not necessarily the	93
	same things.	94
R:	Everyone drives a car now, ten to twenty years ago that wasn't the case. It's the	95
	same with these elective sections, you know, they are going to say why is it	96
	just for a select breed. They are going to say 'If she can ask for an elective	97
	CS, then I'm going to ask for an elective CS'. Social class 5 is now not the	98
	social class 5 it was ten years ago, they all drive cars, they all go on holiday	99
	to Tenerife, they all have an interest in their medical care. They are not	100
	going to believe a doctor just because he says this is what you should be	101
	having.	102

While medicine is broadly regarded as predicated upon scientific principles of objectivity and altruism, moral judgements and evaluations pervade the individual senior team members' perceptions of their clients. Various categorisations or typifications appear in their vocabularies of pregnant women. The consultant and registrar spoke of social class, the consultant also gauges 'what sort of person the patient is' assessing the women's competence in negotiating her preferred treatment options and concluding that the 'educated' patients are the most effective. While individual clients may vary in the degree to which they actually are marked by any of these characteristics, the senior team members are also using these characteristics to distinguish and distance obstetric clients as a group from themselves as medical staff.

The registrar defensively perceives that pregnant women in the NHS are only prepared to trust their obstetricians up to a certain point. This perspective could have serious implications for the clinical work of the team because without the client's concession of trust, a practitioner cannot practise and without a generalised trust a profession loses its authority (Daniel, 1998). It also implies that pregnant women are now beginning to challenge the team members' professional autonomy and authority on an everyday basis.

One element that all clients have in common is that they can pose difficulties for medical staff who, as they see it, are attempting to do their work. Lorber (1975) found that doctors regard as 'good' those patients who do not make trouble, or complain, or interrupt medical routines. There seems to be an unwritten rule operating that is in part consensual and part ideological, that those women who co-operate with medical staff and make minimal demands on their time are 'sensible', whilst those who are uncooperative and interrupt medical routines are 'pessimistic'. The registrar is using an unofficial, moralistic taxonomy of pregnant women. Stein (1990, p. 98) has suggested that 'bad' clients are considered to be non-compliant, demanding and hostile, seeking to control the doctor and question his authority and competence. Therefore making the doctor feel out of control and a 'loser'. These judgements are not being made according to any medical criteria but according to the registrar's own personal, culturally determined values as to how pregnant women should be.

Fragment 13

R: Women want what is fashionable at the time. If NCT were doing a lot of   165
   pushing on natural childbirth that's what they would want at the time. If the   166
   hype at the time is an elective CS, there would be a lot more women coming   167
   for an elective CS. It's the power of the media, the power of peer pressure   168
   and everything else. There are a lot of women out there at the end of the day 169
   who are very sensible and they know that a vaginal delivery is natural. Those 170
   women are always going to still be there. It's going to be those that are   171
   genuinely pessimistic in nature and just don't want a 12-hour labour in pain,   172
   they want the easier route. A lot of women would say yes to an elective CS,   173
   but, a vaginal delivery is natural and I want what is natural. See what I   174
   mean?   175

C: One of the problems is that women generally tend to be very self-centred and   176
selfish but they don't always get the chance to express that or to rectify the   177
situation. But when they are pregnant then somebody has to listen to them (R   178
laughs) they are the centre of attention. The whole obstetric world is set up   179
to focus on the pregnant woman and they are going to take advantage of it.   180
They come along here and they ask questions 'oh where does the Venflon   181
go' and 'how long will I be in the operating theatre?'. I don't think they are   182
really interested at all, it's just that they want to continue to be the centre of   183
attention and the focus of the whole show.   184

In Fragment 13 the consultant obstetrician and the registrar express very low opinions of their obstetric clients. Rather than being perceived as knowledgeable, well informed and able to make their own choices, pregnant women's preferences are trivialised by the registrar who suggests that they 'want what is fashionable at the time'. Furthermore, the pregnant woman's desire for information is defensively perceived by the consultant obstetrician as a desire to blame someone. This phenomenon has been documented elsewhere. Macintyre and Porter (1989) argue that many doctors seem to have a low opinion of their women patients, distrusting them or treating them as ignorant. They also observed that women who asked many questions at the antenatal clinic were likely to be labelled 'anxious'. Hall *et al.* (1985) and McKinlay (1975) reported doctors' lack of appreciation of pregnant women's medical knowledge. The consequences of these medical perspectives are twofold: either women's preferences and requests will not be taken seriously, or they will be dealt with by the obstetricians in such a way that are ignored or not heard.

It would seem from the perspectives of pregnant women held by the consultant obstetrician, that he is adopting an 'old style' masculine model of care which is in accordance with a traditional masculine gender stereotype. His advice to junior colleagues that women tend to be 'self-centred and selfish' is clearly out of step with much current debate on partnership and shared decision-making between professionals and their clients, e.g. Coulter (1999).

Loss of obstetric experience

Obstetrics has been the focus of increasing criticism in recent years. Grant (1997, p. 387) stated:

'There is no doubt that our speciality has received so much scrutiny in the past decade that its very existence is being seriously questioned. Obstetricians are criticised by government commissions for performing too many Caesarean sections and by the legal profession for performing too few ... we are criticised by women for making labour too regimented... We cannot win. It is this unresolved tension over our responsibilities which is so frustrating to obstetricians and accounts for our low morale.'

It is argued by Strauss et al. (1964, p. 4) that at each institutional locale, whether hospital or clinic, the jurisdictional areas of each specialist group have to be adjudicated and negotiated. The division of labour cannot be legislated; it must be worked out at each locale. The obstetric unit and antenatal clinic therefore is a vitally important site, not only for the treatment of clients, but for its bearing upon the destiny and relationships of the specialism of obstetrics. It is here that the professional philosophies are negotiated and transmitted.

In Fragment 14 it is possible to explore aspects of the collective practical reasoning and professional decision-making process that contribute to the development of treatment philosophies. The obstetric team or 'firm' is organised as a traditional three-tier hierarchical structure of consultant obstetrician, registrar and senior house officer, also present are two medical students. This is very much a 'consultant-led' model in which the overall policy and decision-making follows hierarchical lines and is tightly controlled (see also: Seeman and Evans, 1961; Knafl and Burkett, 1975; Bosk, 1979). An important aspect of this subculture concerns the comparatively greater importance placed on clinical as opposed to academic learning and knowledge.

Fragment 14

SHO:	What's going to happen is if the CS rate goes up to 50 per cent, then it's only	46
	going to be the really easy vaginal deliveries that are going to happen. Is it	47
	that in ten years time they'll be saying 'oh no not a vaginal' 'you'd be mad	48
	to do that', if it's a breech you'd think, 'oh my God', and the obstetrician	49
	saying 'I remember doing one of these when I was a young lad'?	50
R:	There's going to be an explosion in sections. For example consultants now,	51
	you can see that the pressure is developing anyway, but they feel they can	52
	put a control on it they think they'll be able to stop it. I don't think they	53
	will be able to stop it; I think they are being very naive if they think they	54
	can. It's been shown, in an article that it's cheaper to do an elective	55
	Caesarean on everyone, sack all the midwives and just do an elective CS on	56
	everyone at 36, 37 weeks. If you're going to have a policy decision of	57
	elective CS on everyone, the overall costs would then be cheaper, you still	58
	have to have a core of team midwifery staff for the pre-term obstetric	59
	problems and whatever else but you can dramatically reduce your daily	60
	core of midwifery staff. Honestly, I am sure we have discussed this	61
	before.	62
Q:	But then, isn't your specialism going to radically alter?	63
R:	It is already, when was the last time I did a Keilands or did a Ventouse? I	64
	used to do them all the time. I'm not saying that CS is wrong, but with that	65
	comes loss of experience. I personally would not attempt to do a Keilands	66
	today because I haven't done a few for a while, do you understand? Why	67
	does C [consultant] section all his breeches? Because he feels most	68
	registrars today aren't as capable of delivering breeches as they were in the	69

	past and for that reason he now feels the lists are higher, the CS rates are	70
	higher. For that reason he feels it's the same problem as with elective CS.	71
C:	Who me, is that's what I think?	72
R:	Yes	73
C:	I think there is a lot to that, it's a very strong argument when you look at	74
	perinatal mortality figures out there on Monday you will see that there	
	are three to	75
	four breech deliveries a month, sometimes there are only two. We have	
	got eight	76
	consultants, three senior registrars, five registrars, a couple of part-time	
	registrars	77
	and a certain number of SHOs who want breech experience. It seems to	78
	me absolutely impossible to have enough experience to maintain breech	79
	delivery skills, especially for those who know how to do it, let alone to	80
	teach people how to do it, it can't be done. It's a self-fulfilling prophecy I	81
	agree and accept that. They will have to be delivered by Caesarean sooner	82
	or later, but I am afraid I am not prepared to stand up in court and say well,	83
	I allowed this trial of breech delivery because my registrar hadn't done very	84
	many.	85

Knafl and Burkett suggest that the group setting in the clinical environment provides ample opportunity for junior staff to become involved in the process of decision-making and to begin acquiring medical judgement. An example of such an occasion is provided here. The senior house officer enters the discussion stating, 'If it's a breech you'd think, "oh my God".' Professionally most of his team colleagues would probably agree with him. What is also eluded to here is the diminishing opportunities for gaining clinical experience and expertise in difficult vaginal deliveries. This is a paradoxical situation for the specialism as it has been argued that a major reason why the Caesarean rate is escalating is because obstetricians have become deskilled (Kitzinger, 1997).

For the team members the registrar's vision of increased demands and pressures being placed on them as practitioners suggests that the core of their clinical obstetric practice and their clinical workload is set to undergo profound changes. The team members' problem is that they now need to reach some definition of what their own therapeutic and management action should be in response to their current clinical dilemma. They need to define their own ideological position that will serve to guide their clinical resolution and practical action.

In line 64 the registrar further shares with his junior colleagues the ambiguities and uncertainties of his clinical practice. In doing so he is providing his audience with a widened, vicarious obstetric experience. He acknowledges his diminishing expertise in the ability to undertake breech deliveries and emphasises to his colleagues his reliance on the personal knowledge and treatment philosophy of the consultant obstetrician who 'sections all of his breeches', 'because he feels most registrars today aren't as capable of delivering breeches as they were in the past'. The personal knowledge and experience of the consultant is treated by the registrar as a warrant for certainty. As also observed by Atkinson (1995, p. 115), the primacy of direct experience is taken by the registrar to guarantee knowledge which the student or practitioner can rely on.

The group context of the pragmatic decision-making specifically affords the junior members of the team with the opportunity to consider and evaluate treatment options without having to assume responsibility for the outcomes. In line 74 the consultant introduces an important organisational factor: there are too many obstetric trainees and insufficient experience available to fulfil their training requirements in relation to breech experience. He concludes therefore, 'they will have to be delivered by Caesarean sooner or later'. However, in assuming responsibility for the team's practical action and treatment philosophy the obstetrician is also placing himself at risk, as Freidson (1988, p. 170) has argued he is, 'always vulnerable to reproach, legal or otherwise'. The obstetrician himself recognises this with his comment, 'I am not prepared to stand up in court and say well I allowed this trial of breech delivery because my registrar hadn't done very many'. The obstetrician is clearly aware that his professional authority, as Freidson has observed, 'teeters between glory and ruin and is prone to claim its glory more because of risk of ruin than because of its accomplishment'.

Being manipulative

It is argued by Freidson (1988, p. 308) that as a profession medicine claims that its mission is to provide a good service to its clientele. The profession asserts what the customer's 'real' wants are by virtue of its special knowledge and, as an 'ethical' occupation, attempts to provide services appropriate to those wants it defines. But in order to exercise its mandate the profession must on occasion provide its clients with services they may not want. In doing so Freidson argues, it must in some way manipulate or exercise control over the client. If medical work is to be performed to the satisfaction of the staff, procedures that minimise interference with their routine and maximise their convenience are required. Asking for something is a client's simplest way of trying to control a professional's work. However, a prominent characteristic that may facilitate professional control is the withholding of information as this can minimise the possibility that the client can exercise control over the way they are treated.

It would seem that the senior team members perceive that they are not able to exert their professional control over negotiations with pregnant women. What is interesting in Fragment 15 is the recourse by the senior team members to defensive rhetoric. They are using a particular sort of vocabulary to account for their social actions. Coffey *et al.* (1996, p. 100) suggest that social actors may be describing events in certain sorts of ways that account for, justify, excuse, or legitimate action or behaviour. The senior team members are justifying their proposed use of manipulative negotiation strategies to their colleagues because they claim, pregnant women are 'manipulating' them and that their 'only defence is to be manipulative back'.

Fragment 15

R: I think that as obstetricians what we need to learn is to start being very   185
    manipulative with the women, because they are being very manipulative   186
    with us. Our only defence is going to be manipulative back because our   187
    normal standard approach which is using logical, factual information and   188
    sense isn't working. It's not going to work. That approach is not going to   189
    work.   190

C: I think this explains why the male obstetrician remains popular. You would   191
    think that all women would want to see a female obstetrician but in fact they   192
    don't. A lot of female obstetricians can see through this, this nonsense and   193
    they won't put up with it at all they are not the least bit interested in it. I am   194
    not being funny, I am being serious, a lot of females see through this and see   195
    the woman is manipulating and they are very unsympathetic.   196

R: The standard approach, being sensible, I think will only take you so far.   197

The registrar initially appeals to his junior audience on the basis that their 'normal standard approach which is using logical, factual information and sense isn't working'. He does not attempt to conceal the moral basis of his comments, but rather demonstrates that their neutral, medical or 'scientific' approach has so far not worked as a justification for more covert negotiation approaches.

More provocative however, are the comments made by the consultant obstetrician. He makes it explicit that he is employing his personal and moral value judgements when categorising pregnant women as 'manipulative' and that these gender-based views reflect his low opinion, suspicion and mistrust of his obstetric clients' motives. He places himself in the role of victim and as someone who cannot 'see through this nonsense' the way a female obstetrician can, implying that pregnant women prefer male obstetricians because they can manipulate them. Central to this argument is the stereotypical view that women are given to complaining and exaggerating their discomforts.

From the senior team members perspectives it would appear that pregnant women now have more power in the obstetrician/client relationship. However, it should not be assumed that obstetricians and their clients are negotiating from equal positions of power. The major dilemma of the doctor/patient relationship is that it is intrinsically unequal. The senior members are talking about pregnant women in a patronising manner that emphasises the low regard in which they are held. If the team members were to treat their clients as moral, rational and intelligent participants this would grant them some independence from their medical authority. They are not seeking mutuality or equality within the obstetrician/client relationship;

they want to remove any advantage that they perceive the pregnant woman has gained so that they may regain control of the encounter. The obstetricians wish their interests to predominate over those of their clients. They are therefore proposing to their junior colleagues that indirect, covert negotiation methods and discursive coping strategies should be adopted in the consultation process as a means to that end.

Hidden agenda

It is now possible to conclude the first descriptive level of the thematic analysis and tentatively answer Wolcott's (1994, p. 12) question of the team narrative data, 'What is going on here?' Situated within this informal narrative is a complex medical story about the everyday work of obstetric practitioners. There are interlinking analytic themes that weave throughout the narrative. There is also a plot line, which has a number of dimensions or layers within it. On an organisation level, conditions and events both internal and external to the clinical environment have changed. Structural factors such as lack of time are having a profound effect on the work of team members in the clinical setting. There are also considered to be too many trainees within the obstetric unit, where there is insufficient clinical experience available to support their training requirements. In the NHS (as opposed to private obstetric care) clients are demanding more of their obstetricians in terms of higher standards of care, but in particular, are requiring more time for further discussions and information.

On a professional level there is a highly uncertain situation developing. Women are requesting elective Caesarean sections and there is now no medical reason not to grant such a request. These changes have brought about a shift in the nature of the practitioner/client relationship. The woman is now perceived to have equal if not greater bargaining power in the negotiation context. However, the senior team members, as professionals, wish to retain the right to control their own work. They are finding the increased demands and expectations of their clients to be frustrating and emotionally draining. These professionals are defensive and perceive that they are now 'in trouble'. Senior team members suggest to their junior colleagues, that it is time to reappraise this clinical dilemma and to reflect on the obstetric team's position regarding treatment ideologies. There is a need to reach some consensus or definition of what the team's therapeutic and management action should be. The senior team members are proposing that there is also a need to explore possible choices as to the team's future clinical action and coping strategies in preparation for negotiating mode of delivery and treatment options with their clients.

Scheff (1968) has emphasised the negotiable nature of interactions and suggests that definitions of reality are produced through interaction. However, he argues, that interactions take place against a background of a 'hidden agenda', known only to the more powerful participant, which compromises information, rules and procedures pertinent to achieving a successful outcome acceptable to the subordinate. In the case of the doctor/client relationship the hidden agenda consists of information about diagnosis, prognosis and treatment, and by controlling access to it, the doctor can maintain control over the encounter and its outcome.

The undisclosed 'hidden agenda' in these circumstances is that, it is not the pregnant woman who is at risk; it is the senior team members who perceive that they are at risk. As obstetricians they risk losing their control of the practitioner/client encounter and therefore their ability to maintain their professional authority when negotiating treatment options. The pragmatic issue for the team members appears to be; what possible resources, interactional practices or discursive strategies could they employ as a means to negotiate their preferred treatment options? The senior team members are advocating the perpetuation of patient uncertainty for as long as possible as a means to protect the obstetrician's professional authority.

Discursive and interactional resources

The second level of the team narrative analysis explores how everyday talk is accomplished between members of the obstetric team. As Atkinson (1995) has argued, medical work and medical knowledge are enacted within an oral culture. He suggests that within the modern teaching hospital physicians and their students repeatedly provide one another with knowledgeable audiences, before whom the practitioner may demonstrate, describe, justify and persuade. Medical knowledge therefore, is grounded in a great deal of talk between colleagues, or between teachers and their students. Atkinson further states that, some of the 'wide range of skills' (90) required to accomplish medical work include rhetorical, embodied skills that are part of the craft knowledge of the experienced practitioner. In large measure they are acquired through the 'apprenticeship' of the junior practitioner. Atkinson notes particularly that it is in the 'backstage' regions of medical settings that medical practitioners consult with each other. As it is here where doctor/doctor interaction constitutes contexts through which medical knowledge and professional judgement are formulated.

Whilst analysing the transcript to explore the way talk was actually used between the team members, it became clear that the senior members were jointly articulating two discourses simultaneously within the narrative. One aimed at the junior members of the team – the professional discourse, the other addressed the obstetric client – the latter in the form of stories and as repeated talk. Sarangi and Roberts (1999, p. 15) suggest that what professionals routinely do as a way of accomplishing their duties and responsibilities can be called the professional discourse and that an apprentice is required to learn the discourse of the profession.

The professional discourse is being employed by the senior team members to socialise and teach their junior colleagues about professional work. They are telling informal stories about routine obstetric events and practice, sharing what they think is significant about it e.g. which clinical tasks have precedence. This tacit, medical knowledge specifically informs the junior members about subsequent clinical action and 'what we do in this team'. In order to achieve this the senior members are skilfully drawing upon a variety of discursive and interactional resources. Their rhetorical skills and competencies are particularly focused upon persuading and justifying to the junior staff, their preferred treatment ideology and approach for the clinical management of their obstetric clients. For example, three-part lists are employed by the senior members to demonstrate how they categorise pregnant women (e.g. Fragment 12, lines 98–100) and quantification is used as an interactional resource to indicate an increase in obstetric workload (e.g. Fragment 8, lines 39–44). The senior members are also using contrastive rhetoric to differentiate between 'us' as professional colleagues and 'them' the obstetric clients.

Fragment 16

R: It is skewed our way when it comes to illness and disease because it's like   282
'I recommend you have this treatment', 'Well, why?' 'Well, if you don't have   283
this treatment you are going to deteriorate this way, and if you do take the   284
treatment the chances are you might still deteriorate but the chances are you   285
won't, so which do you want?' Well, obviously it's skewed our way, we   286
have just convinced her in one blanket statement that has just taken two   287
minutes to explain to the patient, do you know what I mean. So it is skewed   288
our way when it comes to that. That's easy to do, I love that because it's   289
easy and it's like a battle between you that you know you are going to win.   290

The language of resistance and defence permeates their talk about their clients and they arrive at the conclusion that pregnant women want to blame and 'trap' the professional. The metaphor of 'a battle' is specifically used to emphasise this perspective.

The senior members are also giving their version of what it is like to talk to clients as they repeat and rehearse aspects of institutional talk. They are specifically demonstrating to the junior members how they should talk and negotiate treatment options with obstetric clients in the consultation encounter. For example, the registrar is using active voicing to introduce the voice of a client and conduct a 'virtual' consultation in front of his junior audience. This provides the inexperienced junior staff with an opportunity to witness the rehearsal and reconstruction of the more formal institutional discourse. The team members are also jointly negotiating and agreeing about the appropriate amount of information to share with their obstetric clients. It is of particular significance that the rhetoric of risk is used as a shared interactional resource and is extensively promoted by the senior staff as a device that the junior team members should use to rebut and undermine any decisions the pregnant woman may have already made.

> Fragment 17
>
> You're having to deal with that risk. It's a matter of   235
> making a decision on risks and balancing it out. Everyone's got a risk of a   236
> CS and they want to know what that risk is. They'll ask us for the risk and   237
> we'll have to give them a rough guesstimate of that risk. This risk   238
> guesstimate that is given to them really is a guesstimate because we just   239
> have no. ... Each individual person is going to have their own risk. You've   240
> got a lady that's OP, it's a big baby, it's not engaged, there are no figures to   241
> say what her risk of CS is going to be because she is going to be different to   242
> a lady who is not carrying as big a baby, thats head's engaged. That's not an   243
> individual risk, we do it on different things. Do you see what I mean? So   244
> you have to increase the risk slightly or decrease the risk slightly depending   245
> on the clinical situation.   246
> SHO: Round it up?   247
> R: Round it up, yes. Get a four-part figure. She is going to ask for the risk and   248
>   you're going to try to avoid it and she is going to push a bit more and so you   249
>   say fine I'll try to work out a risk and eventually you'll give her a risk and   250
>   she'll say 'I don't like that risk'.   251

Indeed, the senior team members are advocating that the rhetoric of risk be used to construct, assemble and magnify a professional definition of risk in circumstances where none may actually exit for the obstetric client. Even if there are no obstetric problems at all with a woman's pregnancy, the rhetoric of risk is being used to construct birth as a situation of inherent risk requiring expert technical management by obstetricians.

Conclusion

Wolcott (1994, p. 36) considers that the third level of transforming the data, interpretation, is the point 'at which the researcher transcends factual data and cautious analysis and begins to probe into what is to be made of them'. This is where the goal for the researcher is to make sense of what is going on. The team narrative or medical story, gleaned from the backstage area of the antenatal clinic, provides us with an unusual opportunity to explore from an obstetric perspective, the complexity of issues that impact upon the doctor/client relationship. It is a practical story about why particular medical work problems have developed, why they have not been solved, and what the team should be doing to try to solve them.

The team narrative focuses upon the interactional processes of decision-making relating to treatment options, mode of delivery and more specifically, negotiating elective Caesarean section. As the analysis of the micro-level of collegial talk reveals, there appears to be a high level of tension and conflict between the team members and their clients. The team members are using defensive rhetorical and discursive strategies in an attempt to maintain control over their work environment and their relationships with their obstetric clients, who they now perceive have greater power in the negotiation process.

Issues are raised here about the power of information and professional dominance. For the team members the capacity to obscure and conceal information from the obstetric client has become very important. The pregnant woman is being interactionally manipulated into agreeing or even choosing, the course of action that the team members want her to make – a healthy baby delivered by elective Caesarean section. The obstetricians' are not seeking or advising mutuality or equality in the practitioner /client relationship. They do not want to make negotiating treatment options a matter of choice for the woman.

Note

1 This chapter is based on a paper that was published in MIDIRS *Midwifery Digest*, **11** (supplement 2), September 2001, pp. 18–22.

Acknowledgement

The author would like to acknowledge the support of the Northern and Yorkshire NHS Executive, who funded this project through the award of an NHS Executive Regional Research Fellowship 1996/7.

References

Atkinson, P. (1981) *The Clinical Experience: the Construction and Reconstruction of Medical Reality.* Guildford: Gower.

Atkinson, P. (1995) *Medical Work and Medical Talk: The Liturgy of the Clinic.* London: Sage Publications.

Berg, M. (1992) The social construction of medical disposals. Medical sociology and the medical problem solving in clinical practice. *Sociology of Health & Illness*, **14(2)**: 151–80.

Billig, M. (1991) *Ideologies and Beliefs.* London: Sage.

Bosk, C. (1979) *Forgive and Remember: Managing Medical Failure.* Chicago: University of Chicago Press.

Boylan, P.C. (1989) Active Management of Labor: Results in Dublin, Houston, London, New Brunswick, Singapore and Valparaiso. *Birth*, **16(3)**: 114–18.

Coffey, A., Holbrook, B. and Atkinson, P. (1996) Qualitative Data Analysis: Technologies and Representations, *Sociological Research Online*, **1(1)**. Available from: http://www.socresonline.org.uk/socresonline/1/1/4.html.

Coulter, A. (1999) Paternalism or partnership? Editorial in *British Medical Journal*, **319**: 719–20.

Daniel, A. (1998) Trust and medical authority. In A. Petersen and C. Waddell, *Health*

Matters: A Sociology of Illness, Prevention and Care. Buckingham: Open University Press.

Frankel, R. (1990) Talking in interviews: a dispreference for patient-initiated questions in physician–patient encounter. In G. Psathas (ed.), *Interaction Competence.* Lanham, MD: University Press of America.

Freidson, E. (1970) *Professional Dominance: The Social Structure of Medical Care.* Chicago: Aldine.

Freidson, E. (1988) *The Profession of Medicine: A Study of the Sociology of Applied Knowledge.* Chicago and London: University of Chicago Press.

Grant, J.M. (1997) The whole duty of obstetricians. Editorial in *The British Journal of Obstetrics and Gynaecology*, **104**: 387–92.

Hall, H., Macintyre, S. and Porter, M. (1985) *Antenatal Care Assessed,.* Aberdeen: Aberdeen University Press.

Heritage, J. (1997) Conversational analysis and institutional talk. In, D. Silverman (ed.), *Qualitative Research: Theory, Method and Practice.* London: Sage.

Higgins, J. (1988) *The Business of Medicine.* Basingstoke: Macmillan.

Johnson, T. (1972) *Professions and Power.* London: Macmillan.

Kitzinger, S. (1997) A battle for the control of women's bodies. *The Independent*, 22 March.

Knafl, K. and Burkett, G. (1975) Professional socialisation in a surgical speciality: acquiring medical judgement. *Social Science and Medicine*, **9**: 397–404.

Konner, M. (1988) as cited in M. Berg (1992) The social construction of medical disposals. Medical sociology and the medical problem solving in clinical practice. *Sociology of Health and Illness*, **14(2)**: 151–80.

Lazarus, E.S. (1988) Theoretical considerations for the study of the doctor–patient relationship: implications of a perinatal study. *Medical Anthropology Quarterly*, **2(1)**: 34–58.

Linnell, P., Gustavsson, L. and Juvonen, P. (1988) Interactional dominance in dyadic communication: a presentation of initiative-response analysis. *Linguistics*, **26**: 415–42.

Lomas, J. and Enkin, M. (1989) Variations on operative delivery rates. In M. Enkin, M. Keirse and I. Chalmers (eds), *Effective Care in Pregnancy and Childbirth.* Oxford: Oxford University Press.

Lorber, J. (1975) Good patients and problem patients: conformity and deviance in a general hospital. *Journal of Health and Social Behaviour*, **16**: 213–25.

Lupton, D. (1994) *Medicine as Culture: Illness, Disease and The Body in Western Societies.* London: Sage.

Macintyre, S. and Porter, M. (1989) Prospects and problems in promoting effective care at the local level. In M. Enkin, M. Keirse and I. Chalmers (eds), *Effective Care in Pregnancy and Childbirth.* Oxford: Oxford University Press.

McClosky, D. (1998) *The Rhetoric of Economics.* 2nd edn. Wisconsin: University of Wisconsin Press.

McKinlay, J. (1975) Who is really ignorant – physician or patient? *Journal of Health and Social Behaviour*, **16**: 3–11.

Meredith, P. (1993) Patient participation in decision-making and consent to treatment: the case of general surgery, *Sociology of Health and Illness*, **15(3)**: 315–36.

Mishler, E. (1984) *The Discourse of Medicine: Dialectics of Medical Interviews.* Norwood, NJ: Ablex.

Roth, J.A. (1963) *Timetables, Structuring the Passage of Time in Hospital Treatment and Other Careers.* New York: Bobbs Merrill.

Sarangi, S. and Roberts, C. (1999) *Talk, Work and Institutional Order: Discourse in Medical, Mediation and Management Settings.* Berlin: Mouton de Gruyer.

Scheff, T.J. (1966) *Being Mentally Ill: A Sociological Theory.* London: Weidenfeld & Nicolson.

Seeman, M. and Evans, J.W. (1961) Stratification and hospital care: I. The performance of the medical intern. *American Sociological Review*, **26**: 67–80.

Starr, P. (1982) *The Social Transformation of American Medicine*. New York: Basic Books.

Stein, H.F. (1990) *American Medicine as Culture*. Colorado: Westview.

Stevens, R. (1986) The future of the medical profession. In E. Ginsberg (ed.), *From Physician Shortage to Patient Shortage: The Uncertain Future of Medical Practice*. Boulder: Westview.

Strauss, A., Schatzman, L., Bucher, R., Ehrlich, D. and Sabshin, M. (1964) *Psychiatric Ideologies and Institutions*. New York: Free Press of Glencoe, Collier-Macmillan.

Waitzkin, H. and Stoeckle, J. (1972) The communication of information about illness. *Advances in Psychosomatic Medicine*, **8**: 180–215.

Wiles, R., Higgins, J. (1996) Doctor–patient relationships in the private sector: patients' perceptions. *Sociology of Health and Illness*, **18(3)**: 341–56.

Willis, E. (1989) *Medical Dominance: The Division of Labour in Australian Health Care* (revised edition). Sydney: Allen and Unwin.

Wolcott, H. (1994) *Transforming Qualitative Data: Description, Analysis, and Interpretation*. Thousand Oaks, CA: Sage.

CHAPTER 11

Birth Experiences of South Asian Muslim Women: Marginalised Choice within the Maternity Services[1]

NICKY ELLIS

The rationale behind informed choice has been driven by changes within the political arena. The emerging voices of women in the 1990s and other social and political changes gave rise to the publication of *Changing Childbirth* (Department of Health, 1993). The central themes to this policy document were to become known as the Three Cs: Continuity, Choice and Control. Maternity services were charged with making the service more women-focused, and ensuring that high quality and research-based information should be readily available to staff and clients. Since the 1997 White Paper: *The New NHS: Modern, Dependable* (DoH) and *First Class Service* (DoH, 1998) the government programme of health reforms has emphasised quality standards, clinical effectiveness, openness and a culture of active working encompassing service users, the public and health professionals. These policy documents have placed information-sharing and good practice at the centre of good quality care. Women have greater access to information through the Internet, media, soap operas, and health professionals. Subsequently this has given them greater opportunities for choice.

What is informed choice? The development of the relationship between client and midwife is based on trust, respect and caring. In this context Harding (2000) differentiates between 'shared decision-making' and 'informed choice.'

'Shared decision-making' was seen by midwives as being embedded in their role as educators and facilitators in midwifery practice; they saw this as enabling women to share responsibility for their maternity care and take an active part in the decision-making process. Whereas 'informed choice' was described as an information-giving process, to give women an understanding of the options that are available. However Harding found in her study that the information that was given depended on a number of different variables: the situation in which information was given, biases of the information giver, or being aware of the influence they had over their clients. Midwives see informed choice as part of the decision-making process which can be empowering for the woman. Yet the unequal power base can also create dependency (Leap, 2000).

Background

Maternity services and ethnic minority women

> 'The birth of the first child is an important landmark event in the lives of women. No other event has such a dramatic effect which women remember with great clarity and emotion.' (Oakley, 1993)

The last decade has seen a succession of government, and professional publications. The publication of *Changing Childbirth* (DoH, 1993) acknowledged that choice, continuity and control were the areas that women and midwives thought would enhance the experience of birth. This report put the emphasis on women having an individualised package of care. *First Class Service* (DoH, 1998) advocated a quality service for local populations, encouraging partnership between users and health professionals. The Royal College of Midwives' *The Vision* (RCM, 2000) recommends a service that is sensitive to individual needs and reduces inequalities.

These inequalities still exist. The publication of the *Confidential Enquiry into Maternal Deaths* (NICE, 2002) highlights the fact that women from minority ethnic backgrounds and unable to understand English have increased mortality rates, with women from South Asia having the highest risk. Recommendations of the CEMD advise that:

Health professionals who work with disadvantaged groups understand the cultural and social background, and act as advocates for women ... also overcome their own personal and social prejudices and practice in a reflective manner. (NICE, 2001)

Phoenix (1990) and Barj (1995) discuss how the maternity services are discriminatory in the care they deliver. They speak of women from ethnic minorities experiencing stereotyping, discrimination and racism, from a service organised to meet the needs of the white middle class. It is suggested by Neile (1997) that policies and midwifery practice assume that the population is white and English-speaking. Within the birthing culture there appears to be an inflexibility to individualised care when the care is for 'other' women and families. Bowler (1993) studied attitudes of midwives in East London. She confirmed that women from minority backgrounds were frequently stereotyped because of communication difficulties, women were perceived to be non-compliant and to sometimes abuse the service, 'make a fuss about nothing' and lack a maternal instinct.

In Scotland, Bowes and Domokos (1996) found that midwives' negative attitudes towards Pakistani women were expressed in how they delivered care. Some women from this study interpreted their care as being racist.

Katbamna (2000) compared Gujarati and Bangladeshi women using maternity services. The Bangladeshi women were more likely to present late in labour because they anticipated difficulties in an alien hospital environment due to language difficulties and the lack of sensitivity to the needs of the family. However, they were more likely to have normal births with low intervention rates. Whereas the Gujarati women presented early in labour, experienced higher rates of intervention, induction of labour and Caesarean section. Their labour experiences mirrored Sally Inches 'cascade of intervention', and that coupled with lack of cultural sensitivity surrounding the birth they perceived more negative attitudes towards their experiences (Katbamna, 2000).

Theoretical dimensions of race

The theoretical dimensions of race date back to 'scientific racism' in the eighteenth and nineteenth century, which was closely linked with slavery and colonisation. The classification of races was based solely on skin colour and linked black skin with evil, dirt, ignorance and lack of civilisation (Young, 2000). Texts of the time are described as 'biological reductionism' in that race types were organised in a hierarchy and include a sub-species of *homo sapiens* (Fernando, 2002) The anatomists even purported to find biological differences in the skull and brain size. The Darwinian theory in the nineteenth century supported the 'extinction of savage races' because of their inability to change habits (Darwin, 1871). The progress of science has made these early theories scientifically invalid.

There is no rational argument to say that one race is superior to another (Senior and Bhopal, 1994; Sheldon and Parker, 1992). Yet such ideas are often firmly entrenched.

Racism: a conscious or unconscious belief in the superiority of a particular 'race'. Acts of discrimination and unfair treatment whether intentional or unintentional, 'based on this belief'. (Mares *et al.*, 1985)

Racisms are socially constructed: it is physical appearances that people use to define otherness and negative group attitudes and behaviour to such others constitutes racism. Social and economic factors are also important, especially with regard to attitudes which are held collectively and linked into the power structure within institutions (Mullholland and Dyson, 2001). Groups identified as other are easily also identified as posing a threat. The struggles of the collective white workforce to have some control of employment and housing have often been diverted into the social and political exclusion of black people, thus isolating low status groups and reinforcing racist ideas of inferiority and power.

Multiculturalism, and its promotion can also result in strengthening racism. This approach fails to take into account individual differences and changes within groups. It should be recognised that different groups are made up of people of different gender, class, age, and sexual orientation this is where multiculturalism fails. Grouping all Irish people together regardless of where they come from or categorising all Muslims together is disregarding their cultural roots. Stereotyping is more likely with this approach. Bowler (1993) in her study found that midwives stereotyped women into racial categories, and felt that the women's behaviours could be predicted because they belong to a certain ethnic minority group. Some forms of racism are overt i.e. by verbal or physical attacks, others are more subtle and less noticeable. This form of racism has come to be known as *institutionalised racism*.

Institutionalised racism

Midwives care for women from a wide variety of ethnic groups under the umbrella of the NHS. This service was set up in the late 1940s to provide health care free at the point of delivery. Immigration in the thirty years that followed expanded rapidly, but delivery of health care remained entrenched in post-war philosophies of white supremacy

Within the United Kingdom, racial discrimination is illegal. The Race Relations Act (1976) forbids both direct and indirect discrimination on the grounds of colour, nationality, race or ethnic origin. The Macpherson Report (1999) identified that institutionalised racism was prevalent in the Metropolitan Police and highlighted practices that can cause organisations to act unwittingly against the interests of minority groups. The recommendations from Macpherson were that each institution, whether it is health, education or social services should examine its policies to guard against discrimination. The amendment to the Race Relations Act in 2000 broadened the scope of the 1976 Act to include the public sector. Now all public services have a duty to promote equality in the work place. The most recent strengthening of the rights of the individual comes in Articles 9 and 14 of the Human Rights Act 1998, which requires freedom of thought, conscience, and religion. Up to this time religion was excluded from the Race Relations Act.

The UKCC Code of Professional Conduct requires midwives to:

> 'recognise and respect the uniqueness and dignity of each patient and client, and respond to their need for care, irrespective of their ethnic origin, religious belief, personal attributes, the nature of their health problems, or any other factor.'

Yet women whose first language is not English and whose cultural background is not of the majority are more likely to experience maternity care which is inappropriate for their needs. It not just ethnicity but a combination of factors such as social position and spoken language that ensure that their voices remain unheard and reinforce these women's low expectations. This study sought to examine these issues in situations were language was not an obstacle to communication.

Study aims

Whilst the literature has focused on the experiences of women who may not have been fluent in English, I sought to explore the birthing experiences of women from a South Asian Muslim background who were educated in the UK. Specifically, I aimed:

- To explore the experiences of second generation South Asian Muslim women who have been educated in this country, and have no previous experiences of the maternity services.
- To highlight issues of midwifery practice for this specific group of women.

Methodology

The purpose of this study: to examine these South Asian Muslim women's birth experiences, required an ethnographic approach and qualitative data collection methods. Three methods of data collection were chosen.

- Non-participant observation during labour.
- Semi-structured interviews one week after birth.
- The review of a pre-formatted birth-plan.

Access and recruitment

To gain access to women, ethical approval was sought and given by the local NHS Research Ethics Committee.

Recruitment of women took place in the antenatal clinic of the local Maternity Unit. The criteria for women to be approached were as follows:

- Primiparous
- Between the ages of 18 and 35
- Low-risk pregnancy
- Second generation and educated in the United Kingdom
- South Asian Muslim

Women were given information about the research and assurances regarding confidentiality and anonymity. They were then asked to give informed consent if they wished to take part in the study. If consent was given then documentation was made in the woman's handheld records and the hospital notes. This ensured that midwives on the labour ward were aware that I needed to be called when the woman was in labour. Midwives on labour ward were informed about the study. Ten women were recruited to the study. The women's names in the study have been changed to protect their identity.

Data collection and analysis

As a midwife I was already familiar with the structure and culture of a Labour Ward. In order to appreciate Muslim culture I undertook discussions with mothers, their partners, the local Muslim Foundation, and a great deal of background reading into the Koran and the Hadiths. This qualitative study can only be relevant in the geographical context of an NHS labour ward as viewed though the tenets of the Muslim faith and culture. Variation within this community and between individual women are also important. Taking this into account discussions took place with many Muslim women before the study was undertaken. These discussions revealed a broad range of cultural and religious activities though the commonality of Islam links them all.

The initial data was collected by non-participant observation, which was made clear to women during the recruitment period. However, during the observation period on the labour ward I experienced difficulties to remain in the true non-participant observer. On several occasions the women looked at me for clarification of a point the midwife had discussed with them. When they were asked during the interview at home why they asked the researcher, one reply was: 'The midwife was busy anyway, well that was the attitude. So I didn't ask after that.' (Fatima)

The observation process posed further problems on the amount of data that was generated from each session. At the beginning of the study I attempted to document all activity: each eye contact, touch, proximity of people in the room as well as what was being said and the responses. In the final sessions of observation the data recorded was more selective and focused on how women reacted to midwives actions and conversation. These were then followed-up during the interview at home. The observation data was collected in a short hand method with a system of abbreviations. This had the advantage that it was meaningless to others reading it. On one occasion, when I entered the room after visiting the toilet, a midwife hastily replaced my observation on the chair!

After each observation session I also recorded my own feelings and emotions together with some background information. These included general observations on the labour ward. These were at the time of change of shift, in the midwives rest room, which gave a valuable insight into the ambience of the environment. No two days were the same, and appeared to be very dependant on which midwives were working, the levels of experience of staff, the workload of that day, and the midwife co-ordinating the work for that particular shift.

My own inexperience became apparent during the first observation period and I had doubts whether I would be able to carry out the research. Some of these doubts were reflected in my feelings of self-consciousness, and intrusion into what is a very intimate experience. Some midwives appeared to be made very uncomfortable by my presence, though I was never declined on a face-to-face basis. That was manifested in other ways: in the women's notes there was clear documentation that the woman had consented to take part in the study together with my contact details and that I was on 24-hour call for these women. On two occasions I was not contacted. No explanation was forthcoming.

The interviews took place a week later in the women's homes. The supporters who were present at the birth were also present during the interviews. These were mothers, mothers-in-law, husbands, and aunts. The interview focused on the events that I had recorded during the observation period. The main areas of discussion were based on modesty, the presence of males, touch, dress, prayer, ablutions, and staff attitudes.

All the interviews were semi-structured and tape-recorded. Responses of the women were often backed up by the birth supporter, who justified why there is a preference for a particular behaviour. It was difficult, though, to distinguish between the cultural and the religious reasons, when the perceptions are those of a white non-Muslim researcher. Two interviews were conducted with the husbands present. I found it difficult to elicit responses from these women the as husband answered for the women the majority of the time, even though I had increased eye contact and proximity to the women and directed the questions her. Both Hamida and her husband were distressed by what had happened during labour. Her husband vocalised his distress in his account of events with Hamida agreeing with him:

'Nobody explained what was happening. I asked "Can you please tell us …?" I had to repeat this question so many times, every time they did something. I can remember they gave me a lot of medical terms, I asked, "What does that mean?"' (Hamida's husband)

During the interview, Hamida was distressed by the events that happened during labour; so many different men were coming into the room, they then inappropriately touched her, and there was a lack of recognition of the need for modesty by staff. Hamida and her husband were unable to understand why this happened because explanations were not forthcoming from medical and midwifery staff, when explanations were given they were medicalised and difficult to understand. The recall of the events are vivid in the memory especially around significant e.g. vaginal examinations, or changes of staff.

Findings

Understanding a Muslim way of life, the importance of body ideology (Khuri, 2001) and birth customs (Gatrad, 2001) was central to interpreting the data collected during the observation and the interviews, especially when framed within the culture of a busy labour ward. The Five Pillars of Islam are the foundations on which the Islamic Faith is conducted as well as the Shari'a (religious law). A multitude of rituals, such as rites of passage, performance of prayers, purification and covering the body translate to a way of life. From these premises I identified with the women what cultural/religious aspects were important to them. They are as follows:

- Modesty; presence of males, unnecessary intrusions, dress, touch.
- Prayer; ablutions, suitable environment, respect of staff.
- Environment and control.

Data collected during the observation period was analysed for emerging themes. All the women who took part in the study highlighted the above areas as being important.

Modesty

When women were admitted in labour they were given a hospital gown that opens down the back, none of the women refused to put this on, but covered themselves with the long Habara (full length coat) and the Hijab (head scarf) to maintain their modesty. Several women were distressed during the interviews when they were talking about how exposed they were, some partners made attempts to cover their wives. Within Islam women are considered to be immodest if arms, legs and heads are uncovered especially in the presence of males other than their husband. All women covered their heads when they left the room in which they laboured.

The presence of males in the room was also problematic. All women asked for a female doctor, but women doctors were not always available on the labour ward. Some women became distressed when attended by a male doctor especially when the gender of the doctor was not been made clear to them in advance by the midwife.

> 'Then everything changed, everybody started walking in and out without asking permission. I did my best to cover my wife, a couple of guys came in, looked, did nothing and went away. Things changed we didn't have any control at all.' (Hamida's husband)

Later during the same observation period one of the doctors tried to comfort her by touching her neck and arms.

> Hamida: 'I know it's not right for me, I was in such a state I wanted him to get off'.
> Husband: 'All of a sudden he was trying to comfort my wife. He handled her shoulders and he handled her arms. He is a Muslim so he should be aware of touching.'
> Hamida: 'Even in that situation he should have kept touching to a minimum. We had no control.'

Midwives' touch is acceptable if they are female. During medical procedures touch is inevitable, but should be kept to a minimum.

Prayer

One of the Five Pillars of Islam is prayer five times during the day. A necessary symbolic ritual before prayer is purifying the body with washing (ablutions). All secretions of the body are considered to be polluting. Women gained great strengths from prayer during labour. The ritual of vaginal examination during labour is considered a necessity to assess how far labour has progressed. Though the women in the study expected to be examined it was seen as a polluting act, akin to sexual intercourse and menstruation. When women have completed menstruation, had sexual intercourse, or have completed the postpartum period of forty days they take a ritual bath, to cleanse the body of pollution.

> 'I wasn't doing my prayers because I had a internal exam, I needed to wash and do my ablutions.' (Khadija)

None of the women were offered a wash or given a clean jug, which is what they do at home. Khadija felt unable to ask for a jug to wash herself.

Control and the environment

The women perceived their powerlessness and this increased their sense of worthlessness, even though they were the centre of the stage and all the care was focused on them. Only one woman had completed a birth plan. The others said that they were not offered the opportunity to complete a birth plan.

When women had taken a decision about their care and had told the midwife, this was viewed in a negative way by the midwives. Amina asked for information about Vitamin K. She was informed of the different routes of administration and she decided that her baby should have Vitamin K orally. The midwife then was unsure how much the dosage was or when was the correct time to give the drops to baby. Amina agreed to have an injection for the baby because it was less trouble for the staff, though she was unhappy with this.

The woman who had completed a birth plan included her wish not to have males present; this included a male medical student. During her naturally progressing labour, the midwife asked her if she would allow a male medical student to be present. She again declined. Asked again, at the height of a contraction whilst using Entonox, she declined. During the interview a week later her memories were vivid:

'I was under pressure because I was having pains at the same time and then she asked me to think about it. I was sure I was going to say no.'
'I wouldn't have said yes, particularly as it was a male and I had written it down.'
(Amina)

The midwife placed the woman under pressure to comply despite her written and verbally expressed wishes. She also pressed this issue when the woman was not in a situation to answer.

Four women discussed the procedure of vaginal examination, these were analysed into specific areas:

1. Ablutions and prayer
2. Information and consent

Ablutions and prayer

All the women acknowledged that vaginal examinations were necessary.

'They [vaginal examinations] seem to happen all the time, I was dreading it. We are always covered you see. I felt really dirty I couldn't get out of bed to do my ablutions so I was unable to say my prayers. So I read my beads instead.' (Khadija)

Information and consent

'I knew they were going to examine me, but I didn't realise they would keep their fingers in and break my waters with a hook, they didn't tell me that. I was crying, I was so upset.' (Amina)

Though the midwife had consent to examine Amina it is apparent that breaking Amina's membranes was not discussed. She would have appreciated some explanation as to why this needed to be done, and it clearly upset her.

The areas women highlighted during the interviews reflected what was important to them both culturally and from the Muslim perspective. The most important aspects were the cultural context of where the birth was taking place. To understand this, two key issues need to be considered: Racism and racial discrimination and the culture of the environment of birth.

Institutionalised racism

The impact of midwifery practice on women in the study, described during the interviews a week later, was reflected in the comments on the lack of sensitivity. One woman who was admitted during the antenatal period related her experiences on the ward:

> 'There were four of us in the room, you know. We were all chatting. The midwife came to examine one of the other women she asked us to leave the room. When she needed to check me inside [vaginal examination] she didn't ask them to leave. I was so upset, I was crying in pain and embarrassment. But what could I do?' (Hamida)

Hamida felt this humiliation very strongly and was clearly upset when she told me. She expressed her sense of powerlessness and betrayal by the midwife and the other women in her room. The following experience confirms Bowler's (1993) findings.

> 'I was very tired, the other ladies in the room had their breakfasts brought to them in bed. I asked for my breakfast in bed, I asked the nurse to bring me something. She told me to get up and go to the dining room for my breakfast. It wasn't fair. I had also had a baby and I was in pain. What's the point.' (Amina)

Midwives were observed to share information about women from minority groups in a manner which reinforced stereotypes. There was a commonality in the context of these conversations, with one person agreeing with another concerning a particular set of attributes, even though the listener to the conversation has never met the woman. Even outside rooms where the women laboured the stereotyping continued. Van Dijk (1987) in a study on communicating racism claims that everyday talk is prejudiced and prejudice is formed through the social interaction of the dominant group. These midwives demonstrated Van Dijk's assertion that the dominant group have schemata in place which forms the framework for the storage of beliefs and attributes of the prejudiced group. This was illustrated through a chance discussion with a midwife. She was interested in the research I was doing and wanted to share her views with me.

'Well I'm atheist. "They" can do what they like. In my opinion God is all a waste of time. I have no idea what their needs are. They are all Asians so I assume they are all the same.' (Midwife)

'I have very little contact [with them]. I come from a small village with no Asian families and didn't go to school with any.' (Student)

These midwives perceived South Asian women to be lazy. Their conversation, overheard in the coffee room after the incident described by Amina above, stereotyped them thus:

'These women expect to be waited on.' (Midwife)

The organisation of power

One of the key factors in perpetuating racism is power: the power of the institution, the power of midwives and other professionals and the positions they hold within the institution. The medicalisation of birth has determined the context for the birth experiences of the vast majority of women and the status of midwives in this country. Despite the rhetoric of government statements, quoted at the beginning of this chapter, the women in this study experienced institutionalised and medicalised maternity care.

The institutionalisation of birth controlled the childbearing experiences of the women in the study. Women accepted the system and saw no alternative.

'I didn't realise we had a choice, I just let them get on with what they had to do.' (Zainab)

Where there was opportunity for choice, women did not know if they were not told, as was demonstrated when all but one woman recalled no midwife mentioning the possibility of creating a birth plan.

Surveillance

The organisation of power appears to have a direct impact on the experiences of women as consumers of maternity services or as midwives. The shift of birth from the home to the hospital was viewed by Turner (1992) as regulation of the body by the application of scientific medicine. In Foucault's (1973) terms, this centralising of facilities provides the opportunity for the 'medical gaze' to extend the 'surveillance' of labouring women's bodies.

To examine such surveillance the numbers of interruptions during the course of a labour observation was recorded. The midwives 'in charge' (control) of a labour ward would make uninvited appearances to establish what was happening in the rooms where women were labouring. The purpose of these visits was to establish what progress women were making during their labour. If the midwife in charge considered progress to be inappropriate, she reported back to the obstetricians. This is a form of surveillance of the course of labour defined entirely in the medicalised sense of the 'rate of dilation of the cervix' (O'Driscoll *et al.*, 1993), a concept which is also standard in midwifery texts (e.g. Bennett and Brown, 1999). This surveillance was in effect controlling the function of women's bodies. It had a further aspect of observing the midwife assigned to each woman as to whether her behaviour complied with expected norms or whether she was behaving in such a way as could upset the smooth running of the labour ward. Some midwives spoke to me, during my observations, of how they felt they were under scrutiny. Some of the women were also aware of these interruptions and remembered clearly what was said, and that they were not part of that conversation.

The majority of the women in the study experienced normal birth, though the presence of technology, such as continuous electronic fetal heart monitoring, represented another level of surveillance. On the analysis of obstetric knowledge, Arney (1982) stated that:

'Monitoring and surveillance deal with the problem of residual normalcy. Under this regime no distinctions between normal and abnormal exist.'

All eight women were continuously monitored externally though none were being induced or having their labours augmented; only one woman had meconium-stained liquor. All had normal labour yet seven of the eight women had episiotomies.

The relationship between the midwife and woman appears to be controlled by the environment in which birth takes place. The physical layout of a labour suite determines who is allowed access to where (Hunt and Symonds, 1995). Like Sheila Hunt, I observed that midwives were protective of their territory. If a relative came into their rest room inadvertently they were very quickly directed to the appropriate place. The physical layout of the individual rooms also appeared to dictate how women and midwives interacted. The most interesting aspects was how the writing desk was placed in relationship to the position of the delivery bed. This desk was placed opposite the bottom of the bed. Subsequently when midwives were writing in the notes they had their backs turned to the woman. This appeared to limit the communication that took place. A mirror was placed above the sink also opposite the end of the bed. This appeared to ensure that the health professional was able to observe women even when their back was turned. The reflection was of the bed and the occupant. This surveillance continued even though the occupant of the bed was unaware.

Communication

The quality of communication and interpersonal behaviour is dependant on proximity and the non-verbal expressions that the receiver detects. Eye contact, gaze, and distance are integral to effective communication (Argyll,

1983). Within Islamic culture the use of gestures, distance, eye-contact touch have their own meanings (Khuri, 2001). Several instances were observed where the women had instigated a line of conversation which was quickly fore-closed when the midwife turned to write in the woman's notes even though the woman was still seeking to maintain the dialogue. Some examples were observed. A midwife was giving information on the frequency of vaginal examinations and the co-ordinating midwife entered the room and immediately the midwife's attention was on the co-ordinating midwife. The information-giving stopped whilst the two midwives discussed care of the woman with their backs to her. Monitoring equipment also provides a focus away from the woman. During a conversation between a midwife and a woman, when the midwife's gaze was averted from the woman on to the monitor, the conversation ceased and all focused on the technology. The layout of the room also influenced the level of 'surveillance' of the woman. Above the hand washbasin is a mirror, this mirror gives a direct reflection of the occupant on the bed, so with back turned the 'carers' are still able to observe the labouring woman. Whenever a person in a position of authority enters the labour room (e.g. doctor, senior midwife) the focus turns away from the woman and her family. The obstetric notes were usually placed on a wall-mounted table opposite the end of the bed and all midwives kept the notes on this table. When any documentation was required the midwife sat with her back to the woman and her family. This also had the subtle effect of silencing women. By looking at the notes, the midwife ignored all non-verbal communication.

When midwives were seeking information they maintained their attention until the question was answered, but were unlikely to encourage further interaction. Some women were happy with this, others were upset because they viewed it as an unfriendly formal way of seeking further information about what was happening to them. When they perceived the midwives' behaviour as a rebuff, the women quickly reverted back to talking to their supporters in their own language. Thus, both midwives and mothers had another activity, unintelligible to the other actor, in which they engaged when communication between them ceased: writing clinical notes on the midwives' part and speaking in their own language on the mothers' part. Midwives chose when to write in the notes and make themselves clearly unavailable for communication. The women took up conversation with their supporter when the midwife made herself unavailable. Thus the control lay with the midwife.

This behaviour on the midwives' part was an effective way of 'muting' the women. Many felt this keenly.

'Muting' of women is usually described in the literature (e.g. Ardener, 1993) as happening to women where there are theories, structures, or meanings made by men. In this scenario the rules that govern childbirth are made by obstetricians, who are the, largely male, dominant group. The group that the culture purports to serve is the muted group of mothers. The possibility that women will give different meanings to the operations of the service, thus undermining the authoritative body of obstetric knowledge, is resisted by the policies and procedures of the institution and the behaviour of the professionals. Midwives strive to keep a balance between the needs of mothers and colleagues as they interpret them but usually 'go with the flow' of obstetric pressures, especially when the client group are stereotyped as different. Within maternity care there are thus two muted groups; midwives who are muted by the institution within which they work, and women who are muted by midwives and by the institution because of the nature of their own culture.

Similar patterns can be seen the use of language (Ardener, 1975). For women to be heard, their meanings have to be encoded into acceptable male forms. The use of medical terminology by midwives can be viewed as being acceptable to their obstetrician colleagues, and at the same time preserve the mystique that surrounds midwifery; thus maintaining the control. Admission to hospital itself is a ritual in which women are dependant on midwives, but they are also isolated from other labouring women. Kirkham (1983) found when women are isolated in their own rooms they are unable to gain information from other patients and are thus completely dependent upon the midwives.

Some women in the study searched for meanings of events and procedures that happened. Often they were told: 'You'll be fine'. This dismissive statement gave them no information.

Procedures were observed to be carried out without an explanation being given. The procedures included taking blood, rupture of membranes, vaginal examination, cardiotocograph monitoring and episiotomy. By giving no explanation, and assuming the woman's compliance, the midwives did not even seek informed consent and there was no possibility of informed choice on these issues.

To question is to challenge the system, the establishment. During their admission to the labour ward and throughout their labour, these women learnt not to question. Indeed, the midwives' body language left no space for questions. When questioned about this, on interview, the reasons the women gave were that questions might jeopardise the care they were given or the midwife might be unkind to them.

The outcome of women's search for information from the maternity services has been found to be dependant on social class. Women of higher social class tend to be given more information and their questions as less likely to be seen as a threat to the equilibrium of their setting (Cartwright, 1979). Power within the maternity setting is excluded from midwives but, as Kirkham (1996) observed, the power they hold is over the behaviour of their clients. Midwives themselves are muted and they in turn mute women. The women observed in this study appeared to be muted by midwives' behaviour beyond what would be expected in terms of social class. Aisha was upset at the way she was treated:

'They are quite prejudiced, they won't smile at you and you know they don't like you ...At night the other babies went into the nursery, they wouldn't take mine, they were

English ladies when I asked they [night staff] said no ... I was so tired. I didn't want to make a fuss.'

'When I was in labour I didn't want to say anything to them [Aisha was left for a long time on her own]. I was very angry, very angry about that.' (Aisha)

If you are already on the margins of society, from a minority ethnic group, not only are you likely to be muted but discriminated against by the nature of the institution. Care is likely to be substandard and unresponsive as already outlined by Bowler (1993), and knowledge on which care is based also inadequate (Dyson *et al.*, 1996).

Lack of appropriate, individualised care

An important aspect of care that could be perceived as unresponsive was the use of ritualised procedures. The admission process and vaginal examination during labour could both be seen as institutionalised procedures, sometimes but not always necessary. The former is particularly important as it is the woman's first experience of the labour ward and sets the tone for what is to follow. These procedures are concerned with control. Whilst as Sleep (1992) discusses they serve to 'limit the actions of the clinician', they also process the woman as a patient. If these procedures are undertaken without an individualised consideration for the cultural or religious beliefs of a group, they could be considered to contain a form of institutionalised racism. The lack of understanding of the individual's beliefs could be viewed as insulting.

The effects of vaginal examinations, in the cultural context of this group of women, undermined their trust in the midwives. Yet trust is seen as crucial for informed choice (Kirkham, 2000). Some women were unable to pray because they felt dirty. The simple act of asking women what they preferred would have enabled them to be less anxious about the whole procedure, but no choice was offered to any of the women observed. Yet it would have been relatively easy, and not disruptive of labour ward routine, to enable the women to cleanse themselves in a culturally appropriate manner after procedures which were seen as polluting events. The provision of a clean jug for each woman to use for her ablutions would have helped to reduce the anxieties that some women have in labour, especially when prayer is central to the Muslim faith. Prayer for some women gives them the strength to cope with labour. In not allowing them the opportunity to voice their needs, the midwives were denying these women a culturally important coping strategy.

The recognition of the individual is important. There are many different groups of Muslims; Sunni and Shi'ite to name but two. Not to recognise individuality is to deny these women choice. The way information is given will also influence what choice is made. This works in two directions. The women could not make choices because the midwives did not inform them of choices which were available within the clinical system but simply conveyed, by their behaviour, that women should comply, which they did. The midwives could not choose to make available simple resources, such as clean jugs and the privacy to use them, because they did not allow women to give information as to their needs. Given the power of professionals and the situation of labouring women, the responsibility to make informed choice possible must lie with the midwife in the first instance. To make assumptions as to the needs of a particular group of women and to behave so as to deny them the opportunity to express their needs is to deny a basic Human Right and to deny them the right to have control in their lives.

The rhetoric of *Changing Childbirth* (DoH, 1993) and the other reports cited at the beginning of this chapter was not seen in the care given to these women. Midwifery care was not observed or experienced as empowering or facilitating informed choice. No client advocacy was observed or reported. Neither did the midwives listen to these women or give them the opportunity to voice their needs. The women in this study were fluent English speakers and were educated in this country. The problems in communication did not spring from lack of a common language with their carers but from the manner in which they were cared for.

This small study highlighted issues of education for midwifery and medical staff into some of the cultural aspects that impact on women's birthing experiences. Having a planned programme of education for health professionals around communication is fundamental to meeting the cultural and religious needs of the population. This should help to identify the individual needs of the diverse population. I have planned to take this forward in the form of an action research study. This would involve devising a planned programme of education for health professionals, in self-awareness, communication skills and some work on stereotyping and racism. Then I would assess the effectiveness of that education programme on the care and support given to minority ethnic groups by the focus groups made up of consumers that have been cared for by the 'educated' health professional. Feedback from the 'consumer' will then determine how the next cycle of education is delivered. I hope this will go some way to change the negative experiences that were observed in the course of the above research.

Note

1 This chapter is based on research that was part of my Master's degree in Midwifery (Ellis, 2000).

References

Ardener, E. (1993) The nature of women in society. In E. Ardener (ed.) *Defining Females*. Oxford: Berg.

Argyll, M. (1983) *The Psychology of Interpersonal Behaviour*. London: Pelican.

Arney, W.R. (1982) *Power and the Profession of Obstetrics*. Chicago: University of Chicago Press.

Barj, K. (1995) Providing midwifery care in a multicultural society. *Midwifery*, **3(5)**: 271–6.

Bennet, R. and Brown, L. (1999) *A Textbook for Midwives*. London: Churchill Livingstone.

Bowes, A. and Domokos, T. (1996) Pakistani women and maternity care: raising muted voices. *Sociology of Health and Illness*. **18(1)**: 45–65.

Bowler, I. (1993) 'They're not the same as us'. Stereotypes of South Asia descent maternity patients. *Sociology of Health and Illness*, **15(2)**: 157–78.

Cartwright, A. (1979) *The Dignity of Labour*. London: Tavistock.

NICE (2002) *Why Mothers Die, 1997–1999. Confidential Enquiry into Maternal Deaths in the UK*. London: National Institute for Clinical Excellence.

Darwin, C. (1871) *The Descent of Man*. London: Murray.

Department of Health (1993) *Changing Childbirth: Report of the Expert Maternity Group*. London: HMSO.

Department of Health (1997) *The New NHS: Modern, Dependable*. London: HMSO.

Department of Health (1998) *First Class Service: Quality in the New NHS*. London: HMSO.

Douglas J. (1995) Developing anti-racist health promotion strategies. In R. Bunten, S. Nellete and R. Burrows (eds), *The Sociology of Health Promotion*. London: Routledge.

Dyson, S., Fielder, A. and Kirkham, M. (1996) Midwives' and senior students' knowledge of haemoglobinpathies in England. *Midwifery* **12**: 23–30.

Ellis, N. (2000) *'What's all the fuss about? Yes that's the sort of attitude I got': Perceptions of childbirth experience by second generation English-speaking Muslim women*. Unpublished MA dissertation. De Montfort University, Leicester.

Fernando, S. (2002) *Mental Health, Race and Culture*. London: Palgrave.

Flint, C. *Teams and Caseloads*. London: Butterworth Heinemann.

Foucault, M. (1973) *The Birth of the Clinic*. London: Tavistock.

Gatrad, A.R. and Sheikh, A. (2001) *Muslim Birth Customs Archives of Diseases in Childhood* (Fetal and Neonatal edition), **84(1)**: F6–8.

Harding, D. (2000) Making choices in childbirth. In Leslie Page (ed.) *The New Midwifery*. London: Churchill Livingstone.

Hunt, S. and Symonds, A. (1995) *The Social Meaning of Midwifery*. London: Macmillan.

Inch, S. (1982) *Birthrights*. London: Paladin.

Katbamna, S. (2000) *Race and Childbirth*. Buckingham: Open University Press.

Khuri, F. (2001) *The Body in Islamic Culture*. London: Al Saqi Books.

Kirkham, M. (1983) Admission in labour: teaching the patient to be patient? *Midwives Chronicle*, Feb (1983) 44–5.

Kirkham, M. (1996) Professionalisation past and present: with women or with the powers that be? In D. Kroll (ed.), *Midwifery Care for the Future*. London: Baillière Tindall.

Kirkham, M. (2000) How can we relate? In idem (ed.) *The Midwife–Mother Relationship*. Basingstoke: Palgrave Macmillan.

Leap, N. (2000) The less we do, the more we give. In M. Kirkham (ed.) *The Midwife–Mother Relationship*. London: Palgrave Macmillan.

Macpherson, W. (1999) *Thr Stephen Lawrence Enquiry: Report of an Enquiry by Sir William Macpherson of Cluny*. London: HMSO.

Mares, P., Henley, A. and Baxter, C. (1985) *Health Care in Multiracial Britain*. Cambridge: National Extension College.

Miles, R. (1982) *Racism and Migrant Labour*. London: Routledge & Kegan Paul.

Mulholland, J. and Dyson, S. Sociological theories of race and ethnicity. In L. Culley and S. Dyson (eds), *Ethnicity and Nursing Practice*. Basingstoke: Palgrave Macmillan.

Neile, E. (1997) Control for black and ethnic minority women: a meaningless pursuit. In M. Kirkham and E. Perkins (eds), *Reflections on Midwifery*. London Baillière Tindall.

Oakley, A. (1993) Birth as a normal process. In *Essays on Women, Medicine and Health*. Edinburgh: Edinburgh University Press.

O'Driscoll, K., Meagher, D. and Boylam, P. (1993) *Active Management of Labour.* London: Mosby.

Phoenix, A. (1990) Black women and maternity services. In J. Garcia, R. Kilpatrick, M. Richards (eds), *Politics of Maternity Care.* Oxford: Clarendon Press.

Royal College of Midwives (2000) *The Vision 2000.* London: Royal College of Midwives.

Senior, P.A. and Bhopal, R. (1994) Ethnicity as a variable in epidemiological research. *British Medical Journal,* **309**: 327–30.

Sheldon, T. and Parker, H. (1992) Race and ethnicity in health research. *Journal of Public Health Medicine,* **14(2)**: 104–10.

Sleep, J. (1992) Research and the practice of midwifery. *Journal of Advanced Nursing,* **17**: 1465–71.

Turner, B. (1992) *Regulatory Bodies: Essays in Medical Sociology.* London: Routledge.

UKCC. (1993) *Midwives Code of Practice.* London: UKCC.

Van Dijk, T. (1987) *Communicating Racism: Ethnic Prejudice in Thought and Talk.* London: Sage.

Young, L. (2000) Imperial culture. In Les Back and John Solomos (eds), *Theories of Race and Racism: A Reader.* London: Routledge.

CHAPTER 12

The Misleading Myth of Choice: The Continuing Oppression of Women in Childbirth[1]

TRICIA ANDERSON

Chapter Contents

■ Compulsion, not choice

■ Control, not choice

■ Damaged midwives, damaged women

■ The end of the story

I am deeply troubled by the stories of several pregnant women in whose care I have recently been involved.

Lisa was pregnant with twins; she had had a previous successful home birth and felt confident in her body's ability to give birth to her twin babies, both of whom were cephalic and growing well.

Joanne's baby was lying in a breech position at 39 weeks; like Lisa she had had a previous lovely home water birth, and felt sure that her body could give birth to its breech baby without difficulty.

Teresa had had a previous elective Caesarean section, but this time around wanted to labour and give birth in water, as she believed it would help her relax.

All three women had a firm belief in the normalcy of childbirth as a natural, physiological process which women's bodies have evolved to do over generations, and confidence in their strong, healthy bodies to do it well. They were all well informed and aware of the increased potential for possible difficulties with VBAC, breech and twin births, but equally well informed of the increased health risks associated with routine intervention and elective Caesarean section.

With this in mind, the three women had thoughtfully made their informed choices: what they all wanted was to be in a hospital setting to give birth, with facilities for obstetric and paediatric support immediately on hand should they or their babies need it. However, they wanted to labour freely, and give birth without interference, most likely on their hands and knees. They wanted midwifery care and support in as much of a home birth atmosphere as could be managed. All three were clear that, unless complications occurred, they did not want a medical-style birth, with routine venflon, cardiotocography, lithotomy, epidural, Syntocinon and so forth in a room full of strangers. If complications were to occur, however, they would willingly accept medical guidance and help.

Quite a reasonable choice, I thought. But no…

Their choice was denied them. *They were not allowed it.* They were told in no uncertain terms by an assortment of midwifery managers, supervisors and obstetricians that if they came into hospital they would have to do it the medical way. Full stop. That if they crossed the labour ward threshold they would have to follow hospital protocols and rules. (In one hospital they approached, all women with twins are required to labour in the operating theatre.) That it would depend on the obstetric registrar on duty, who probably would only know how to assist such births with women in lithotomy, and that it would be up to *him* on the day. They would not countenance any alternative. Community midwives were not supported to undertake the women's intrapartum care at home unless they absolutely refused to come into hospital: an unpredictable confrontation that the women did not want to risk.

They were thus faced with two unpalatable choices, neither of which they wanted. Either they would have to succumb to the medical approach, which is all that the NHS maternity services seem to offer for women with these variations of normal pregnancies. Or, if there was one available in their area and if they could afford it (two very big 'ifs'), they could have their babies at home with independent midwives: which they felt was not the safest place for them and where they did not want to be.

There is a third possible choice, which Jean Robinson of AIMS writes is becoming worryingly more and more common, particularly in women who cannot afford or find an independent midwife: they could decide to birth alone at home without help (Robinson, 2002), making their lack of genuine choice and access to supportive NHS care a significant health issue of public health and safety.

The illusion that there is any meaningful choice in contemporary childbirth or that maternity care is woman-centred lies shattered. Even the well-meaning supervisor of midwives who tried to help could not tackle the power and influence of the obstetric hegemony. 'Well, I suppose they might agree to Lisa not labouring in theatre…' was about as far as she could go. I cannot begin to describe the harassment and un-evidence-based shroud-waving these women were made to endure. A major stumbling block seemed to be limitations of the shift system; one consultant said he might be willing to support Joanne, but he could not expect the on-call registrar to do so (and he wasn't prepared to go on-call himself). The midwives clearly felt themselves to be under the control of their obstetric masters; they felt unable to offer to care for Lisa, Joanne or Teresa themselves without medical approval.

Why can't NHS maternity services offer more in the way of support and genuine choice to these women? Is what they want so unreasonable?

Compulsion, not choice

As Katz Rothman (1990) writes, 'while new technology opens up some choices, it closes down others. The new choice is often greeted with such fanfare that the silent closing down of the door on the old choice goes unheeded. As "choices" become available, they all too rapidly become *compulsions* to "choose" the socially endorsed alternative'. An example of this would be the 'choice' to have a very large family – a choice frowned upon in this era of contraception when a couple are only supposed to have the children they can afford. The theory of informed choice down at grassroots level transforms into the practice of enforced compliance with the recommended choice; in this case, a medically managed birth.

She continues: 'For those whose choices meet the social expectations, for those who want what the society wants them to want, the experience of choice is very real.' But for those who want to make other, alternative choices, the ideology of choice disappears in the twinkling of an eye.

From the experiences of Lisa, Joanne and Teresa it is absolutely clear that full power and control of women in childbirth still resides unequivocally within the patriarchal, bureaucratic, obstetric institution. Feminism stands helpless at the entrance to the maternity hospital: the oppression of women continues unchecked inside. Choice is an empty promise; a smokescreen behind which the patriarchal medical model churns relentlessly on.

Control, not choice

Were we naive? Over twenty years ago, Richards pointed out the central problem: 'Pushing for alternatives in maternity care... fails to comes to grips with the central issues of who is in control' (Richards, 1982). In a hierarchical, bureaucratic NHS that works to a technocratic model as outlined by Davis-Floyd (2001), the expectation that a humanistic charter for change to woman-centred, individualised maternity care such as *Changing Childbirth* (Department of Health, 1993) would succeed without challenging the ruling hegemony was doomed to disappointment and failure. The NHS emphasises the standardisation of care pathways rather than an individualised approach; the supremacy of technology over shadows women's voices; and bureaucracy and fear of litigation trample over their wishes and dreams. Only certain 'choices' are sanctioned. Care remains firmly institution-centred; in the case of these three women, the interests of the staff and the institution were of more concern to everyone while the wishes of the women were seen as an irritation. As Weber pointed out at the beginning of this century, the needs of the institution will always outweigh the needs of the individual (Weber, 1995). The midwives' allegiance throughout was clearly to their employer – the institution, rather than to the individual women.

'It has become increasingly recognised that "*choice*" is too narrow a concept to encapsulate the broad-based social changes needed to enhance women's autonomy and control' (Carter, 1995). The rhetoric of women's choice, writes Sheila Kitzinger, 'ignores the sales pressure put on them to chose one place of birth or kind of care than another, the power of the medical system compared with the relative powerlessness of women having babies, and what amounts to emotional blackmail' (Kitzinger, 1991). Lisa, Joanne and Teresa had all been subject to this form of oppression as repeated attempts were made to manipulate them into acquiescing to the obstetricians' choice: a medically managed, hospital-centred delivery.

'Many women's acceptance that birth should be in a hospital and that the use of technology is desirable, has been influenced by obstetricians who convey this message with all their power and authority' (Miles, 1991). The only people whose interests are served by perpetuating the danger/risk model of childbirth are the obstetricians, and, increasingly, the new specialty of obstetric anaesthesia. Of course some term breech and twin births get into difficulties (which is why even Mary Cronk, the UK's most prominent midwifery breech expert, recommends hospital as the preferred place of birth (Cronk, 2002)), but where is even the mention of the vast majority who have no problems, and who prior to the 1960s would have been born at home (Leap and Hunter, 1993; Allison, 1996)? Much of the angst around these births is associated with factors to do with prematurity and congenital abnormality, not presentation; the greatest risk of uterine rupture occurs through inappropriate use of Syntocinon and prostaglandin (Enkin, Keirse *et al.*, 2000), and yet they are all muddled up in one 'high risk' bundle which is used to frighten women into acquiescing to obstetric control, using their babies' well-being as a threat. One of the major restrictive features of the technocratic paradigm of healthcare is its intolerance of other ways of thinking (Davis-Floyd, 2001). As far as the obstetric team are concerned, there is nothing to discuss: there is no alternative.

Despite *Changing Childbirth* (DoH, 1993), very little has changed in the last ten years, when Miles wrote the following description of the institutionalisation of pregnancy and birth. 'A woman, finding herself pregnant, finds also that a regime of antenatal care is laid down for her, that she is expected to report regularly during pregnancy to a clinic or surgery and undergo medical check-ups and tests, and that quite early in the pregnancy arrangements are made for the birth to take place in a particular hospital where she will duly go to have her baby delivered under professional supervision and with whatever medical monitoring and intervention is thought appropriate' (Miles, 1991). If she does not choose to follow the path laid down for her, she is labelled a trouble-maker, and, in extreme cases, is excluded from mainstream maternity services unless she agrees to conform.

This may seem far-fetched. But a letter written by a Supervisor of Midwives recently to a pregnant woman planning a home birth after a previous Caesarean section confirms that this withdrawal of services does occur. 'You do have a legal right to refuse to accept professional advice and to refuse the treatment offered to you and your baby. However, if you choose to do that, then the responsibility for what happens to you and your baby rests entirely with you… In conclusion, I therefore regret that we are unable to offer you a home delivery service. We remain willing and able to provide you with the necessary care and support that you and your baby need in hospital.' (At the time of writing this case is ongoing and therefore must remain anonymous.)

This notion that the NHS provides a service only when it suits them is further confirmed in a letter to MPs written by John Hutton, Minister of State at the Department of Health on 17 October 2002 in response to enquiries concerning midwifery insurance. In particular, the last two paragraphs read:

> 'The Government supports a woman's right to choose where and how to give birth, bearing in mind the need to safeguard both mother and baby and taking into account the overall needs of the local community. You may be interested to note that the NHS does provide a home birth facility *wherever this is possible and clinically appropriate*.' (My emphasis)

Who decides what is clinically appropriate, and since when has this been statutory grounds for the provision or withdrawal of NHS midwifery services? This is a chilling example of state control of women and the creeping erosion of their rights. There are a number of women who, for various reasons, choose not to enter a maternity hospital to give birth. Their reasons may range from a fear or distrust of authority, previous bad experiences at the hands of the NHS maternity services or Social Services, previous traumatic personal experiences such as sexual abuse or domestic violence, or personal, religious or cultural belief systems. The Department of Health has a responsibility for the health of the public, and is required to provide health services to all people, not just those who are compliant and fit into a predetermined mould. The notion that the NHS might decline to provide skilled midwifery services for such women puts them and their babies at extreme risk. Giving birth alone without trained help – which has been proven to be the most 'high risk' option – should not be the only course open to them. This is like something out of the Victorian era. Indeed, providing these women with sensitive midwifery services should be an NHS priority for the safety of mother and baby. The notion that an NHS home birth service should only be provided when it is deemed 'clinically appropriate' reveals a complete lack of insight into the realities of many women's lives, and is another sinister instance of using the so-called 'safeguarding' of mother and baby as currency to enforce women's compliance.

The suppression of midwives and the oppression of pregnant women has a long, long history, from the Middle Ages to the present day. Even the 1902 Midwives' Act, being 'celebrated' this year may not be such a cause for rejoicing, as Jean Donnison reminds us through the quotations given in her history of the struggle for control over childbirth (Donnison, 1988):

> 'If it were possible, I would have every woman attended to by a duly qualified medical man, but as this cannot be, public safety and humanity demand legislative action to enable poor women to know whether those who call themselves midwives are safely competent.' (Dr Aveling, *Nursing Notes*, 1891)

> 'The Boards to which the duty of regulating the registration and examination of midwives is assigned are to consist of medical men of standing who will be likely to impress their limitations upon them.' (*Lancet*, 26 May 1890)

> 'In order to "police" the boundaries between midwifery and medical practice, it was imperative that the medical profession had supremacy.' (*British Medical Journal*, 1873)

The suppression of midwives within the UK has recently reached new heights. At the end of September 2002, the UK Nursing and Midwifery Council concluded a consultation period as to whether carrying professional indemnity insurance should be a mandatory or ethical requirement for all nurses and midwives. This resulted in a statement that all nurses, midwives and health visitors in the UK are 'advised by their regulatory body to maintain adequate indemnity insurance cover to protect patients and themselves' (Nursing and Midwifery Council, 2003). Yet, at the time of writing, there is quite simply no insurance available for midwives who work outside of the NHS. Independent midwives – that is to say, all midwives outside that which is sanctioned by the ruling hegemony of contemporary NHS maternity services – cannot do what their statutory body advises. Women who want anything other than standard NHS-sanctioned care will either have to conform, opt for an uninsured service or give birth alone. In another, equally sinister development, the NHS Clinical Services Negligence Trust – the central Trust that pays out money when claims are won against the NHS – is increasingly dictating how maternity services should operate, setting out what policies they should follow and so forth. This is a service-led agenda at its most blatant. These are frightening times.

Damaged midwives, damaged women

In terms of supremacy, little has changed: it is clear that the obstetricians remain the ultimate policy- and decision-makers. Except that now 'midwives have also been drawn into the female conspiracy where women conspire against women' (Murphy-Black, 1995). 'That women control other women by colluding with men, either implicitly or explicitly, has been demonstrated time and time again in the maternity hospitals of this country' (Kirkham, 1999). 'The really sad aspect of this is that it is often done in the name of "being a good midwife"; that is, blindly following the rules designed for the needs of the institution rather than the needs of the individual' (Murphy-Black, 1995). Now the obstetricians can, on occasion, step back and be Mr Nice-Guy; the midwives have become the agents of oppression and control. The midwives do their dirty work for them. It was first and foremost midwives who told Lisa, Joanne and Teresa that they could not have the choices they wanted. The Nursing and Midwifery Council's Code of Professional Conduct (NMC, 2002) states that midwives must protect and support the health of individual clients, which 'indicates clearly the expectation that the practitioner will act as an advocate on behalf of clients' (UKCC, 1989). There was scant evidence of any midwives acting as advocates on behalf of the three women: the few that tried were quickly shot down by other, more senior midwives.

> 'Many senior nurses behave in such a heartless and insulting way … it is hard to believe that they have been through similar experiences themselves. But therein perhaps lies the key; the experience of becoming a nurse and rising through the ranks leaves so many scars that self-protection is the only route most people can follow. Insecurity, lack of confidence, lack of assertiveness and the often unrealistic expectations of other people may provoke a very natural human response of defensiveness, so that at least on the outside one can appear indestructible.' (Salvage, 1985)

Jane Salvage wrote this about the nursing profession nearly twenty years ago, but it applies equally to midwifery. A generation of midwives who have been damaged in this way have learnt how to appear hard and 'indestructible' – perhaps the only way that they can enforce policies that they know are wrong.

It is currently impossible for the maternity team to meet the needs of women like Lisa, Joanne and Teresa unless the ruling hegemony is seriously challenged, and there are no signs that this is happening.

The end of the story

And what of the three women?

They all gave birth – at home – with ease, with the support of various independent midwives. Lisa's twins were a boy and girl, weighing 7lb and 8lb 1oz respectively; Joanne's breech baby was a girl weighing 7lb 7oz; Teresa got her much-wanted water birth. With the new clause in the NMC Code of Conduct, care such as this would only be possible where midwives were willing to act against the advice of their statutory body, and practise without insurance. The tyranny of the medicalisation of childbirth thus increases.

Will the Lisas and Joannes of the next decade give up the fight and have their legs put up in stirrups, or will they birth alone at home? Those may be the only 'choices' they have left.

And, if any of their babies had struggled or died, at whose door would you lay the blame?

Note

1 The following chapter first appeared in a slightly shortened format as an article in the MIDIRS *Midwifery Digest*, **12(3)**, 405–7. We are grateful to MIDIRS for giving us permission to reproduce it here.

References

Allison, J. (1996) *Delivered at Home*. London: Chapman & Hall.

Carter, J. (1995) *Feminism, Breasts and Breastfeeding*. Basingstoke: Macmillan.

Cronk, M. (2002) Personal communication.

Davis-Floyd, R. (2001) The technocratic, humanistic and holistic paradigms of childbirth. *International Journal of Gynecology and Obstetrics*.

Department of Health (1993) *Changing Childbirth*. London: HMSO.

Donnison, J. (1988). *Midwives and Medical Men: A History of the Struggle for the Control of Childbirth*. New Barnet: Historical Publications.

Enkin, M., Keirse, M. *et al.* (2000) *A Guide to Effective Care in Pregnancy and Childbirth*. Oxford: Oxford University Press.

Katz Rothman, B. (1990) *Recreating Motherhood: Ideology and Technology in a Patriarchal Society*. New York: Norton.

Kirkham, M. (1999) The culture of midwifery in the NHS in England. *Journal of Advanced Nursing*, **30**: 3.

Kitzinger, S. (1991) *Home Birth and Other Alternatives to Hospital*. London: Dorling Kindersley.

Leap, N. and Hunter, B. (1993)*The Midwife's Tale*. London: Scarlet Press.

Miles, A. (1991) *Women, Health and Medicine*. Milton Keynes: Open University Press.

Murphy-Black, T. (1995) Comfortable men, uncomfortable women. In: T. Murphy-Black (ed.), *Issues in Midwifery*. Edinburgh: Churchill Livingstone.

Nursing and Midwifery Council (2002) *Code of Professional Conduct*. London: NMC

Nursing and Midwifery Council (2003) Press release 17 Jan. http://www.nmc-uk.org/nmc/main/pressStatements/newIndemnityClauseForCode.html

Richards, M. (1982) The trouble with 'choice' in childbirth. *Birth*, **9(4)**: 253–60.

Robinson, J. (2002) High-risk clients. *British Journal of Midwifery*, **10(2)**: 109.

Salvage, J (1985) *The Politics of Nursing*. London: Butterworth Heinemann.

United Kingdom Central Council for Nursing and Midwifery (1989) *Exercising Accountability*. London: UKCC.

Weber, M. (1995) *The Protestant Ethic and the Spirit of Capitalism*. Reprinted 1995, London: Roxbury Publishing Company. (Published in London (1930) by Allen & Unwin. Original edition in German 1904–5, revised edition 1920.)

CHAPTER 13

Choice and Bureaucracy

MAVIS KIRKHAM

> **Chapter Contents**
>
> ▪ Identifying choices
>
> ▪ The choices which are taken for granted
>
> ▪ Definitions
>
> ▪ Making choices
>
> ▪ The package of care and its implications
>
> ▪ Unequal interactions
>
> ▪ Consent and choice
>
> ▪ Control of professional work
>
> ▪ Control of one's own experience
>
> ▪ Balancing caring
>
> ▪ Is partnership possible?
>
> ▪ Culture, scale and choice
>
> ▪ Choices and processes
>
> ▪ The future

This book is about individuals, organisations and how they interact. Individual women have babies, usually attended by one or more midwives and sometimes by doctors. These individuals are enmeshed within the organisation of maternity services which provides resources and technical and organisational back-up to those involved in births whilst placing many pressures upon them.

Organisational pressures influence both the choices people wish to make and the choices they feel able to act upon. Nadine Edwards (Chapter 1) and Tricia Anderson (Chapter 12) describe individual women and their search for maternity care which supported the choices they saw as best for themselves

and their families. They made compromises so as not to alienate NHS professionals, or opted out into the care of independent midwives (an option very
much under threat at present). Valerie Levy (Chapter 3) examines midwives'
struggle to balance the many pressures upon them as they 'facilitate informed
choice' for women. Helen Stapleton describes examples of midwives putting
themselves in isolated and vulnerable positions in order to honour women's
choices but overall the pressure on midwives to 'go with the flow' was almost
irresistible (Chapter 5). Other chapters show how the nature of the flow is
created and adjusted.

Maternity services fit Lipsky's definition of a street-level bureaucracy of
'public service workers who interact directly with citizens in the course of
their jobs, and who have substantial discretion in the execution of their work'
(Lipsky, 1980, p. 3). Lipsky's analysis fits the situation described in many
chapters in this book.

> 'Ideally, and by training, street-level bureaucrats respond to the individual needs or char-
> acteristics of the people they serve or confront. In practice, they must deal with clients
> on a mass basis, since work requirements prohibit individualised service ...At best,
> street-level bureaucrats invent benign modes of mass processing that more or less
> permit them to deal with the public fairly, appropriately, and successfully. At worst, they
> give in to favouritism, stereotyping, and routinising – all of which serve private or
> agency purposes.' (Lipsky, 1980, p. xii)

Informed choice is important within policy statements on maternity services. Yet it remains at the level of rhetoric and informed compliance (BMJ,
2002) appears to serve the purposes of the maternity service. Informed
choice was an explicit aim in *Changing Childbirth* (Department of Health,
1993), together with control and continuity of care for childbearing
women. None of these aims, set for the year 1998, were achieved, though
they still appear in policy documents. In a real sense they are organisation-
ally impossible within the prevailing constraints of the maternity services
bureaucracy. Department of Health policy may contain the rhetoric of
informed choice but policy is also forged in the practice of midwives and
obstetricians:

> 'the routines they establish, the devices they invent to cope with uncertainties and
> work pressures, effectively *become* the public policies they carry out.' (Lipsky, 1980,
> p. xii)

Chapters in this book shed light upon several aspects of the dilemma whereby
maternity services perform in a manner which is contrary to the declared aims
of the Department of Health. The descriptions of the experience of childbearing women and staff show how the aim of informed choice is just one
issue amongst many more powerful pressures which lead them to 'go with the
flow' of service routines.

Identifying choices

Normative practice means that many choices are made by default. It was an interesting aspect of evaluating the MIDIRS *Informed Choice* leaflets (Kirkham and Stapleton, 2000 and Chapters 5 and 6) to find that some of the choices identified as the subject of leaflets were not treated as choices in practice. Women were often given leaflets about place of birth and ultrasound scanning after they had been booked for a hospital birth and had received several scans as part of normal practice without these events being treated as occasions for choice. The following two quotations, from a service user and a midwife, in our informed choice study, illustrate the 'reality gap' in the perception of choice from different positions:

'When I declined the dating scan, the receptionist said: "Oh, I'll just go and see if you're *allowed*." [woman's emphasis] That did annoy me, you're not allowed this, you're not allowed that... I didn't have a dating scan and I had a hassle over it right up to the end.' (Service user, control site)

'I don't think they [service users] understand they have a choice and can say no. I think they just go along with it because it's the accepted thing to do.' (Midwife, control site)

The local constraints on choice were such that the vast majority of women complied with suggested interventions and thus choice was often communicated as an ultimatum, with consent assumed rather than being explicitly sought. It was often only in the context of the research agenda, and sometimes long after the decision-making event, that women became aware that other options existed. (Kirkham and Stapleton, 2000, p. 100)

Occasions for choice are defined by the service. Unless they are well read and articulate and assertive, women are unlikely to formulate their own questions. This is particularly true for women pregnant for the first time.

'Having not gone through a pregnancy before, I didn't know what questions to ask. I was being led by what they told me. I didn't really know what I was doing, just used to turn up for my appointments and luckily everything was all right. I didn't know what I should be asking.' (Focus group 5; Kirkham and Stapleton, 2001, p. 114)

Women are particularly unlikely to ask about options which staff did not tell them about, as Valerie Levy demonstrates with water birth (Chapter 3).

Strategies for gaining women's compliance with normal practice can be presented as choices between treatments without the option of refusal. In our study Vitamin K provided a good example, as women's requests to know about that routine injection were often answered with a choice as to whether the baby should have Vitamin K by injection or by mouth. Having Vitamin K was normal practice. Similarly, choice concerning the oxytocic injection routinely given at delivery was often presented as a choice between Syntometrine and Syntocinon, not the choice between active and physiological management of the third stage of labour (Kirkham and Stapleton, 2001). Thus choice is reconfigured to fit in with clinical practice and options are narrowed.

Where women wish to make choices which are not defined by the service, they often feel that they cannot voice them even when achieving their choice would involve a relatively small change in professional behaviour. Nicky Ellis (Chapter 11) demonstrates this with regard to some Muslim women's need to wash between vaginal examinations and prayer. The power differences ensure that such needs are rarely voiced. Clinical priorities and failure to identify with those seen as 'other' prevent staff from asking about such women's needs (Lipsky, 1980) and manifest in such circumstances as racism.

The choices which are taken for granted

Many habits and choices are deeply embedded in our way of life. Practices and preferences which are normal for the individual can be problematic within a bureaucracy such as the NHS.

Medical authority is deeply embedded in life in this country. One of the meanings the Collins Dictionary gives for 'care' is 'protective or supervisory control: as in the care of the doctor'. It can be seen as part of such supervisory control that there are medically defined right choices. It is, therefore, not surprising that many women do not feel they have choices. Low expectations with regard to informed choice may explain the relatively high level of informed choice perceived in Alicia O'Cathian's baseline survey (Chapter 4). Yet there is also dissatisfaction with this situation which has let to documents such as *Changing Childbirth* (Department of Health, 1993) and the rhetoric of informed choice.

Admission to hospital can no longer be seen as implying 'general consent' to hospital policy. Barbara Hewson describes in Chapter 2 how this approach is being criticised and is changing in Ireland. Yet maternity services have professional agendas and each encounter between professional and client consists of many small procedures to which choice or consent is largely assumed.

Clearly there are many tensions where ways of life do not fit with NHS practice, and where service users take seriously the rhetoric of health policy which does not fit with NHS reality. In a diverse population and a consumer-orientated society such tensions are likely to be frequent. The pressures to 'go with the flow' should not be underestimated but there are ripples and eddies.

Definitions

I have not been able to find a widely accepted definition of informed choice and hope this is because the term speaks for itself. Meg Wiggins and Mary Newburn (Chapter 7) state essentials:

> 'If women are to be fully involved in decisions about their care then they need to have a sense that alternative courses of action can be taken, that these are equally accessible, and to have reliable information about the advantages and disadvantages so that they can make informed choices.'

Helen Stapleton (Chapter 5) quotes a range of very different statements as to what professionals and women understood by the term informed choice. Alicia O'Cathain's questionnaire contained a central question and a number of supporting questions to assess women's perceived degree of informed choice (Chapter 4).

All the definitions agree that we must know of options in order for choice to be possible. Information is clearly fundamental to informed choice. Yet information exists and is used within a social context.

Making choices

Weighing up and sussing out

Before making choices we need information. The difficulty of weighing up the existing evidence around key areas of decision-making in pregnancy was the reason for the creation of the MIDIRS *Informed Choice* Leaflets (see Chapter 4 and Carne, 2002). Such information is complex to weigh as is demonstrated in Chapter 9 with regard to elective Caesarean section. Personal and ethical issues for staff also influence the information given to women (see Chapter 3).

There is also ample evidence that childbearing women seek to validate their existing knowledge and to weigh up knowledge from different sources before making decisions. This is an example concerning breastfeeding:

> 'My health visitor was giving advice and, I must admit, I like to test the water and see if someone else will give me the same advice.' (Mother quoted in Trewick, Ellis and Kirkham, 2001, p. 59)

This process was clearly demonstrated in Meg Wiggins and Mary Newburn's study (Chapter 7), where women participated in group discussion of evidence based information and felt that these exchanges 'made a difference' to them. This opportunity to consider their own and others' reaction to the contents of the MIDIRS leaflets may account for the greater use of that information in this study compared with our large trial of the same leaflets in normal clinical practice which did not include discussion (Kirkham and Stapleton, 2001).

Important figures in a mother's life have a particular influence upon decision-making. This is acknowledged with regard to infant feeding (e.g. Duddridge, 2000) and many breastfeeding initiatives now focus on educating partners or grandparents. Knowledge and advice from key members of a woman's social network are often strengthened by normative practice within her community: 'what people like us usually do', and moral decisions as to what constitutes a 'good' mother, woman or partner (Murphy, 1999).

Infant feeding information may not always be adequate but, after the weighing up process, decision-making is within the control of the woman in that she will be primarily responsible for feeding the baby. Decisions which require action by service providers are more complex. Where there is one local maternity service the normative social practice of using that service serves as introduction to the normative clinical practices within that service. With centralisation of services and uniformity of practice, women may perceive few options.

Shopping around

Users of health services are increasingly portrayed as consumers or clients rather than patients. Consumers make choices and shop around. The situation in health care can be somewhat different.

Glaser (1972) used the term 'comparative shopping' to describe situations where a layperson has many choices of experts and can sample and compare them over time. Lack of time in a pregnancy limits such choice, in labour it renders many choices impossible. Such limitations mean that 'it is dissatisfaction with the suitability of a current resource that drives women to search for other possibilities' (Wuest, 2001, p. 179) rather than an initial desire to shop around.

Comparative shopping is only possible where other services are available. The recent centralisation of maternity services limits options. In Sheffield there used to be three maternity units, small GP units and a considerable number of home births. Now there is one maternity hospital and a few home births. In some areas choice is available for some women within the NHS, for instance in circumstances where home births or birth centre care is available. However, Nadine Edwards demonstrates (Chapter 1) how women booked for home births can still feel limited in their choices and make compromises to please their midwives.

Chapters 1 and 12 give us some insight into the lack of choice within the NHS which led some women to book with independent midwives late in their pregnancy. This is only possible where the women's aims and choices can be fulfilled by midwives and independent midwives are available. Private obstetric care may enable some women to make choices acceptable to obstetricians, such as Caesarean section (see Chapter 9). Julia Simpson's data suggests that private obstetrics may give more discussion but no more options (Chapter 10). Non-NHS care brings the issue of price into choice.

Taking risks or opting out

In the USA Judith Wuest found that 'When women know that there are suitable resources to support their caring but find them unavailable, they may simply dismiss the possibility, but many become *risk takers.*' She gives examples of complex negotiations, expenditure that a family may not be able to afford, or organising a 'safe and attended' but illegal home birth. In this country home birth is not illegal but I have known of women choosing birth at home without professional attendance rather than accept local NHS constraints on their choices. It seems reasonable to say that they are taking risks in desperation. Power is exercised whenever risk is cited as a reason for denying options to women. The drawing of boundaries of what is acceptable to service providers clearly demonstrates the limitations on the choices available to women. Since professional care exists to make birth safer, the risks defined by those institutions appear to mainly concern perceived risk to their service, not their clients.

Where midwives offer care to women who have made choices which place them outside what the maternity service sees as acceptable, they endeavour to offer the women a safer option than birthing without professional attendance. Yet midwives in such circumstances are often treated as having opted out of the system themselves and can find themselves in very vulnerable positions with regard to their employers or supervisors.

Going with the flow

In our study (Kirkham and Stapleton, 2001), the choices women made largely reflected the policies of the local unit and the preferences of health professionals, particularly obstetricians. This observation reflects what has been described elsewhere: 'For many patients, what happens to them depends more on locally accepted practice than rigorous clinical evidence'; hence the phrase 'geography is destiny' (Farrell and Gilbert, 1996, p. 21).

Going with the flow was seen by midwives and obstetricians as a logical response to the pressures upon them within a hierarchical and under-resourced service. Some professionals were seen to go against the flow to facilitate choice but few women experienced such facilitation (Kirkham and Stapleton, 2001).

The package of care and its implications

The design of antenatal care has great implications for women's choices. The offer of a package of care by professionals carries an assumption that it is designed to be of maximum value for clients. This issue has been discussed mainly with regard to antenatal screening.

'Despite an intended neutrality the very act of offering Down's syndrome screening … intrinsically puts forth the assertion that possession of this knowledge will be beneficial and empowering. In other words the potential damage of mandatory offering is that the process of making the offer of a test can appear to the mother to be compulsion.

Women come to perceive screening as an integral part of antenatal care and feel a responsibility to have it.' (Robins, 2002)

This pressure is increased where there is government endorsement, as in targets for screening, which can 'display a distinctly authoritarian dynamic' (see Chapter 2). In Barbara Hewson's view 'informed choice is being sacrificed' in such screening policies. Tricia Anderson speaks of 'compulsion not choice' and describes options being withdrawn as new, usually more technical, options become part of the regime of care (Chapter 12).

Maternity care has been becoming more packaged and more technical for many years now. Technical skills and equipment justify and support professional prestige, though skills are also being lost (see Chapter 10). The 'technocratic imperative' (Davis-Floyd, 1994) is very powerful and the professionally endorsed 'right choice' is usually the option for technology.

The package of care is also, inevitably, associated with the professionals offering the care and women's need for good relationships with their carers. James Robins, a consultant obstetrician, finds this as at odds with the concept of informed choice:

'It may be that a fully informed choice is not possible in the antenatal setting. An offer that is made under conditions that take advantage of a woman's vulnerabilities, when she is hoping for good care and attention and does not want to be seen to disappoint her obstetrician, midwife or general practitioner, does not respect her voluntariness. The woman may fear covertly expressed suggestions of rejection by the professional staff when she wants to be seen to be doing the best for her baby. Her resistance is weakened by her desire for the complete antenatal care package, (which is after all almost exclusively organised around the provision of prenatal screening tests – in itself a presumption of acceptance.)' (Robins, 2002)

Childbearing women are motivated to do the best for their baby. Thus the provision of a package of care defined by experts together with women's sympathising in silence with busy staff ('you don't like to ask') serve to produce compliance rather than choice.

The rules of the game

There have been patterns and regimes of antenatal care for as long as antenatal care has been offered as a service. I remember being taught as a student midwife, thirty years ago, how often women were to be seen antenatally and the professional agenda for each visit. Similar teaching continues today. Custom and practice was, and is, very powerful, whether it concerns how often women are seen antenatally or how often they are examined in labour. There is little evidence to support these habits. Where there is research comparing such regimes, the research is based upon normal practice compared with a, usually cheaper, variation. All options could not possibly be researched but habits become transmuted into good or even 'evidence based' care (Kirkham and Stapleton, 2001).

There are now many pressures towards standardised care. The Department of Health links *The Essence of Care* with benchmarking (Department of Health, 2001). Consistent care, in this sense, is needed if services are to be equitable. Yet this is concerned with the client's environment and services, it is not concerned with the more personal issues of relationships or choices.

We live in a world of rules or near-rules. Policies, procedures, guidelines and evidence-based care, as derived from randomised controlled trials, all apply to the average childbearing woman. Yet all childbearing women are individuals. Respecting their need for control of their situation (Green, Coupland and Kitzinger, 1988) and nurturing their specialness improves outcomes but does not fit with the bureaucracy of large-scale maternity services. 'Guidelines quickly become claimed as "standard practice" – which is then passed on to students as midwifery knowledge ... A great deal of power is given to Guidelines ... this impacts on how far a midwife can 'stray' from the dominant medicalised culture of birth' (Banks, 2001). Guidelines, policies and procedures rapidly fossilise into rules. They also extend increasingly widely. A new word has entered our vocabulary, 'proceduralisation', used to describe circumstances where written procedures exist for all eventualities. I have recently heard claims that home birth or birth centre care has been proceduralised in particular NHS Trusts!

Insurance

The issue of insurance adds another dimension to proceduralisation and the norms/rules of practice. The Clinical Negligence Scheme for Trusts, the central body which settles claims won against the NHS, now lays down specific risk management standards which NHS maternity services should follow (NHS Litigation Authority, 2002). The option of moving to a different CNST Level has considerable economic implications for Trusts and has a deep impact upon the nature and extent of proceduralisation. Thus the economic interests of the service can serve to define many 'right' choices. Ironically, along with many other aspects of risk management, CNST requirements are now being seen as a rationale for informed choice (Carne, 2002).

The Nursing and Midwifery Council, the UK statutory body for nurses and midwives, has recently considered whether all nurses and midwives should be required to carry professional indemnity insurance. In January 2003 a statement was issued:

'All nurses, midwives and health visitors in the UK are now being advised by their regulatory body to maintain adequate indemnity insurance cover to protect patients and themselves.' (Nursing and Midwifery Council, 2003).

Yet no insurance is currently available for independent midwives anywhere in the world. Many efforts have been made to negotiate such cover with insurance companies, some of which I have been involved in. In such negotiations, insurance companies proposed considerable proceduralisation and massive fees but the negotiations still did not come to fruition.

Fear

In Holly Richards' view 'birth simultaneously encompasses the three events that civilised societies fear – birth, death and sexuality' (Richards, 1993). There is much truth in this statement and such fear and our response of technical control has been discussed by many authors (e.g. Davis-Floyd, 1994; Taylor, 1996).

We now have a fourth fear, litigation. In our study we found that fear of litigation cast a dark shadow for obstetricians and other health professionals, many of whom volunteered that they worked 'with a lot of fear around'. A number of respondents expressed the opinion that it was fear of litigation, rather than the striving for standards of excellence, which was currently the primary motivation for change in the maternity services (Kirkham and Stapleton, 2001).

For childbearing women and professionals fear often leads to a need for control in an attempt to ensure that what is most feared cannot happen. As Susan Bewley and Jayne Cockburn examine in Chapter 8, this can distort what is seen as informed choice. They stress the need not just to accept requests for Caesarean section (CS) as informed choices. They see a real 'danger in not recognising fears and phobias, but renaming them "requests"'. In a technological era when fear of birth is growing (Green, 2002) it must be important that 'if deep and genuine fears are driving the request for CS, then doctors must address them sensitively' (Chapter 8), not just accept them as choices to be accepted or refused. Honouring fear-driven requests simply as choices avoids difficult and time-consuming, but nevertheless vital aspects of care for individual women. Caesarean section 'may give an illusion of control (to mother and surgeon), but miss what is really going on and make postnatal adaptation worse' (Chapter 8).

Unequal interactions

Time and knowledge

Many women do not know what to expect when they encounter maternity services in their first pregnancy. They make choices and gather information in a limited timeframe. This situation can be exacerbated by pressures for women to make some important decisions at administratively defined, but not clinically necessary, points in time. Some decisions need to be made at a specific gestation, but decisions as to place of birth or length of postnatal hospital stay, for example, are often made in early pregnancy for purely administrative reasons. Thus experience and knowledge gathered later cannot inform such decisions.

Obstetricians, midwives and service managers have had many years of education concerning their specialism. They have had time to consider and be socialised into its practice and values. This imbalance in expertise and in time to learn is respected by women and manifest, therefore, as an imbalance in power. Without definite and strategically planned help to overcome this imbalance, informed compliance is likely to continue.

The immediate pressures of time in consultations prevent women questioning professional staff who might otherwise be seen as useful sources of information and discussion. Our impression in so many consultations was of midwives so pressured that they did not give the women time to speak (Kirkham and Stapleton, 2001). Thus midwives dominated their interaction with women. Most women we observed did not ask for further information. 'You don't like to ask, the midwives are so busy' is a statement which recurs in many studies of women's views of maternity services. There is also the difficulty of framing the right questions when a woman's understanding and knowledge may be limited and the consultation rushed. The pressures upon the midwife's time and the many things the midwife felt she must say therefore resulted in action which robbed women of their time and their voice. In such an unequal situation, where most clients tried so hard to please, the 'asymmetry between the consulting patient's time' and that of the health professional is 'both functional and symbolic' (Frankenberg, 1992, p. 1). Most professionals took this imbalance for granted. Where women endeavoured to take time and voice their concerns they risked alienating professionals on whom they felt very dependent.

It is significant to note the time allowed for antenatal booking consultations and other midwife antenatal consultations in a Trust with the specific aim of 'enabling women to work towards continually making their own informed decisions' (Chapter 8, Figure 8.1). These time allocations, which Jill Demilew includes in 'organisational factors supporting informed choice', are very different from those in many other NHS Trusts and represent a strategic allocation of resources to this end.

Information and knowledge: sources and control

Choice can only be made where the individual has knowledge of options. Yet the information made available by midwives and obstetricians is mostly framed so as to support the locally defined right choices. We certainly observed information being withheld from women who were not trusted to make the right choices (Kirkham and Stapleton, 2001).

As maternity care is resourced and organised, it would be impossible to respond in a sensitive way to all the women. Clinics only end and the service is only possible because most women don't ask. But this does not mean they do not want to know (Wiggins *et al.*, 2000). The service is unequal in the information it makes available to women. Only by processing many women rapidly and relatively silently can staff make time for the few who do ask. Those who

ask questions are usually the more articulate and educated (Kirkham and Stapleton, 2001). Barbara Hewson explains how, from a legal viewpoint, specific
questions must be answered (Chapter 2). Thus the inverse care law (Hart,
1971; Kirkham *et al.*, 2002) is perpetuated and legally reinforced! Midwives do
stereotype women in terms of their information needs; it is a coping mechanism.
Only by judging many as not wanting or needing information, explanation or
support can the time be made available to explain to others. Thus the practice
differs from the rhetoric and midwives continue to cope.

Where women are unhappy with choices offered, they feel a great need for
information to support unconventional decisions. It is unusual for NHS
professionals to give women information on alternatives to what the service
offers and many women speak of having to find out for themselves. In
discussing this difficult process, women tended to use metaphors of military
conflict, seeking information 'to arm' or 'to defend' themselves against the
system (Chapter 1, and Kirkham and Stapleton, 2001).

Information can be presented so as to ensure compliance or it can be used
to facilitate choice. This depends upon the aims of the practitioner which in
turn derive from their context. The MIDIRS *Informed Choice* Leaflets did not
facilitate informed choice in the normal practice setting of our trial (Chapter
4) but some of the same leaflets did facilitate change after they had been used
in discussion on a smaller scale (Chapter 7). The level of strategic planning for
informed choices described by Jill Demilew in Chapter 8 is certainly unusual.
Yet she still describes 'a huge gap with working reality' and the need for 'new
knowledge and new competencies in professional practice' in order for
women's informed choice to become reality.

Types of information: evidence and experience

The information offered by midwives and obstetricians is usually constructed
from a professional viewpoint in order to demonstrate convincing reasons for
the desired 'right' choice. The concept of evidence based practice is not value-
free. 'Evidence that reinforces notions of authoritative knowledge' is likely to
be favoured by professionals (Stewart, 2001; Kirkham and Stapleton, 2001).

Information and likely subsequent decisions by women may be standardised by staff creating a 'package' of verbal information which is delivered in a
similar manner to most women, or by giving leaflets without discussion. Yet
before deciding to undergo something, it is reasonable to wish to know what
to expect during and after the experience. This is just the category of information which women find is missing. Despite the rising Caesarean section rate
and the intense debate around this, Helen Stapleton gives a long list of information women needed before their elective Caesareans but were not given
(Chapter 5).

Woman have been found to value and rely upon embodied knowledge from
their own personal experience or which they see others close to them acting
upon and reproducing in their daily lives (Hoddinott, 1999; Trewick, Ellis

and Kirkham, 2002; Chapter 7). Yet professionals tend to see themselves as dispensing knowledge as clinical evidence not as personal or professional experience. In our study women often said to the midwife 'What would you do?' Most midwives interpreted this as avoiding the responsibility associated with decision-making and quickly moved the responsibility back to the woman with the phrase, 'It's your choice ....'. It is noteworthy that midwives were frequently heard to use the word 'discuss' as in 'Here are some leaflets about things we have discussed'. Yet the term was persistently used when the woman had neither been asked her opinions nor had her concerns expressed (Kirkham and Stapleton, 2001). Such concerns were often experiential.

> 'They don't "discuss" things with you. They "tell" you things. They tell you what to do. Like you're still at school... With breastfeeding, they told me all the advantages and disadvantages but I know them already. I wanted to know what it would "feel" like ... about feeling embarrassed and if it would hurt for long. My mum couldn't help me on that. She'd bottle-fed all of us.' (16-year-old respondent: Stapleton *et al.*, 2002)

Where informal, equal, conversational exchange was experienced it was valued by women as 'sharing' of life experiences, 'normal' two-way conversation which could lead to trust. A few midwives spoke of such conversation as important to them but this was rare (Kirkham and Stapleton, 2001). Such conversation has been identified in neonatal nursing as 'shifting the locus of control', 'minimising power differentials between nurses and women' (Fenwick, Barclay and Schmied, 2001, p. 589) and 'promoting collaboration and engendering a sense of maternal control' (p. 591). These achievements feature large in midwifery rhetoric but the conversation which facilitated them was rarely observed in practice (Kirkham and Stapleton, 2001).

Communication skills

In recent years there has been increased emphasis on communication skills in medical and midwifery education. Professionals also feel real pressure to give information and record that they have done this in case they are challenged. In such pressurised circumstances it is perhaps not surprising that women perceive midwives as 'telling not listening' (Chapter 1) or 'checking not listening' (Kirkham and Stapleton, 2001). The absence of listening in such so-called communication is striking, though understandable in its context. If 'communication' only concerns clinical evidence and is one way, there is no opportunity for it to be made relevant to the individual or placed in the context of experience.

As a midwife who pioneered 'communication' as part of the midwifery curriculum, it saddens me that listening is so rare. We appear to have created a skill of 'communication' without relationship. This is doubtless the result of highly fragmented clinical care but fits none of the definitions of communication as an essentially two way activity.

The building of trust appears not to be seen as part of communication skills. This area of education has itself become fragmented.

Consent and choice

Several chapters in this book discuss informed consent. Until recently informed consent rather than informed choice was a key concept in maternity care, as it is in every area of medical care.

Consent to treatment

Consent concerns a decision to accept or refuse what is offered by an expert, usually a course of treatment or investigations. The term is concerned with illness: where a medical problem is perceived and an accurate diagnosis is needed followed by treatment to prevent further ill health or even death. Such a concept does not see birth as a natural process or consider the many paths which may be chosen by childbearing women. Choosing not to accept a medical package does not mean, for most childbearing women, that disaster will follow.

The concept of consent comes from the medical model of illness, where the main actor is the professional. The concept of choice comes from a social model where the main actor, the childbearing woman, bears her child within a social context. Department of Health publications over the last decade have adopted, to varying degrees, the discourse of the social model. The service has, however, changed little in its hierarchical and bureaucratic structure apart from becoming more centralised. Professionals are quick to adopt the language of official policy and therefore speak of choice. The policy enacted in practice, however, is largely concerned with consent to medically defined 'treatments'. The language of the obstetricians in Julia Simpson's chapter is significant here.

With the development of the concept of risk management through screening, consent to a medically endorsed screening package is encountered by women very early in pregnancy. The concepts of diagnosis and treatment thus become routine with all their implications of professional power.

Ethics and consent

Susan Bewley and Jayne Cockburn, both consultant obstetricians, address the ethical complexity of informed choice concerning the topical issue of Caesarean section requests (Chapter 9). They examine 'the difficult interplay between safety and choice' in terms of outcome statistics for mothers and babies, of individual's fears and anxieties and wider issues for present and future families, all within the context of what is seen as good mothering and good professional practice. Their conclusion is not to specify an ethically right answer but to make ten recommendations, the first of which is to listen to women. Thus good practice is portrayed as flexible and negotiated with women in the light of their underlying concerns. It may however involve several medical specialisms.

Brenda Ashcroft, a midwife teacher, takes a viewpoint which sees professional clinical judgement as the ethical denominator, not as open to negotiation and concludes:

> 'All demands for clinically unsound treatment can safely be ignored, as the midwife must always act in the best interests of the woman according to her clinical judgement.' (Ashcroft, 1998, p. 505)

The woman retains the right to 'withhold her consent' (Ashcroft, 1998, p. 505) but the professionals retain the power to define the service offered. Thus the situation described in Chapter 12 is ethically justified and the wider context of women's decision-making is not addressed.

In the context of antenatal screening, a study by social scientists casts light on midwives' lack of control around informed choice. 'Promoting informed choice is commonly recognised as the chief purpose and benefit of prenatal screening, its very presence being viewed as a key way in which the process can be distanced from eugenics' (Williams, Alderson and Farsides, 2002a, p. 743). Yet the views of those responsible for such screening raised many doubts as to whether informed choice could be achieved and saw 'the expansion of screening, which might further compromise informed choice, as an inevitable and inexorable process over which they had little, if any, control.' (Williams, Alderson and Farsides, 2002a, p. 743).

Given the pressures to comply with services offered, Barbara Hewson sees Department of Health policies of universal screening, which are as lacking in explanation at the policy level as they are at the practice level, as displaying 'a distinctly authoritarian dynamic, and they treat adults like children' (Chapter 2). As a barrister, she sees the current situation in practice – our attempts to implement Department of Health directives – as unethical and legally unsound. 'Cursory or 'routine' testing procedures, which involve a few quick questions and giving a leaflet to someone, will not withstand hostile legal scrutiny' (Chapter 2):

> 'Both the DoH and the RCM had advised midwives that they need spend only a "few minutes" in pre-test discussion. One is forced reluctantly to the conclusion that neither the DoH or the RCM intended that the pregnant woman should give properly informed consent to HIV screening. This is tantamount to being a compulsory scheme, the legality of which must be doubtful.' (Chapter 2)

Thus the bureaucratic pressures, which lead us to speak the language of informed choice whilst processing women hurriedly towards predetermined targets, have put the service in a position which does not engage with women (Ashcroft, 1998) or which infantalises them and is legally doubtful. Such a situation must be reconsidered at a policy level and by NHS Trusts.

Control of professional work

Routine

Routines can be comforting in difficult circumstances. As George Eliot observed:

> 'We do not expect people to be deeply moved by what is not unusual … tragedy in frequency … our frames could hardly bear much of it.' (Eliot, 1871/1980, p. 226)

What is true of tragedy applies equally to many other emotional aspects of childbearing women's encounters with maternity services. The organisation of services in ways which protect staff from anxiety can be seen throughout institutional health care (Menzies, 1970). Yet the 'frequency' only applies to the professional, because women have few children and maternity services are organised to present professionals with frequent, specialised tasks. The operation of routines thus serves as an important professional coping mechanism for staff confronted by the problem of managing work stresses (Lipsky, 1980, pp. 85–6). It also creates predictability which would not be possible were each childbearing woman to think through all her options and make her own choices whilst experiencing her own family's happiness or tragedy. Where time and resources are in short supply, predictability becomes very important.

> 'Routinisation operates on two levels. At the level of the individual, it provides for ontological security in the predictability of events. At a collective level, routinisation is critical to the workings of institutions which exist by virtue of the continued reproduction of routines.' (Frolich, Corin and Potvin, 2001, p. 788)

These two levels are mutually reinforcing in clinical practice where the predictable behaviours of all concerned 'are part and parcel of this implicit, routinised, practical logic of everyday life' (Williams, 1995, p. 598). Routinisation, in its inflexibility, can also be justified as fair and therefore serve to ration limited resources such as professional time: 'set procedures designed to insure regularity, accountability, and fairness … protect workers from client demands for responsiveness' (Lipsky, 1980, p. 100). Where clients are treated as individuals, routines are inappropriate.

Thus plans, guidelines, procedures and care pathways fossilise as rules which define and reassure the staff who operate them. This can be reinforced by the concept of evidence and the randomised controlled trial (RCT) as the research gold standard. RCTs are immensely useful, but always create a range of questions as to how far, in slightly different circumstances, they still provide evidence for practice. Routine practices and guidelines together can limit the asking of the uncomfortable, but crucial questions for clinical practice and future research. Many questions are triggered by any query as to what extent the guidelines or the evidence fit an individual woman; routine prevents such questions being asked.

Thus women are 'steered' and 'swayed' towards making the right choices as demonstrated in Chapters 1, 3 and 5. Informed compliance is usually achieved whatever it is called. Staff do not always act so as to insulate themselves from anxiety or relationship with clients. Altruism does occur and some staff put themselves in very vulnerable positions with regard to their own hierarchy to support some women in their choices. Most 'develop techniques to salvage service and decision-making values within the limits imposed by the structure of the work' building 'conceptions of their work and of their clients that narrow the gap between their personal and work limitations and the service ideal' (Lipsky, 1980, p. xiii).

Medicine retains the ultimate power to steer in its assumption of the power to define safety. Despite the statement in *Changing Childbirth* that 'safety is not an absolute concept' (Department of Health, 1993), this medical 'final say' is widely enacted as coercion, as examined in Chapter 1.

Control of one's own experience?

A woman's caring for her foetus is part of her wider web of caring for her family (Edwards, 2002), whereas professional maternity care is defined and limited in its focus and its timespan. In Carol Gilligan's work (1982) the 'hierarchy' and the 'web' identify the different male and female imagery of relationships. Any one image must oversimplify. Yet this is a useful tool where women are considering safety in terms of a family and all its relationships now and in the future and obstetricians feel they carry the ultimate responsibility for the foetus until it is delivered.

> 'Thus the images of hierarchy and web inform different modes of assertion and response: the wish to be alone at the top and the consequent fear that others will get too close; the wish to be at the centre of connection and the consequent fear of being too far out on the edge. These disparate fears of being stranded and being caught give rise to different portrayals of achievement and affiliation, leading to different modes of action and different ways of assessing the consequences of choice.' (Gilligan, 1982/1993, p. 62)

The senior obstetricians who speak in Julia Simpson's chapter clearly convey their need to be 'alone at the top' in decision-making, even when dealing with trends that come from within their profession but which can be projected as coming from without (Chapter 9). The women whom Nadine Edwards studied (Chapter 1 and Edwards, 2002) wished to maintain their many connections with family and with midwives. When professionals' response to their choices left these women with 'fears of being stranded' they often sacrificed their carefully chosen preferences. Such sacrifice may be seen as necessary but is nevertheless sacrifice.

Carol Gilligan identified caring as crucial to women's concepts of self and of morality. Caring is an active process and such nurturing through caring is linked to the development and sense of personal autonomy of the carer

(Noddings, 1984; Abel and Nelson, 1990; Wuest, 2001). Nadine Edwards sees decision-making as integral to self-esteem (Chapter 1).

Balancing caring

Midwives and mothers in this book convey the precariousness of their caring position because of the need to balance the many calls upon them. The 'precarious ordering of caring' (Wuest, 2001) is demonstrated for mothers in Nadine Edwards' chapter and for midwives in Valerie Levy's chapter. Senior obstetricians are to some extent protected by the power of their position, yet where they enter into relationships, they too take risks which can upset their balance (Kirkham and Stapleton, 2001). The efforts of such balancing acts lead to the setting of boundaries and to 'fraying connections'.

> 'Fraying connections reflect the contradictions in the emotional, cognitive, relational, and material aspects of caring and occur between women and those for whom they care and those on whom they rely for help. Fraying connections are evident in daily struggles, altered prospects and ambivalent feelings.' (Wuest, 2001)

Many fraying connects can be found within this book.

Midwives are in a particularly precarious position as 'piggy in the middle' (Murphy-Lawless, 1991), balancing the needs of medicine and management and those of the women in their care.

Is partnership possible?

The behaviour of professionals is a logical response to their situation. Routinisation and failure to relate to individual clients are coping mechanisms which enable professionals to get through the work and balance conflicting pressures. Socially, this is a parallel response to that of their clients who smoke as 'something for themselves' when life offers them little else (Graham, 1993, p. 32). The consoling 'something' which obstetricians and midwives seek for themselves is their professional status, which isolates them further from their clients, making informed choice even less possible. In each case – professionals who know best and women who smoke – exhortations that individuals should or must change their coping behaviour are likely to be futile without real change in their context. We therefore need to question how change in context is possible.

Robbie Davis-Floyd and Flora Mather (2002) usefully outline three paradigms of health care that 'heavily influence contemporary childbirth'. These are 'the technocratic model of medicine, the humanistic (biopsychosocial) model of medicine and the holistic model of medicine'. They conclude that:

'If midwives and their obstetrical collaborators could apply appropriate technologies in combination with the values of humanism and the spontaneous openness to individuality and energy chartered by holism, they could in fact create the best obstetrical/midwifery system the world has ever known.' (Davis-Floyd and Mather, 2002, p. 506)

This work provides an inspiring vision and helps practitioners to clarify their aims. The rhetoric of the many policy statements that have been influenced by a social model of birth are moving towards a more humanistic model. Yet these models and paradigms give no guidance as to how the reality of service delivery can be changed, and how we may move from the present fearful bureaucracy to such an ideal situation. Meanwhile midwives continue to apply technology which they know to be inappropriate, such as routine electronic fetal heart monitoring in normal labour, because it is expected in their place of work.

Given the difficulty professionals, especially midwives, have in balancing the many pressures upon them, it is logical that they are likely to give more attention to women and relate better with them where the other pressures are less.

Culture, scale and choice

If we are to create strategies to improve maternity care we need first to identify where things are better currently and learn from these circumstances how we may bring about improvement.

Scale

Where maternity care is on a small scale, relationships are very different. The smallest scale of care must be an individual midwife booking a woman for a home birth. Whilst the bureaucracy of the large NHS Trust which usually employs community midwives can affect the relationships between woman and their community midwife (see Chapter 1), the context of home birth does change care, especially where relationships can develop. Where independent midwives book women they do not have an employee relationship with the bureaucracy and the absence of this power relationship can greatly enlarge the options for women (see Chapter 12). Such situations give women and midwives much more power and control of their situation. For these reasons, and many others, the options of home birth inside and outside the NHS must be defended and preserved.

Within larger maternity services, care can be provided so that women receive continuity of care from one or two midwives with whom they can build relationships. These relationships then become important and sustaining for all concerned (e.g. Sandall, Davies and Warwick, 2001; Flint, 1993; Page, 1994), in contrast to the fragmented nature of most maternity care. Here again, where midwife and mother know each other, trust can develop and options widen.

There are clearly differences between large hospitals and small units. These are demonstrated in Chapter 6 and in many studies (e.g. Churchill and Benbow, 2000 and Kirkham, 2003). In small units midwives are removed from many of the immediate pressures ever present in large hospitals. Birth centres work within a social rather than a medical model of birth. Doctors and managers are not immediately present, clients are few and local and, without the passive option of epidural anaesthesia, women have to cope with their labours. In these circumstances the midwife/mother relationship becomes very important and the midwife's key role is to support the woman in coping with her childbearing as best she can. Thus the woman takes a more active and central role which makes different options possible. Kate Griew (2003) sees the birth centre environment as making it possible for midwives to 'truly listen'. From this listening there follows a different use of language with less jargon, less instruction and a focus on support for the woman rather than the use of language which protects the midwife. Birth centres are noted for the excellent communication within and without the unit (NHS Management Executive, 1993).

There are real differences in how power is exercised in birth centres compared with hospitals. Birth centre midwives take greater personal responsibility than in hospitals and are protected from neither the anxiety nor the emotional rewards of their relationships with women. This is identified as 'carrying the can' and 'real midwifery' (Hunter, 2000 and 2003) which midwives find rewarding, though challenging in terms of their relationship with the hospital to which they may have to refer women. The potential for 'sharing power' and for the mutual empowerment of mothers and midwives can be realised within the smaller and simpler structures of birth centres. Rather than midwives being piggy in the middle and women feeling coerced, a 'positive spiral' of mutual support is being strategically nurtured in some birth centres (Jones, 2000). Mutual empowerment does not fit with hierarchical structures and it is therefore important that there are alternatives where it is possible to realise the rhetoric of maternity care.

In birth centres midwifery care can be personalised and given in response to the individual needs of women and their families. Marion Hunter draws from her research a list of the 'additional skills' required by midwives providing intrapartum care in small units in New Zealand.

- Being confident to provide intrapartum care in a low technology setting.
- Being comfortable to use embodied knowledge and skills to assess a woman and her baby as opposed to using technology.
- Being able to let labour 'be' and not interfere unnecessarily.
- Being confident to avert or manage problems that might arise.
- Being willing to employ other options to manage pain without access to epidurals.
- Being solely responsible for outcomes without access to on-site specialist assistance.
- Being confident to trust the process of labour and be flexible with respect to time.
- Being a midwife who enjoys practising what the participants call 'real midwifery'.
  (Hunter, 2000, p. 143)

This list is strikingly different to the usual lists of midwifery skills or competencies. The flexibility inherent in these skills make a range of options possible and choices can therefore be heard, though their range is limited to what is possible in the birth centre. The skills on this list are all states of 'being', statements regarding the midwife's self and her use of self, rather than tightly defined manual or intellectual skills. These are skills for relationships not for narrowly defined tasks.

Where midwives work as individuals in relationships with women, or where their contact with colleagues is limited, their 'primary reference group' (Lipsky, 1980, p. 47) becomes their clients (Stapleton, Duerden and Kirkham, 1998; Hunter, 2003). This radically changes midwives' relationships, protecting them to varying extents from institutional pressures and enabling mutually supportive relationships to develop with clients. In this relatively protected situation it is possible to develop more flexible and resilient support structures (Stapleton, Duerden and Kirkham, 1998; Jones, 2000) which enhance confidence, options and trust. In New Zealand this situation has been brought about strategically from a national level by the implementation of the midwifery partnership model of care. This has led to a real shift in power.

'Partnership involves a shift of power from the health professional to the woman in the same way that the midwife's allegiance moves from the hospital or doctor to the woman as she supports her and stands alongside her through the process of pregnancy and childbirth.' (Pairman and Guilliland, 2003, p. 229)

Trust and risk

Trust is highly significant here. The woman booked in a birth centre, or planning a home birth learns 'to trust her body' and the midwife to 'trust her own judgement' (Kirkham, 2003) as well as to trust each other and the process of labour. Trust is infectious and the midwife's trust is conveyed to the woman. This is more difficult but not impossible in a hospital setting. Chapters 8 and 9 give us glimpses of circumstances where women's voices may be heard in highly medicalised settings.

In the culture of large maternity units there is a striking lack of either trust between midwives or of professional trust in clients (see Chapter 6). Clients are, however, expected to trust professionals and the maternity service to act in their best interests as defined by that service. This makes choice a somewhat passive process.

Risk is highlighted in modern society (Furedi, 1997) and modern obstetrics. Increasingly we strive to define risks and fear taking them. Many of the acknowledged areas of choice in maternity care are also defined as areas of risk where technical procedures are employed to reveal or avoid that risk. This is exemplified in antenatal screening. Thus 'risk increasingly becomes the lens through which choice is filtered' (Lippman, 1999) and the right choice is seen as the avoidance of risk. The concept of risk inevitably engenders fear which can corrode trust.

Choice as the embodiment of risk?

There is a viewpoint which sees 'choice as a risk to women's health' (Lippman, 1999). This statement focuses our attention on the social and economic construction of choice. Seeing choice as an individual selecting from a menu hides the fact that service users do not construct the menu and find it extremely difficult to make choices outside the menu.

What appears to be a personal choice, such as screening for Down's syndrome, is taken in the social context of inadequate social support and resources for such children and their families (Shakespeare, 1998) and the stigmatising of both disabled children and their parents who, 'could have known better' if they had accepted screening. Here again there is little information for parents on 'what it would be like' to have an affected child, but details are provided on the degree of risk to the individual woman of having such a child (Williams, Alderson and Farsides, 2002b). The identification of a foetus with Down's syndrome has been identified as a risk because such identification is possible and commercial interests support the technology involved, not because it is identified as a fear by parents.

Abby Lippman lists the 'trends that may contribute to structural constraints on choice today'. These include changing concepts of risks and risk management which 'frame the body as a site of "virtual pathology"', changing programmes of testing, changing concepts of normality and changing concepts of responsibility with emphasis on individual '"self-reliant" choice' (Lippman, 1999, p. 283–4). Thus it can be claimed that choice is a 'social construct that makes people feel free even in a context of oppression' (Gregg, 1995, p. 27 quoted and explored in Chapter 1).

Choices and processes

Nicky Leap usefully brings together the issues of choice and trust:

> 'There is a fragile element within the notion we call 'informed choice'. Apart from the potential for decision-making that is biased by the person doing the informing, there are many situations in which no amount of information will clarify the decision process for women. Instead of giving women lists of possibilities and options to choose from, a "wait and see – keep your eyes open" policy is arguably more useful. In antenatal groups and with individual women, I have found that, in many situations, raising the notion of "uncertainty" has led to more fruitful discussion than pursuing the idea of "informed choice". Embracing uncertainty sometimes brings a sense of calm, a sense that what will be, will be. This is not about engendering a passive fatalism but more about enabling women to learn to trust that they will cope with whatever comes their way. Working through these issues is particularly important in a culture that privileges the notions of "choice" and "control".' (Leap, 2000, p. 5)

Such an approach assumes a relationship within which such discussions can take place. It echoes Susan Bewley and Jayne Cockburn's efforts to understand women's fears (Chapter 9). Linking the need for trust and the presence of uncertainty in all childbearing highlights the need for on-going dialogue to extend what is seen as possible rather than choice from a set menu. This is possible in on-going relationship whether between women and midwives or women and obstetricians. Keeping options open is also a process over time. This echoes the emphasis of the GMC on informed consent as a process, not a one-off event, which is examined by Barbara Hewson in Chapter 2. Yet our research revealed considerable organisational pressures to record choices as taken. Thus preferences expressed by women at the booking visit were often taken as firm decisions and only rarely did these decisions appear to be revisited later in pregnancy (Kirkham and Stapleton, 2001, p. 101). This exemplifies the manner in which choice, presented as a series of predefined options, may give an 'illusion of control' (Chapter 9) whilst limiting possibilities.

Embracing uncertainty is, however, contrary to the main pressures of both modern society (Furedi, 1998) and the bureaucracies within which most maternity care takes place (Lipsky, 1980). Even within very thorough strategic planning towards informed choice, Jill Demilew found that 'few professionals appeared to be absolutely comfortable with sharing uncertainty about various interventions and being able to easily articulate relative risks and benefits of these interventions' (Chapter 8).

The future

The complex, frustrating situation around informed choice conveyed in this book is deeply unsatisfactory. It is riven with contradictions, not least those between the rhetoric of Department of Health policy and the policy forged in under-resourced and bureaucratic practice.

The answer is not to urge professionals to implement the rhetoric. I have used Lipsky's work as a theoretical thread throughout this Chapter to demonstrate that the problem is structural. The behaviour of all concerned is logical within a public service bureaucracy, it is not the fault of individual midwives or obstetricians. The rhetoric does not work because of the context.

Changing the values and philosophy of a bureaucracy is a massive undertaking, even with good will and reasonable resources (see Chapter 8). Bureaucracies can be broken down into small units where relationships protect on-going choices, as in continuity of midwifery care schemes within some NHS Trusts (e.g. Sandall, Davies and Warwick, 2001; Allen, Dowling and Williams, 2001; Flint, 1993; Page, 1994) or as is national policy in New Zealand (Guilliland and Pairman, 1995).

If we are to develop better ways of taking decisions and women are to be involved in their childbearing on their terms, profound change is called for in the organisation and resourcing of maternity services. This would involve debate and strategising which acknowledged powerful opposing trends in society. This is necessary for the future retention of midwives (Ball, Curtis and Kirkham, 2002) and for the experience of women. Meanwhile, it is vital that options in maternity care are kept open, publicised and developed. There is a direct parallel between the diverse needs of women and of staff.

The contradictions within our present unsatisfactory system need to be understood so that they can be worked upon. This book is offered as a contribution to that understanding.

References

Abel, E. and Nelson, M. (eds) (1990) *Circles of Care*. Albany, NY: State University of New York Press.

Allen, I., Dowling, S.B. and Williams, S. (2001) *A Leading Role for Midwives? Evaluation of Midwifery Group Practice Development Projects*. London: Policy Studies Institute.

Ashcroft, B. (1998) Choices in childbirth: myth or reality. *British Journal of Midwifery*, **6(8)**: 502–6.

Ball, l., Curtis, P. and Kirkham, M. (2002) *Why Do Midwives Leave?* London: Royal College of Midwives.

Banks, M. (2001) But whose art frames the questions? *The Practising Midwife*, **4(9)**: 34–5.

British Medical Journal (2002): Editor Choice: Informed compliance. *British Medical Journal*, **3249(7338)**: 621.

Carne, V. (2002) Informed choice – a solution to health information delivery challenges of the 21st century. *MIDIRS Midwifery Digest*, **12(4)**: 440–4.

Churchill, H. and Benbow, A. (2000) Informed choice in maternity care. *British Journal of Midwifery* **8(1)**: 41–7.

Davis-Floyd, R. (1994) Culture and Birth: The technocratic imperative. *International Journal of Childbirth Education* **9(2)**: 6–7.

Davis-Floyd, R. and Mather, F.S. (2002) The technocratic, humanistic, and holistic paradigms of childbirth. *MIDIRS Midwifery Digest* **12(4)**: 500–6.

Department of Health (1993) *Changing Childbirth*, London: HMSO.

Department of Health (2001) *The Essence of Care: patient-focused benchmarking for healthcare practitioners*. London: Department of Health.

Duddridge, E. (2000) The influence of grandparents on infant-feeding choice. *British Journal of Midwifery* **8(5)**: 302–4.

Edwards, N. (2002) *Women's experiences of planning home births in Scotland. Birthing Autonomy*. Unpublished Phd, University of Sheffield.

Eliot, G. (1871/1980) *Middlemarch*. Harmondsworth: Penguin.

Farrell, C. and Gilbert, H. (1996) *Health Care Partnerships*. London: King's Fund.

Fenwick, J., Barclay, L. and Schmied, V. (2001) 'Chatting': an important clinical tool in facilitating mothering in neonatal nurseries. *Journal of Advanced Nursing*, **33(5)**: 583–93.

Flint, C. (1993) *Midwifery Teams and Caseloads*. Oxford: Butterworth-Heinemann.

Frankenberg, R. (1992) (ed.) *Time, Health and Medicine*. London: Sage.

Frolich, K.L., Corin, E. and Potvin, L. (2001) A theoretical proposal for the relationship between context and disease. *Sociology of Health and Illness*, **23(6)**: 776–97.

Furedi, F. (1997) *Culture of Fear: Risk-taking and the Morality of Low Expectation*. London: Cassell.

Gilligan, C. (1982, 1993 edition) *In a Different Voice: Psychological Theory and Women's Development*. Cambridge, MA: Harvard University Press.

Glaser, B. (1972) *Experts versus Laymen: A Study of the Patsy and the Subcontractor.* Mill Valley, CA: Sociology Press.

Graham, H. (1993) *When Life's a Drag: Women, Smoking and Disadvantage.* London: HMSO.

Gready, M., Newburn, M., Dodds, R. and Guage, S. (1995) *Birth Choices – Women's Expectations and Experiences.* Report of a research project – choices: childbirth options, information and care in Essex. National Childbirth Trust.

Green, J.M., Coupland, V.A. and Kitzinger, J.V. (1988) *Great Expectations: A Prospective Study of Women's Expectations and Experiences of Childbirth.* University of Cambridge: Child Care and Development Unit.

Green, J.M. (2002) Verbal presentation of findings of Greater Expectations Study. University of Sheffield: Society for Reproductive and Infant Psychology Conference.

Gregg, R. (1995) *Pregnancy in a High-Tech Age: Paradoxes of Choice.* New York and London: New York University Press.

Griew, K. (2003) Birth Centres in Australia. In M. Kirkham (ed.), *Birth Centres: A Social Model for Maternity Care.* Oxford: Butterworth-Heinemann.

Guilliland, K. and Pairman, S. (1995) *The Midwifery Partnership: A Model for Practice.* Dept of Nursing and Midwifery, Victoria University of Wellington.

Hart, T.L. (1971) The inverse care law. *Lancet,* **1**: 405–12.

Hoddinott, P. (1999) *Why don't some women want to breastfeed and how might we change their attitudes? A qualitative study.* Unpublished PhD, University of Wales College of Medicine, Cardiff.

Hunter, B. (2003) *Emotion Work in Midwifery.* Unpublished PhD. University of Wales, Swansea.

Hunter, M. (2000) *Autonomy, clinical freedom and responsibility: the paradoxes of providing intrapartum midwifery care in a small maternity unit as compared with a large obstetric hospital.* Unpublished MA, Massey University, Palmerston North, New Zealand.

Hunter, M. (2003) Autonomy, clinical freedom and responsibility: the paradoxes of providing intrapartum midwifery care in a small maternity unit as compared with a large obstetric hospital. In M. Kirkham (ed.), *Birth Centres: A Social Model for Maternity Care.* Oxford: Butterworth Heinemann.

Jones, O. (2000) Supervision in a midwife-managed birth centre. In M. Kirkham (ed.), *Developments in the Supervision of Midwives.* Manchester: Books for Midwives Press.

Kirkham, M. (2003) (ed.) *Birth Centres: A Social Model for Maternity Care.* Oxford: Butterworth Heinemann.

Kirkham, M. and Stapleton, H. (eds) (2001) *Informed Choice in Maternity Care: An Evaluation of Evidence-based Leaflets.* NHS Centre for Reviews and Dissemination, University of York.

Kirkham, M., Stapleton, H., Curtis, P. and Thomas, G. (2002) The inverse care law in antenatal midwifery care. *British Journal of Midwifery,* **10(8)**: 509–13.

Leap, N. (2000) The less we do, the more we give. In M. Kirkham (ed.) *The Midwife–Mother Relationship.* London: Macmillan.

Lippman, A. (1999) Choice as a risk to women's health. *Health, Risk and Society,* **1(3)**: 281–91.

Lipsky, M. (1980) *Street-Level Bureaucracy: Dilemmas of the Individual in Public Services.* New York: Russel Sage Foundation.

Menzies, I.E.P. (1970) *The Functioning of Social Systems as a Defence Against Anxiety.* London: Tavistock.

Murphy, E. (1999) 'Breast is Best': Infant-feeding decisions and maternal deviance. *Sociology of Health and Illness,* **21(2)**: 187–208.

Murphy-Lawless, J. (1991) Piggy in the middle: the midwife's role in achieving woman-controlled childbirth. *Irish Journal of Psychology*, **12(2)**: 198–215.

NHS Litigation Authority (2002) *Clinical Negligence Scheme for Trusts: Clinical Risk Management Standards for Maternity Services*. London: NHSLA.

NHS Management Executive (1992) *A Study of Midwife- and GP-led maternity units*. London: Department of Health.

Noddings, N. (1984) *Caring: A Feminine Approach to Ethics and Moral Education*. Berkeley: University of California Press.

Nursing and Midwifery Council (2003) Press release 17 Jan. http://www.nmc-uk.org/nmc/main/pressStatements/newIndemnityClauseForCode.html

Page, L. (1994) *Effective Group Practice in Midwifery*. Oxford: Blackwell Science.

Pairman, S. and Guilliland, K. (2003) The New Zealand experience. In M. Kirkham (ed.) *Birth Centres: A Social Model for Maternity Care*. Oxford: Butterworth-Heinemann.

Richards, H. (1993) Cultural messages of childbirth: the penetration of fear. *International Childbirth Education Association Journal*, 7(**3**): 2.

Robins, J.B. (2002) Compliant behaviour in the antenatal setting. *British Medical Journal* http://bmj.com/cgf/eletters/324/7338/639.

Sandall, J., Davies, J. and Warwick, C. (2001) *Evaluation of the Albany Midwifery Practice*. London: Kings College.

Shakespeare, T. (1998) Choices and rights: eugenics, genetics and disability equality. *Disability and Society*, **13**; 665–81.

Stapleton, H., Duerden, J. and Kirkham, M. (1998) *Evaluation of the Impact of the Supervision of Midwives on Professional Practice and the Quality of Midwifery Care*. London: English National Board for Nursing and Midwifery.

Stapleton, H., Kirkham, M., Thomas, G. and Curtis, P. (2002) Language use in antenatal consultations. *British Journal of Midwifery*, **10(5)**: 273–7.

Stewart, M. (2001) Whose evidence counts? An exploration of health profesionals' perceptions of evidence-based practice, focusing on the maternity service. *Midwifery* **17**: 279–88.

Taylor, M. (1996) An ex-midwife's reflections on supervision from a psychotherapeutic viewpoint. In M. Kirkham (ed.) *Supervision of Midwives*. Hale: Books for Midwives Press.

Trewick, A., Ellis, D. and Kirkham, M. (2001) *Evaluation of the Breastfeeding Telephone Helpline in Doncaster*. Sheffield: University of Sheffield, School of Nursing and Midwifery.

Wiggins, M., Singh, D., Newburn, M. and Burbridge, R. (2000) In D. Singh and M. Newburn (eds), *Access to Maternity Information and Support*. London: National Childbirth Trust.

Williams, C., Alderson, P. and Farsides, B. (2002a) Too many choices? Hospital and community staff reflect on the future of prenatal screening. *Social Science and Medicine*, **55**: 743–53.

Williams, C., Alderson, C. and Farsides, B. (2002b) What constitutes balanced information in the practitioners' portrayals of Down's Syndrome? *Midwifery*, **18**; 230–7.

Williams, S.J. (1995) Theorising class, health and lifestyles: can Bourdieu help us? *Sociology of Health and Illness*, **17**: 577–604.

Wuest, J. (2001) Precarious ordering: towards a formal theory of women's caring. *Health Care for Women International*, **22**:1–2, 167–193.

Index